Cross Cultural Psychiatry

In loving memory of
Micaela Morales Herrera

I am home in heaven, dear ones,
Oh, so happy and so bright!
There is perfect joy and beauty
in this everlasting light.
All the pain and grief is over,
every restless tossing passed.
I am now at peace forever,
safely home in heaven at last.
Did you wonder I so calmly
trod the valley of the shade?
Oh, but Jesus' love illumined
every dark and fearful glade.
And he came himself to meet me
in that way so hard to tread,
and with Jesus' arm to lean on,
could I have one doubt or dread?
Then you must not grieve so sorely,
for I love you dearly still.
Try to look beyond earth's shadows,
pray to trust our father's will.
There is work still waiting for you,
so you must not idly stand.
Do it now, while life remaineth
you shall rest in Jesus' land.
When that work is all completed,
he will gently call you home.
Oh, the rapture of that meeting,
oh, the joy to see you come!

Cross Cultural Psychiatry

Edited by

John M. Herrera
Eli Lilly and Company
Indianapolis, USA

William B. Lawson
Indiana University School of Medicine
Indianapolis, USA

and

John J. Sramek
California Clinical Trials
Beverly Hills, USA

This publication was supported by educational grants from
Eli Lilly and Company
and
Janssen Pharmaceutica

JOHN WILEY & SONS

Chichester • New York • Weinheim • Brisbane • Singapore • Toronto

Other Wiley Editorial Offices

John Wiley & Sons, Inc., 605 Third Avenue,
New York, NY 10158-0012, USA

WILEY-VCH Verlag GmbH, Pappelallee 3,
D-69469 Weinheim, Germany

Jacaranda Wiley Ltd, 33 Park Road, Milton,
Queensland 4064, Australia

John Wiley & Sons (Asia) Pte Ltd, 2 Clementi Loop #02-01,
Jin Xing Distripark, Singapore 129809

John Wiley & Sons (Canada) Ltd, 22 Worcester Road,
Rexdale, Ontario M9W 1L1, Canada

Library of Congress Cataloging-in-Publication Data

Herrera, John M.
    Cross cultural psychiatry / John M. Herrera, William B. Lawson,
John J. Sramek.
        p. cm.
    Includes bibliographical references and index.
    ISBN 0-471-98587-2
        1. Mental illness—Chemotherapy—Cross cultural studies—
Congresses.   2. Psychiatry, Transcultural—Congresses.
    3. Psychopharmacology—Cross cultural studies—Congresses.
    I. Lawson, William B.   II. Sramek, John J.   III. Title.
    [DNLM: 1. Mental Disorders—drug therapy congresses.   2. Mental
Disorders—ethnology congresses.   3. Cross Cultural Comparison
congresses.   4. Psychopharmacology congresses.   WM 402 H565c 1999]
    RC483.H47   1999
    616.89—dc21
    DNLM/DLC
    for Library of Congress   98–40979
                                                                 CIP

British Library Cataloguing in Publication Data

A catalogue record for this book is available from the British Library

ISBN 0-471-98587-2

Typeset in 10/12pt Baskerville from the author's disks by Mayhew Typesetting, Rhayader, Powys
Printed and bound in Great Britain by Biddles Ltd, Guildford and King's Lynn
This book is printed on acid-free paper responsibly manufactured from sustainable forestry, in which at
least two trees are planted for each one used for paper production.

Contents

Contributors

Kathy Akiyama, MD *Assistant Clinical Professor, Department of Psychiatry, University of California at San Francisco, San Francisco, CA 94143, USA*

Scott Andersen, MS *Assistant Senior Statistician, Eli Lilly and Company, Indianapolis, IN 46285, USA*

Milagros Bravo, PhD *Associate Professor, Department of Graduate Studies, University of Puerto Rico, Puerto Rico*

Diane Buckingham, MD *Truman Medical Center, Private Practice, Overland Parks, KS 66210, USA*

Peter Chu, MD *Assistant Clinical Professor, Department of Psychiatry, Mount Sinai School of Medicine, Elmhurst Hospital Center, Elmhurst, NY 11373, USA*

Michelle Clark, MD *Associate Clinical Professor, Department of Psychiatry, University of California at San Francisco, San Francisco, CA 94143, USA*

Yasmine Collazo, MD *Assistant Clinical Professor, Department of Psychiatry, Mount Sinai School of Medicine, Elmhurst Hospital Center, Elmhurst, NY 11373, USA*

Neal R. Cutler, MD *Director, California Clinical Trials, Beverly Hills, CA 90211, USA*

Albana M. Dassori, MD *Assistant Professor, Department of Psychiatry, University of Texas Health Science Center, San Antonio, TX 78284, USA*

Jorge Dávila, MD *Attending Psychiatrist, San Ignacio Hospital, Bogota, Columbia*

Nang Du, MD *Assistant Clinical Professor, Department of Psychiatry, University of California at San Francisco, San Francisco, CA 94143, USA*

Timi Edeki, MD, PhD *Department of Internal Medicine, University of Louisville, Louisville, KY 40202, USA*

Edyta J. Frackiewicz, PharmD *Research Pharmacologist, California Clinical Trials, Beverly Hills, CA 90211, USA*

Man C. Fung, MD, FACP *Clinical Research Physician, Pharmacovigilance and Epidemiology, Eli Lilly and Company, Indianapolis, IN 46285, USA*

Kenneth K. Gee, MD *Assistant Clinical Professor, Department of Psychiatry, University of California at San Francisco, San Francisco, CA 94143, USA*

Peter J. Guarnaccia, MD   *Associate Professor, Department of Human Ecology, Rutgers University, New Brunswick, NJ 08901, USA*

David C. Henderson, MD   *Associate Director of Psychotic Disorders, Erich Lindemann Mental Health Center, Freedom Trial Clinic, Boston, MA 02114, USA*

John M. Herrera, PhD   *Clinical Research Specialist, Eli Lilly and Company, Indianapolis, IN 46285, USA*

James J. Hudziak, MD   *Assistant Professor, Department of Psychiatry, University of Vermont College of Medicine, Burlington, VT 05405, USA*

Dilip V. Jeste, MD   *Professor, Department of Psychiatry & Neuroscience, University of California, San Diego, La Jolla, CA 92093, USA*

Stanford S. Jhee, PharmD   *Research Pharmacologist, California Clinical Trials, Beverly Hills, CA 90211, USA*

Rajinder Judge, MD   *Medical Director, Eli Lilly and Company, Indianapolis, IN 46285, USA*

Kenneth Kwong, MD, PhD   *Clinical Research Physician, Eli Lilly and Company, Indianapolis, IN 46285, USA*

Jonathan P. Lacro, PharmD   *Assistant Clinical Professor, Department of Psychiatry, University of California, San Diego, La Jolla, CA 92093, USA*

William B. Lawson, MD, PhD, FAPA   *Professor, Department of Psychiatry, Indiana University School of Medicine, Indianapolis, IN 46202, USA*

Freda Lewis-Hall, MD   *Director, Lilly Center for Women's Health, Eli Lilly and Company, Indianapolis, IN 46285, USA*

Keh-Ming Lin, MD, MPH   *Professor, Department of Psychiatry, Harbor-UCLA Medical Center, Torrance, CA 90502, USA*

Laurie Lindamer, PhD   *Assistant Project Scientist, University of California, San Diego, La Jolla, CA 92093, USA*

Francis Lu, MD   *Clinical Professor, Department of Psychiatry, University of California at San Francisco, San Francisco, CA 94143, USA*

Rick A. Martinez, MD   *Associate Medical Director, Janssen Pharmaceutical Inc., Titusville, NJ 08560, USA*

Salvador Mata, MD   *Attending Psychiatrist, Jose Maria Vargas Hospital, Caracas, Venezuela*

Guido Mazzotti, MD   *Attending Psychiatrist, Instituto Nacinal de Salud Mental, Lima, Peru*

Ricardo P. Mendoza, MD   *Professor of Psychiatry, Department of Psychiatry, Harbor-UCLA Medical Center, Torrance, CA 90502, USA*

Alexander L. Miller, MD *Professor of Psychiatry, Department of Psychiatry, University of Texas Health Science Center, San Antonio, TX 78284, USA*

Rodrigo Munoz, MD *President, American Psychiatric Association Clinical Professor of Psychiatry, University of California, San Diego, La Jolla, CA 92093-0924, USA*

Ilena M. Norton, MD *Assistant Professor, University of Colorado, Denver Health Medical Center, Denver, CO 80262, USA*

Samuel O. Okpaku, MD, PhD, MRCPI, FRCPC *Clinical Professor of Psychiatry, Vanderbilt University School of Medicine, Nashville, TN 37203, USA*

Alfonso Ontiveros, MD *Attending Psychiatrist, Instituto Nacinal de Salud Mental, Lima, Peru*

Jorge Ospina, MD *Attending Psychiatrist, San Vicente de Paul Hospital, Medellin, Columbia*

Antonio Pacheco, MD *Attending Psychiatrist, Centro de Orientacion y Docncia las Palmas, Caracas, Venezuela*

Moramay Palacios, MD *Clinical Project Management Associate, Eli Lilly and Company, Indianapolis, IN 46285, USA*

Edmond H. Pi, MD *Director of Consultation and Liaison Service, Department of Psychiatry, University of Southern California Medical Center: Hospital Place, Los Angeles, CA 90033, USA*

John Plewes, MD *Clinical Research Physician, Eli Lilly and Company, Indianapolis, IN 46285, USA*

Luis F. Ramirez, MD *Associate Professor-Vice Chairman, Department of Psychiatry, Case Western Reserve University, Cleveland, OH 44106, USA*

Emile Risby, MD *Clinical Research Psychiatrist, Department of Psychiatry, DeCamp Crisis Center, Decater, GA 30030, USA*

Ecaterina Rotaru, MD *Study Coordinator, Department of Psychiatry, Mount Sinai School of Medicine, Elmhurst Hospital Center, Elmhurst, NY 11373, USA*

Maritza Rubio-Stipec, MA *Department of Psychiatry, University of Puerto Rico, San Juan, Puerto Rico 00936, USA*

Lawrence P. Rudiger, PhD *Research Fellow, Department of Psychiatry, University of Vermont, Burlington, VT 05405, USA*

Sigfried Ruiz, MD *Assistant Clinical Professor of Psychiatry, Mount Sinai School of Medicine, Elmhurst Hospital Center, Elmhurst, NY 11373, USA*

Delia Saldaña, PhD *Clinical Assistant Professor of Psychiatry, University of Texas Health Science Center, San Antonio, TX 78284, USA*

Erina Shavers, PharmD   *Clinical Research Administrator, Eli Lilly and Company, Indianapolis, IN 46285, USA*

Michael W. Smith, MD   *Assistant Professor, Department of Psychiatry, Harbor-UCLA Medical Center, Torrance, CA 90502, USA*

Lonnie R. Snowden, PhD   *Professor, School of Social Welfare, University of California, Berkeley, CA 94720, USA*

John J. Sramek, PharmD   *Director of Research, California Clinical Trials, Beverly Hills, CA 90211, USA*

Raymond Tam, MD   *Assistant Clinical Professor, Department of Psychiatry, Mount Sinai School of Medicine, Elmhurst Hospital Center, Elmhurst, NY 11373, USA*

Roy Tamura, PhD   *Senior Research Scientist, Eli Lilly and Company, Indianapolis, IN 46285, USA*

Pierre V. Tran, MD   *Clinical Research Physician, Eli Lilly and Company, Indianapolis, IN 46285, USA*

Scott Van Sant, MD   *Clinical Research Psychiatrist, DeCamp Crisis Center, Decater, GA 30030, USA*

Marcio Versiani, MD   *Attending Psychiatrist, Federal University Rio De Janeiro, Brazil*

Hsiao-hui Wu, MS   *Clinical Research Associate, Eli Lilly and Company, Taipei, Taiwan*

Introduction

Rodrigo A. Munoz

University of California, San Diego, La Jolla, CA, USA

The demographic changes occurring in the USA have brought most psychiatrists to the realization that cultural competence will remain an issue for all involved in clinical work. Clinical competence is no longer an abstract issue. It refers to specific diagnostic and therapeutic strategies that apply to individuals belonging to different cultures. In the case of the group to which I belong, the Hispanics, the clinically competent psychiatrist will know that disorders tend to have a somatic presentation, that patients tend to harbor strong prejudices against mental illness and its treatment, that patients tend to abandon treatment before a proper regimen has been established, that patients abandon most treatments when the first signs of recovery appear, and that pessimism and fatalism about the illness often interfere with treatment.

Doctors Herrera, Lawson, and Sramek have assembled a very distinguished panel of researchers that present most of the issues relevant to those interested in practicing the best psychiatry in the USA of the future. This comprehensive edition begins with chapters on pharmacogenetics and pharmacodynamic modeling. Next, focus turns to the more clinical implications of differential drug response among ethnic and racial groups. Subsequent sections review cross cultural diagnostic issues and treatment considerations in the management of schizophrenia and affective disorder. These sections include exciting information on novel antipsychotics and the results of comparative antidepressant clinical trials conducted in Latin America and the Far East. Inpatient psychiatric treatment of ethnic minorities is a late and innovative section theme. The text concludes with sections dedicated to gender issues in cross cultural psychiatry and the psycho-pharmacological treatment of children and adolescents, an often neglected area of concerns. My personal regards are extended to the editors and contributing authors for their preparation of this most important and informative text.

Acknowledgments

Planning of this text began with a symposium entitled Diversity in Psychopharmacology, presented at the American Psychiatric Association annual meeting in 1995 and supported by an unrestricted educational grant from Eli Lilly and Company. In 1996, planning continued with a Grand Rounds presentation series, entitled Cross Cultural Psychopharmacology, delivered to the Department of Psychiatry at Elmhurst Hospital Center (an academic affiliate of the Mount Sinai School of Medicine, New York), and supported by an unrestricted educational grant from Janssen Pharmaceuticals. In 1997, John Wiley & Sons completed their editorial review and formal invitations were issued to contributors. Suffice it to say, the editors wish to express their appreciation to these organizations for making this collection possible.

The editors and contributing authors also wish to acknowledge the invaluable assistance of Teresa S. Williams in coordinating editorial activities. Teresa's diligence has been most delightful. The assistance of Robert Massing, Beth Montano and Cheryl Maynard is also appreciated.

Basic Mechanisms

1

Ethnicity and the Pharmacogenetics of Drug-Metabolizing Enzymes

Ricardo P. Mendoza, Michael W. Smith and Keh-Ming Lin

Department of Psychiatry, Harbor-UCLA Medical Center, Torrance, CA, USA

INTRODUCTION

Ethnic and interindividual differences in drug response have long been recognized and reported in the literature [1–4]. Variability in the rate of biotransformation of medications has largely been theorized to underlie these differences but it is only in the last two decades that objective information has emerged to support these speculations. Investigators in the field of pharmacogenetics (the study of idiosyncratic drug responses having a hereditary basis) have led the search for substantiating evidence and have focused their efforts on the cytochrome P-450 isozyme system, which plays a pivotal role in the metabolism of most medications used in medicine and psychiatry today [5, 6]. Early research assessed the functional expression (phenotype) of key cytochrome P-450 (CYP) metabolizing enzymes and identified polymorphic variability; that is, several forms of the same enzyme were shown to exist and the frequency with which they occurred varied among ethnic populations. Most recently, utilizing methodologies developed by molecular biologists for the analysis of genetic structure (genotyping), researchers have clearly identified ethnic-specific mutations in these drug metabolizing enzymes [2, 7–9]. These ethnic-specific mutations in the CYP system correspond to varying efficiencies in drug metabolism among members of different ethnic minority populations and, in general, enzyme mutations appear to play a crucial role in interindividual differences in response to medications.

In this chapter we will closely examine the relationship of pharmacogenetics and ethnicity. We first review the literature regarding genetic variations in the drug-metabolizing enzymes and the differences in the catalytic activity of these enzymes among ethnic minority populations. Genetic mutations in drug-metabolizing enzymes do not singularly determine drug response, however; we therefore also summarize the data that shows how environmental factors, especially diet, can

Cross Cultural Psychiatry. Edited by John M. Herrera, William B. Lawson and John J. Sramek.
© 1999 John Wiley & Sons Ltd.

powerfully influence the activity and efficiency of the drug-metabolizing enzymes. Given the demographic shifts occurring in the population of the USA, American psychiatrists will be routinely involved in the pharmacological management of patients from ethnic minorities and so we make every effort to address the clinical implications of these findings for practicing psychiatrists. In light of recent data demonstrating the extent of the morbidity, and even mortality, associated with adverse drug responses [10] we underscore the need for the proper clinical application of genotyping and phenotyping methodologies to more accurately predict response to the administration of medications.

THE PHARMACOGENETICS OF DRUG-METABOLIZING ENZYMES

More than 20 xenobiotic-metabolizing P-450 enzymes have been identified in humans [2, 11]. Among these CYP2D6, CYP2C19, CYP1A2 and CYP3A3/4 appear to be the most clinically relevant for the practice of psychiatry and have been the major focus of pharmacogenetic research [12]. CYP2D6 and CYP2C19 clearly demonstrate polymorphic variability. Simply stated, when several forms of the same enzyme exist within a given population, individuals who are administered a substrate that is metabolized by the enzyme will fall into one of two groups: poor metabolizers (PMs) and extensive metabolizers (EMs). With respect to CYP2D6 and CYP2C19, the percentage of PMs of enzyme substrates varies considerably across ethnic groups [13]. Although no distinct polymorphisms have been demonstrated for CYP1A2 and CYP3A3/4, dramatic ethnic differences in their activities have been reported [14–16].

CYP2D6

CYP2D6 was the first P-450 isozyme to be identified and has been the focus of intense investigation since the 1970s [2, 11, 13]. Much of our current knowledge regarding the complexity of drug metabolism and the nature of drug–drug inter-actions stems from research with CYP2D6. Early phenotypic studies clearly established that PMs lacked the ability to metabolize known CYP2D6 substrates. The rate of PMs varies substantially across ethnic groups, ranging from 6–10% in Caucasians [2, 9, 13] to less than 1% among Asians [9, 13]. Recent genotyping studies utilizing both restriction fragment-length polymorphisms (RFLP) [17] and allele-specific polymerase chain reaction (PCR) assays [18] identified a number of mutations that are associated with poor metabolizer status in Caucasians. Among these, CYP2D6A, CYP2D6B and CYP2D6D are the most important [19–21]. CYP2D6B accounts for approximately 70% of Caucasian PMs [19, 22, 23], the remaining 30% being divided between CYP2D6A and CYP2D6D. The CYP2D6D genotype is caused by a total deletion of the gene and appears to occur at similar frequencies in different ethnic groups [24]. In contrast, both CYP2D6B and CYP2D6A genotypes are extremely rare outside of Caucasian populations and the CYP2D6B genotype appears to be largely responsible for the higher rate of PMs in Caucasians than in Asians [25–27] and African Blacks. Although a previous study, of small sample size, identified a PM rate of 4.5% among Mexican Americans [Lam, personal communication 1991], a more recent pharmacogenetic investigation of 97 Mexican Americans showed a PM rate of 1% [28]. This rate is similar to that found among Asian populations; however, the genotyping results from this study revealed that the allele frequency of CYP2D6B was closer to that for Caucasians. This finding may reflect the heterogeneity and genetic admixture reported among Mexican mestizo populations which is the result of European Spaniard inbreeding after their conquest of Mexico [29].

A large degree of interindividual variability, usually more than 100-fold, has been demonstrated in CYP2D6 EMs in all ethnic groups [2, 13]. In Caucasians, intermediate metabolizing efficiency (greater than PMs but less than EMs) is explained in part by the existence of heterozygotes for the mutations CYP2D6B, CYP2D6A and CYP2D6D; these are more frequently found among Caucasians. Another mutation, CYP2D6C, was recently identified in Caucasian subjects and is associated with slower metabolism [30]. The allelic frequency of this mutation, however, is extremely low. As previously stated, with the exception of the CYP2D6D genotype, the A, B and C mutations are rarely found in non-white populations. The low rate of penetration in ethnic minority groups of alleles known to produce PM status among Caucasians would suggest that members of these populations should demonstrate high CYP2D6 activity and require higher dosages of medication. However, the clinical literature indicates this is not the experience of most practitioners involved in the pharmacological management of ethnic minorities. In fact, most studies in Asians [25, 31–33] and African Blacks [34–42] show that members of these groups require lower dosages. This apparent discrepancy between phenotype and genotype across ethnic lines was recently resolved by the discovery of the CYP2D6J and CYP2D6Z mutations, which confer intermediate or slow metabolizer (SM) status in Asians and African Blacks that, respectively, possess these mutations. CYP2D6J occurs at an extremely high frequency in Asians (47–70%) [31, 33, 42], while the allele frequency of CYP2D6J is quite low in both Caucasians [43] and Mexican Americans [28].

The CYP2D6Z mutation is ostensibly responsible for the slowing of enzyme activity in African Blacks [42]. Interestingly, this mutation has also been shown to metabolize different CYP2D6 substrates (sparteine and debrisoquine) with varying degrees of efficiency. This has led to discrepancies in the results of phenotyping studies among African Blacks when different probe compounds are used in phenotyping protocols by different investigators [34–42]. The significance of this finding remains undetermined and the prevalence of this newly identified mutation among African Americans or other ethnic minority groups has not yet been examined.

Although many of the mutations previously discussed are the result of deletions and substitutions of the enzymatic genetic code and result in absent or limited enzyme efficiency, several recent studies have identified a mutation that produces multiple copies of the CYP2D6 gene and 'supra extensive metabolism' (SEM) of CYP2D6 substrates [44]. The mutation commonly associated with this condition, CYP2D6L2 (denoting the existence of two copies of the CYP2D6L gene), has been detected using a combination of RFLP and PCR methods among 7% of Spaniards residing in Spain [44], but in only 1% of Swedes living in Sweden [45]. The allele frequency of this mutation has not yet been determined in any other population groups.

CYP2C19

Phenotyping studies conducted in 1984 [46–48] established the polymorphic nature of mephenytoin hydroxylase (CYP2C19). It soon became apparent that the phenotype of this enzyme also varies substantially across ethnic groups, from approximately 3% in Caucasian groups in Western Europe and North America to more than 20% in most East Asian populations. As CYP2C19 is involved in the metabolism (demethylation) of certain psychotropics such as diazepam and tricyclic antidepressants, the higher PM rate in Asians has been proposed as a possible mechanism for the slower rate of metabolism of these drugs that has been reported in this population [13, 52]. Other ethnic minority groups have been less well studied: although an earlier study (based on a small sample size) showed a PM rate of 18.5% among older African Americans [49], a study being conducted by Edeki [personal communication] suggests a PM rate in this group comparable to those reported in Caucasians, African Blacks, and younger African Americans [50, 51]. The discrepancy of these findings in Black population subgroups would indicate the need for additional research. A PM rate of 14% for CYP2C19 was recently discovered among a fairly large sample of Mexican Americans [Lin, personal communication]. This finding approximates the frequency established in Asian populations and would suggest the possibility of slower benzodiazepine and tricyclic antidepressant metabolism among Latino patients.

The underlying genetic mechanisms responsible for the CYP2C19 polymorphism were characterized only recently [53, 53]. In one study [54] two mutations, CYP2C19m1 and CYP2C19m2, accounted for 100% of PMs among Japanese subjects. The CYP2C19m2 isozyme appears to be specific to Asians because it was not found in any of the Caucasian subjects, whereas the CYP2C19m1 genotype explained 83% of PMs in Caucasians. Recent studies among Zimbabweans [42] and African Americans [51] support the ethnic specificity of the CYP2C19m2 mutation; the majority of PMs in these populations were homozygotic for CYP2C19m1. Similarly, in a recent study of 100 Mexican American subjects, the only one who was PM was also homozygous for m1 and had an allele frequency of only 0.5% for the m2 mutation [55].

CYP1A2 and CYP3A3/4

In contrast to CYP2D6 and CYP2C19, CYP1A2 and CYP3A3/4 do not appear to be under primary genetic control and no polymorphic variability has, as yet, been identified. CYP1A2 is involved in the metabolism of various commonly prescribed medications [2], including theophylline, propranolol, phenacetin and caffeine, as well as psychotropics such as imipramine [56], clomipramine, fluvoxamine [57], clozapine [58, 59] and olanzapine [60]. CYP1A2 is highly inducible and consequently exhibits large interindividual variability secondary to differential exposure to various environmental agents, including indoles contained in cruciferous vegetables such as brussels sprouts and cabbage [61] and the polycyclic aromatic hydrocarbons generated by cigarette smoking and charcoal-broiling of beef [62–64]. Because it is highly inducible, it is reasonable to expect CYP1A2 activity to vary substantially across ethnic/cultural groups with divergent dietary habits [13–14].

Representing more than 50% of the P-450 enzymes in the liver, CYP3A3/4 is involved in the metabolism of a large number of xenobiotics, endogenous substances (for example steroid hormones) and medications, including psychotropics such as triazolo-benzodiazepines, diazepam, nefazodone, carbamazepine, and verapamil [2]. Initial reports regarding the possibility of polymorphic variability of this enzyme [65] have not been borne out, but its activity does exhibit a large degree of interindividual variability, probably due to the existence of natural substrates serving as inhibitors and inducers of the enzyme. As with CYP1A2, similar non-genetically regulated mechanisms may be responsible for the lower CYP3A3/4 activity reported in a number of non-White populations, including Asian Indians [65], Japanese, and Mexicans [66]. To the best of our knowledge, CYP3A3/4 has not been examined in ethnic minority populations in the USA.

ENVIRONMENTAL AND DIETARY EFFECTS ON P-450 ENZYME ACTIVITY

In addition to being under genetic control, at least some of the CYP enzymes are quite sensitive to various enzyme-inducing and inhibiting agents, including environmental toxins (such as nitrosamines in cigarette smoke and polluted air), alcohol, circulating hormones, and an exhaustive list of drugs [67, 68]. Cimetidine is just one example of a potent CYP enzyme-inhibiting agent that has been shown to produce reductions in the clearance of many pharmacoactive compounds [69]. Less well known and appreciated is the influence of diet on the metabolism of various drugs [64, 70, 71]. Several studies have demonstrated that dietary manipulations significantly alter the pharmacokinetics of many drugs [69–71], including acetaminophen, antipyrine, propranolol, hexobarbital, phenacetin, oxazepam, and theophylline. For example, a change from a high protein diet to one rich in carbohydrates for a period of 1 to 2 weeks resulted in a 30% reduction in the clearance of theophylline.

In addition, although no similar effect has been well documented in humans, alterations in dietary fat content have resulted in significant changes in the metabolic efficiency of the CYP system in animals [64, 69, 72].

The relationship between dietary practices, ethnicity, and variability in drug response was first reported upon by Branch *et al.* [73], who compared the rate of antipyrine biotransformation in three study cohorts. A significantly longer anti-pyrine half-life was discovered among Sudanese living in their home villages than in Sudanese residing in Britain or in Caucasian British subjects. Of the three groups, only the last two metabolized antipyrine at similar rates, suggesting that environmental factors such as diet were responsible for the observed pharmaco-kinetic differences. Similar findings were reported in studies involving Asian Indians living in India, Asian Indian immigrants in Britain, and Caucasian British subjects [73–75]. A follow-up study reported that those Asian Indian immigrants who retained their dietary habits as lactovegetarians demonstrated pharmacoki-netic profiles similar to Asian Indians living in their home country, whereas the pharmacokinetic profiles of those who became meat eaters were indistinguishable from the British Caucasian subjects [74]. More recently, and consistent with the above findings, a study showed that Asian Indians were also much slower metabolizers of nifedipine [65].

The CYP isozymes most likely to be involved in mediating macronutrient dietary influences on drug response are CYP1A2 and CYP3A3/4 [68]. These enzymes are highly inducible and are responsive to environmental influences. However, there is no empirical data to substantiate this speculation—and further, although the activities of CYP2D6 and CYP2C19 are thought to be largely genetically regulated, the influence of diet on these important enzymes has not been rigorously tested.

The extent to which diet can influence drug metabolism and pharmacologic response must be further clarified. It is conceivable that if diet can significantly influence the extent of metabolism, as the studies cited would suggest, then dietary interventions might be instituted along with pharmacotherapy to increase or decrease the metabolism of particular drugs through certain metabolic pathways. This has clinical implications because metabolites produced from varying pathways may be linked with more or less adverse effects and even medical morbidity [75–77]. To illustrate, corn is the main dietary staple of many Hispanic subgroups and quercitin, the main flavonoid ingredient that is found in corn, has been shown to dramatically increase the frequency and severity of side-effects of nifedipine administration [78]. The need to downwardly adjust nifedipine dosages in this population group would seem apparent. In a similar fashion, an understanding of customary ethnocultural dietary practices and their unique effects on drug bio-transformation might afford us additional opportunities to dynamically manipulate our pharmacological treatment to achieve better outcomes with members of different ethnic groups. In addition to these clinical considerations, dietary mani-pulations with patients receiving medications may have pharmacoeconomic implications. A recent study demonstrated that cyclosporin levels were dramatically increased in patients who were concomitantly administered grapefruit juice [76, 77]. Since the per-pill costs of many of today's newer generation psychoactive compounds often prove prohibitive, dietary inhibitors and inducers could also be employed to limit pharmacy costs.

THE IMPORTANT ROLE OF PHARMACOGENETIC RESEARCH AND FUTURE DIRECTIONS

Continued pharmacogenetic research on the CYP isozymes is important for a number of reasons in addition to their role in drug metabolism. The pharmacologic information that is accumulating about the metabolic pathways of medications used in medicine and psychiatry allows clinicians to better predict drug–drug interactions [79, 80]. This is especially important in ethnic minorities where herbal preparations are widely used. Many herbal preparations and natural compounds (for example, ginseng) are inducers and inhibitors of the CYP enzyme system and questions regarding their use should be included in any evaluation of cross cultural patients. Evidence is also mounting that CYP isozyme phenotypes and genotypes may be associated with risks for certain medical conditions [2]. For example, CYP2D6 PMs are less likely to develop lung cancer [81–83] and bladder cancer [84–86], but may be more susceptible to the development of conditions such as systematic lupus erythematosus [87], Parkinson's disease [88], neuroleptic malignant syndrome [89], and tardive dyskinesia [90]. This, coupled with the information regarding identification of ethnic specific mutations, may ultimately enhance our ability to predict the risk for developing certain cancers and other medical conditions in different ethnic minority populations.

More recently, pharmacogenetic researchers have explored the level of CYP isozymes in the central nervous system. The information obtained has led to a greater understanding of the complexity of the issues involved in an area of growing concern—substance abuse: extensive metabolizers of CYP2D6 have been reported as more prone to substance abuse [91]. This finding appears to hold true not only for those illicit substances that are metabolized by the CYP2D6 enzyme—such as amphetamine, codeine, hydrocodone, methylenedioxymethamphetamine (MDMA), and morphine—but also for those that clearly are not established substrates (cocaine, nicotine, alcohol). These findings suggest the existence of a central mechanism underlying the relationship of CYP2D6 metabolism and the phenomenon of addiction [92, 93]. This hypothesis is strengthened by recent reports of the existence of CYP2D6 in the brain [94, 95].

The discovery of CYP2D6 in the central nervous system has also been speculatively linked with differences in pain tolerance [96] and is consistent with the data concerning the central mechanisms possibly involved in drug addiction. The significance of these findings for the prevention and treatment of substance abuse among ethnic minority populations remains unexplored.

CONCLUSION

Innovation, followed by success in the field of pharmacogenetic research, has validated what many practitioners involved in the medication management of ethnic minorities have long suspected—that patients of color often respond differently than Caucasians to pharmacologic compounds. The pharmacogenetic data that has emerged during the last two decades regarding the CYP enzyme system in general, and specifically the CYP2D6 enzyme, has firmly established the molecular biological basis of these clinically observed differences. We now know of ethnic-specific mutations in at least two CYP enzymes which account for a broad range of metabolic efficiencies—absent to intermediate to extensive to supra-extensive.

Much of the pharmacogenetic data has, however, focused on discrete ethnic minority populations residing outside the USA [2, 13]. As a result, the phenotypic and genotypic status of these enzymes among ethnic minority patients in this country is largely unknown. Only recently has this research been extended to US resident African Americans and Mexican Americans. In addition, although many studies have been conducted among Caucasians, thus providing stable estimates, data for most ethnic minority groups has been based on only one or two studies of relatively small sample sizes. These studies require replication, especially with samples from different geographic locations, to ensure generalizability.

Although mutational isoforms have not yet been identified for other important CYP drug-metabolizing enzymes, the search for the etiology of observed ethnic differences in these cases has highlighted the importance of the environment, especially diet and hormonal influences, in shaping pharmacologic responsiveness. Psychoactive compounds are clearly metabolized via multiple pathways and by several drug-metabolizing enzymes. Certain critical pathways may produce more metabolites that are toxic with the potential for medical morbidity. In the future we may see increasing sophistication in the dynamic manipulation of diet and other drugs to facilitate the metabolism of medications through 'preferred routes' to enhance therapeutic outcomes.

To date, phenotyping and genotyping have largely been regarded as research tools and methodologies. It would appear the time has arrived to establish the appropriate use of these methodologies in the clinical arena in order to better individualize our pharmacotherapeutic approach to patients of all color. As health-care costs continue to rise, despite managed care, research protocols aimed at identifying the potential for cost savings and establishing the effectiveness of these tools to predict pharmacologic response in the natural world must be initiated.

ACKNOWLEDGMENTS

This study, from the Research Center on the Psychobiology of Ethnicity and the Department of Psychiatry, UCLA School of Medicine, Harbor-UCLA Medical Center, was supported in part by the Research Center on the Psychobiology of Ethnicity MH47193.

REFERENCES

1. Kalow W. 1990. Pharmacogenetics: past and future. *Life Sci* **47**: 1385–97.
2. Kalow W. 1992. *Pharmacogenetics of Drug Metabolism*. New York: Pergamon Press.
3. Mendoza R, Smith MW, Poland RE, Lin KM, Strickland TL. 1991. Ethnic psychopharmacology: The Hispanic and Native American perspective. *Psychopharmacol Bull* **27**: 449–61.
4. Strickland TL, Rangananth V, Lin KM, Poland RE, Mendoza R, Smith MW. 1991. Psychopharmacologic considerations in the treatment of Black American populations. *Psychopharmacol Bull* **27**: 441–8.
5. Alvan G. 1991. Clinical consequences of polymorphic drug oxidation. *Fundament Clin Pharmacol* **5**: 209–28.
6. Gram LF, Brosen K, Sindrup S, Skjelbo E, Nielsen KK. 1992. Pharmacogenetics in psychopharmacology: Basic principles and clinical implications. *Clin Neuropharmacol* **15** (Suppl 1 Pt A): 76A–77A.
7. Islam SA, Wolf CR, Lennard MS, Sternberg MJ. 1991. A three-dimensional molecular template for substrates of human cytochrome P450 involved in debrisoquine 4-hydroxylation. *Carcinogenesis* **12**(12): 2211–19.
8. Gonzalez FJ, Skoda RC, Kimura S, Umeno M, Zanger UM, Nebert DW et al. 1988. Characterization of the common genetic defect in humans deficient in debrisoquine metabolism. *Nature* **331**: 442–6.
9. Gonzalez F. 1989. The molecular biology of cytochrome P450s. *Pharmacol Rev* **40**: 243–88.
10. Lazarou J, Pomeranz BH, Corey PN. 1998. Incidence of adverse drug reactions in hospitalized patients: a meta-analysis of prospective studies. *JAMA* **279**(15): 1200–5.
11. Meyer U, Zanger U, Grant D, Blum M. 1990. Genetic polymorphisms of drug metabolism. *Adv Drug Res* **19**: 307–23.
12. Gonzalez F, Nebert D. 1990. Evolution of the P450 gene superfamily: animal–plant 'warfare' molecular drive and human genetic differences in drug oxidation. *Trends Genet* **6**: 182–6.
13. Lin KM, Poland RE, Nakasaki G. 1993. *Psychopharmacology and Psychobiology of Ethnicity*. Washington DC: American Psychiatric Press.
14. Relling MV, Lin JS, Ayers GD, Evans WE. 1992. Racial and gender differences in *N*-acetyltransferase, xanthine oxidase, and CYP1A2 activities. *Clin Pharmacol Ther* **52**(6): 643–58.
15. Ashan CH, Renwick AG, Macklin B, Challenor VF, Waller DG, George CF. 1991. Ethnic differences in the pharmacokinetics of oral nifedipine. *Br J Clin Pharmacol* **31**: 399–403.
16. Palma-Aguirre JA, Gonzalez-Llaven J, Flores-Murrieta FJ, Castaneda-Hernandez G. 1997. Bioavailability of oral cyclosporine in healthy Mexican volunteers: evidence for interethnic variability. *J Clin Pharmacol* **37**(7): 630–4.
17. Skoda RC, Gonzalez FJ, Demierre A, Meyer UA. 1988. Two mutant alleles of the human cytochrome P-450db1 gene (P450C2D1) associated with genetically deficient metabolism of debrisoquine and other drugs. *Proc Natl Acad Sci USA* **85**(14): 5240–3.
18. Heim M, Meyer UA. 1990. Genotyping of poor metabolisers of debrisoquine by allele-specific PCR amplification. *Lancet* **336**(8714): 529–32.
19. Meyer UA. 1996. Overview of enzymes of drug metabolism. *J Pharmacokinet Biopharm* **24**(5): 449–59.
20. Heim MH, Meyer UA. 1992. Evolution of a highly polymorphic human cytochrome P450 gene cluster: CYP2D6. *Genomics* **14**(1): 49–58.
21. Eichelbaum M, Gross AS. 1990. The genetic polymorphism of debrisoquine/sparteine metabolism—clinical aspects. *Pharmacol Ther* **46**(3): 377–94.

22. Dahl ML, Johansson I, Palmertz MP, Ingelman-Sundberg M, Sjoqvist F. 1992. Analysis of the CYP2D6 gene in relation to debrisoquine and desipramine hydroxylation in a Swedish population. *Clin Pharmacol Ther* **51**: 12–17.
23. Kagimoto M, Heim M, Kagimoto K, Zeugin T, Meyer UA. 1990. Multiple mutations of the human cytochrome P450IID6 gene (CYP2D6) in poor metabolizers of debrisoquine: Study of the functional significance of individual mutations by expression of chimeric genes. *J Biol Chem* **265**(28): 17209–14.
24. Masimirembwa CM, Johansson I, Hasler JA, Ingelman-Sundberg M. 1993. Genetic polymorphism of cytochrome P450 CYP2D6 in Zimbabwean population. *Pharmacogenetics* **3**(6): 275–80.
25. Bertilsson L, Lou YQ, Du YL, Liu Y, Kuang TY, Liao XM *et al.* 1992. Pronounced differences between native Chinese and Swedish populations in the polymorphic hydroxylations of debrisoquine and *S*-mephenytoin. *Clin Pharmacol Ther* **51**(4): 388–97.
26. Lou YC, Ying L, Bertilsson L, Sjoqvist F. 1987. Low frequency of slow debrisoquine hydroxylation in a native Chinese population. *Lancet* **2**(8563): 852–3.
27. Yue QY, Bertilsson L, Dahl-Puustinen ML, Sawe J, Sjoqvist F, Johansson I, Ingelman-Sundberg M. 1989. Disassociation between debrisoquine hydroxylation phenotype and genotype among Chinese. *Lancet* **2**, 870.
28. Mendoza R, Wan Y, Poland RE, Smith M, Lin KM. CYP2D6 Polymorphism in a Mexican American Population: Relationship Between Genotyping and Phenotyping (submitted for publication).
29. Vargas-Alarcon G, Garcia A, Bahena S, Melin-Aldana H, Andrade F, Ibanez-de-Kasep G *et al.* 1994. HLA-B alleles and complotypes in Mexican patients with seronegative spondyloarthropathies. *Ann Rheum Dis* **53**(11): 755–8.
30. Tyndale R, Aoyama T, Broly F, Matsunaga T, Inaba T, Kalow W *et al.* 1991. Identification of a new variant CYP2D6 allele lacking the codon encoding Lys-281: possible association with the poor metabolizer phenotype. *Pharmacogenetics* **1**(1): 26–32.
31. Wang SL, Huang JD, Lai MD, Liu BH, Lai ML. 1993. Molecular basis of genetic variation in debrisoquine hydroxylation in Chinese subjects: Polymorphism in RFLP and DNA sequence of CYP2D6. *Clin Pharmacol Ther* **53**: 410–18.
32. Dahl ML, Yue QY, Roh HK, Johansson I, Sawe J, Sjoqvist F, Bertilsson L. 1995. Genetic analysis of the CYP2D locus in relation to debrisoquine hydroxylation capacity in Korean, Japanese, and Chinese subjects. *Pharmacogenetics* **5**(3): 159–64.
33. Yokota H, Tamura S, Furuya H, Kimura S. 1993. Evidence for a new variant CYP2D6 allele CYP2D6J in a Japanese population associated with lower in vivo rates of sparteine metabolism. *Pharmacogenetics* **3**: 256–63.
34. Eichelbaum M, Woolhouse NM. 1985. Inter-ethnic difference in sparteine oxidation among Ghanaians and Germans. *Eur J Clin Pharmacol* **28**(1): 79–83.
35. Woolhouse NM, Eichelbaum M, Oates NS, Idle JR, Smith RL. 1985. Dissociation of co-regulatory control of debrisoquine/phenformin and sparteine oxidation in Ghanaians. *Clin Pharmacol Ther* **37**(5): 512–21.
36. Lennard MS, Tucker GT, Woods HF, Silas JH, Iyun AO. 1989. Stereoselective metabolism of metoprolol in Caucasians and Nigerians—relationship to debrisoquine oxidation phenotype. *Br J Clin Pharmacol* **27**(5): 613–16.
37. Iyun AO, Lennard MS, Tucker GT, Woods HF. 1986. Metoprolol and debrisoquine metabolism in Nigerians: lack of evidence for polymorphic oxidation. *Clin Pharmacol Ther* **40**(4): 387–94.
38. Lennard MS, Tucker GT, Woods HF, Iyun AO, Eichelbaum M. 1988. Stereoselective 4-hydroxylation of debrisoquine in Nigerians. *Biochem Pharmacol* **37**: 97–8.
39. Sommers DK, Moncrieff J, Avenant J. 1988. Polymorphism of the 4-hydroxylation of debrisoquine in the San Bushmen of southern Africa. *Human Toxicology* **7**(3): 273–6.

40. Woolhouse NM. 1986. The debrisoquine/sparteine oxidation polymorphism: evidence of genetic heterogeneity among Ghanaians. *Progr Clin Biol Res* **214**: 189–206.
41. Woolhouse NM, Andoh B, Mahgoub A, Sloan TP, Idle JR, Smith RL. 1979. Debrisoquin hydroxylation polymorphism among Ghanaians and Caucasians. *Clin Pharmacol Ther* **26**(5): 584–91.
42. Masimirembwa C, Bertilsson L, Johansson I, Hasler JA, Ingelman-Sundberg M. 1995. Phenotyping and genotyping of S-mephenytoin hydroxylase (cytochrome P450 2C19) in a Shona population of Zimbabwe. *Clin Pharmacol Ther* **57**(6): 656–61.
43. Armstrong M, Fairbrother K, Idle JR, Daly AK. 1994. The cytochrome P450 CYP2D6 allelic variant CYP2D6J and related polymorphisms in a European population. *Pharmacogenetics* **4**(2): 73–81.
44. Dahl ML, Johansson I, Bertilsson L, Ingelman-Sundberg M, Sjoqvist F. 1995. Ultra-rapid hydroxylation of debrisoquine in a Swedish population. Analysis of the molecular genetic basis. *J Pharmacol Exp Ther* **274**(1): 516–20.
45. Agundez JA, Ledesma MC, Ladero JM, Benitez J. 1995. Prevalence of CYP2D6 gene duplication and its repercussion on the oxidative phenotype in a white population. *Clin Pharmacol Ther* **57**(3): 265–9.
46. Kupfer A, Preisig R. 1984. Pharmacogenetics of mephenytoin: a new drug hydroxylation polymorphism in man. *Eur J Clin Pharmacol* **26**(6): 753–9.
47. Kupfer A, Preisig R. 1983. Inherited defects of hepatic drug metabolism. *Semin Liver Dis* **3**(4): 341–54.
48. Kupfer A, Desmond PV, Schenker S, Branch RA. 1982. Stereoselective metabolism and disposition of the enantiomers of mephenytoin during chronic oral administration of the racemic drug in man. *J Pharmacol Exp Ther* **221**(3): 590–7.
49. Pollock BG, Perel JM, Kirshner M, Altieri LP, Yeager AL, Reynolds CF III. 1991. S-mephenytoin 4-hydroxylation in older Americans. *Eur J Clin Pharmacol* **40**(6): 609–11.
50. Evans WE, Relling MV, Rahman A, McLeod HL, Scott EP, Lin JS. 1993. Genetic basis for a lower prevalence of deficient CYP2D6 oxidative drug metabolism phenotypes in black Americans. *J Clin Invest* **91**: 2150–4.
51. Edeki TI, Goldstein JA, de Morais SM, Hajiloo L, Butler M, Chapdelaine P, Wilkinson GR. 1996. Genetic polymorphism of S-mephenytoin 4'-hydroxylation in African-Americans. *Pharmacogenetics* **6**(4): 357–60.
52. Bertilsson L, Kalow W. 1993. Why are diazepam metabolism and polymorphic S-mephenytoin hydroxylation associated with each other in white and Korean populations but not in Chinese populations? *Clin Pharmacol Ther* **53**(5): 608–10.
53. Goldstein JA, de Morais SM. 1994. Biochemistry and molecular biology of the human CYP2C subfamily. *Pharmacogenetics* **4**(6): 285–99.
54. de Morais SM, Wilkinson GR, Blaisdell J, Nakamura K, Meyer UA, Goldstein JA. 1994. The major genetic defect responsible for the polymorphism of S-mephenytoin metabolism in humans. *J Bio Chem* **269**(22): 15419–22.
55. Smith M, Lin KM, Mendoza R, Wan Y, Poland RE. CYP2C19 Polymorphism in a Mexican American population: Relationship between genotyping and phenotyping (submitted for publication).
56. Lemoine A, Gautier JC, Azoulay D, Kiffel L, Belloc C *et al.* 1993. Major pathway of imipramine metabolism is catalyzed by cytochromes P-450 1A2 and P-450 3A4 in human liver. *Mol Pharmacol* **43**(5): 827–32.
57. Nielsen KK, Flinois JP, Beaune P, Brosen K. 1996. The biotransformation of clomipramine in vitro, identification of the cytochrome P450s responsible for the separate metabolic pathways. *J Pharmacol Exp Ther* **277**(3): 1659–64.
58. Brosen K. 1995. Drug interactions and the cytochrome P450 system. The role of cytochrome P450 1A2. *Clin Pharmacokinet* **29**(Suppl 1): 20–5.

59. Linnet K, Olesen OV. 1997. Metabolism of clozapine by cDNA-expressed human cytochrome P450 enzymes. *Drug Metab Dis* **25**(12): 1379–82.

60. Ring BJ, Catlow J, Lindsay TJ, Gillespie T, Roskos LK, Cerimele BJ *et al*. 1996. Identification of the human cytochromes P450 responsible for the in vitro formation of the major oxidative metabolites of the antipsychotic agent olanzapine. *J Pharmacol Exp Ther* **276**(2): 658–66.

61. Kall MA, Clausen J. 1995. Dietary effect on mixed function P450 1A2 activity assayed by estimation of caffeine metabolism in man. *Hum Exp Toxicol* **14**(10): 801–7.

62. Conney AH, Pantuck EJ, Kuntzman R, Kappas A, Anderson KE, Alvares AP. 1977. Nutrition and chemical biotransformations in man. *Clin Pharmacol Ther* **22**(5 Pt 2): 707–20.

63. Conney AH, Pantuck EJ, Hsiao KC, Kuntzman R, Alvares AP, Kappas A. 1977. Regulation of drug metabolism in man by environmental chemicals and diet. *Fed Proc* **36**(5): 1647–52.

64. Yang CS, Brady JF, Hong JY. 1992. Dietary effects on cytochromes P450, xenobiotic metabolism, and toxicity. *FASEB J* **6**(2): 737–44.

65. Ahsan CH, Renwick AG, Waller DG, Challenor VF, George CF, Amanullah M. 1993. The influence of dose and ethnic origins on the pharmacokinetics of nifedipine. *Clin Pharmacol Ther* **54**(3): 329–38.

66. Castaneda-Hernandez G, Hoyo-Vadillo C, Palma-Aguirre JA, Flores-Murrieta FJ. 1993. Pharmacokinetics of oral nifedipine in different populations. *J Clin Pharmacol* **33**(2): 140–5.

67. Clark W, Brater D, Johnson A. 1988. *Goth's Medical Pharmacology* 12th edition. St. Louis: CV Mosby.

68. Okey A. 1992. *Enzyme induction in the cytochrome P-450 system*. New York: Pergamon Press.

69. Anderson KE, McCleery RB, Vesell ES, Vickers FF, Kappas A. 1991. Diet and cimetidine induce comparable changes in theophylline metabolism in normal subjects. *Hepatology* **13**: 941–6.

70. Anderson KE, Conney A, Kappas A. 1982. Nutritional influences on chemical biotransformations in humans. *Nutr Rev* **40**: 161–9.

71. Anderson KE. 1988. Influences of diet and nutrition on clinical pharmacokinetics. *Clin Pharmacokinet* **14**: 325–46.

72. Anderson KE, Kappas A. 1991. Dietary regulation of cytochrome P450. *Annu Rev Nutr* **11**: 141–67.

73. Branch R, Salih S, Homeida M. 1978. Racial differences in drug metabolizing ability: a study with antipyrine in the Sudan. *Clin Pharmacol Ther* **24**: 283–6.

74. Desai NK, Sheth UK, Mucklow JC. 1980. Antipyrine clearance in Indian villagers. *Br J Clin Pharmacol* **9**: 387–94.

75. Fraser H, Mucklow J, Bulpitt C, Kahn C, Mould G, Dollery C. 1979. Environmental factors affecting antipyrine metabolism in London factory and office workers. *Br J Clin Pharmacol* **7**: 237–43.

76. Yee GC, Stanley DL, Pessa LJ, Dalla Costa T, Beltz SE, Ruiz J, Lowenthal DT. 1995. Effect of grapefruit juice on blood cyclosporin concentration. *Lancet* **345**(8955): 955–6.

77. Hollander AA, van Rooij J, Lentjes GW, Arbouw F, van Bree JB, Schoemaker RC *et al*. 1995. The effect of grapefruit juice on cyclosporine and prednisone metabolism in transplant patients. *Clin Pharmacol Ther* **57**(3): 318–24.

78. Palma-Aguirre JA, Nava Rangel J, Hoyo-Vadillo C, Girard-Cuesy ME, Castaneda-Hernandez G, Arteaga-Granados E, De Mucha-Macias R. 1994. Influence of Mexican diet on nifedipine pharmacodynamics in healthy volunteers. *Proc West Pharmacol Soc* **37**: 85–6.

79. Gram LF, Brosen K. 1992. Drug interactions and pharmacokinetic risk factors when

using antidepressants in the medically ill patients. *Clin Neuropharmacol* **15**(Suppl 1 Pt A): 642A–3A.
80. Gram LF, and Fredricson-Overo K. 1972. Drug interaction: Inhibitory effect of neuroleptics on metabolism of tricyclic antidepressants in man. *BMJ* **1**: 463–5.
81. Benitez J, Ladero JM, Jara C, Carrillo JA, Cobaleda J, Llerena A *et al*. 1991. Polymorphic oxidation of debrisoquine in lung cancer patients. *Eur J Cancer* **27**: 158–61.
82. Caporaso NE, Shields PG, Landi MT, Shaw GL, Tucker MA, Hoover R *et al*. 1992. The debrisoquine metabolic phenotype and DNA-based assays: implications of misclassification for the association of lung cancer and the debrisoquine metabolic phenotype. *Environ Health Perspect* **98**: 101–5.
83. London SJ, Daly AK, Leathart JB, Navidi WC, Carpenter CC, Idle JR. 1997. Genetic polymorphism of CYP2D6 and lung cancer risk in African-Americans and Caucasians in Los Angeles County. *Carcinogenesis* **18**(6): 1203–14.
84. Benitez J, Ladero JM, Fernandez-Gundin MJ, Llerena A, Cobaleda J, Martinez C *et al*. 1990. Polymorphic oxidation of debrisoquine in bladder cancer. *Ann Med* **22**: 157–60.
85. Kaisary A, Smith P, Jaczq E, McAllister CB, Wilkinson GR, Ray WA, Branch RA. 1994. Genetic predisposition to bladder cancer: ability to hydroxylate debrisoquine and mephenytoin as risk factors. *Cancer Res* **20**: 5488–93.
86. Roots I, Drakoulis D, Brockmoller J. 1992. Polymorphic enzymes and cancer risk: concepts, methodology, and data review. In: Kalow W, ed. *Pharmacogenetics of Drug Metabolism*. New York: Pergamon Press, pp. 815–41.
87. Baer AN, McAllister CB, Wilkinson GR, Woosley RL, Pincus T. 1986. Altered distribution of debrisoquine oxidation phenotypes in patients with systemic lupus erythematosus. *Arthritis Rheum* **29**(7): 843–50.
88. Martinez C, Agundez JA, Gervasini G, Martin R, Benitez J. 1997. Tryptamine: a possible endogenous substrate for CYP2D6. *Pharmacogenetics* **7**(2): 85–93.
89. Iwahashi K. 1994. CYP2D6 genotype and possible susceptibility to the neuroleptic malignant syndrome [letter]. *Biol Psychiatry* **36**(11): 781–2.
90. Arthur H, Dahl ML, Siwers B, Sjoqvist F. 1995. Polymorphic drug metabolism in schizophrenic patients with tardive dyskinesia. *J Clin Psychopharmacol* **15**(3): 211–16.
91. Otton SV, Schadel M, Cheung SW, Kaplan HL, Busto UE, Sellers EM. 1993. CYP2D6 phenotype determines the metabolic conversion of hydrocodone to hydromorphone. *Clin Pharmacol Ther* **54**(5): 463–72.
92. Sellers EM, Otton SV, Busto UE. 1991. Drug metabolism and interactions in abuse liability assessment. *Br J Addiction* **86**(12): 1607–14.
93. Wu D, Otton SV, Sproule BA, Busto U, Inaba T, Kalow W, Sellers EM. 1993. Inhibition of human cytochrome P450 2D6 (CYP2D6) by methadone. *Br J Clin Pharmacol* **35**(1): 30–4.
94. Kalow W, Tyndale RF. 1992. Debrisoquine/Sparteine monooxygenase and other P-450's in brain. In: Kalow W, ed. *Pharmacogenetics of Drug Metabolism. International Encyclopedia of Pharmacological Therapy*. London: Pergamon Press, pp. 649–56.
95. Tyndale RF, Sunahara R, Inaba T, Kalow W, Gonzalez FJ, Niznik HB. 1991. Neuronal cytochrome P450IID1 (debrisoquine/sparteine-type): potent inhibition of activity by (–)-cocaine and nucleotide sequence identity to human hepatic P450 gene CYP2D6. *Mol Pharmacol* **40**: 63–8.
96. Sindrup SH, Brosen K, Bjering P, Arendt-Nielson L, Larsen U, Angelo HR, Gram LF. 1991. Codeine increases pain thresholds to copper vapor laser stimuli in extensive but not poor metabolizers of sparteine. *Clin Pharmacol Ther* **49**: 686–93.

2

Genetic Polymorphism of Drug Oxidation

Timi Edeki

University of Louisville, Louisville, KY, USA

INTRODUCTION

In the past three decades a number of genetic defects in the way the body handles drugs have been discovered. These defects may be responsible for unusual drug reactions and can be divided into two types [1]:

1. Those due to altered pharmacokinetic handling of the drug—that is, the effect of the body on the drug.
2. Those which are due to altered tissue responsiveness and hence are pharmacodynamic in origin—that is, the effect of the drug on the body.

`Acetylation and oxidation are two areas of drug metabolism in which genetic polymorphism has been extensively studied. One of the earliest references to oxidative drug polymorphism was by Kutt [2], who described deficient p-hydroxylation of phenytoin. Interethnic variation in the metabolism of phenytoin has been reviewed in a recent publication [3]. Shahidi [4] reported a pedigree of two sisters who exhibited defective o-de-ethylation of phenacetin and were much more sensitive to methemoglobinemia than normal subjects. Unfortunately these early observations were not followed up in more detail. In the past decade interest in genetic polymorphism of drug oxidation has been renewed, with the discovery of monogenic control in the oxidative metabolism of the antihypertensive drug debrisoquine [5] and of sparteine, a drug with both oxytocic and antiarrhythmic properties [6]. Progress in this field has been enhanced by the discovery, identification and characterization of different cytochrome P-450 (CYP) enzymes [7]. The main focus of this chapter is the genetic polymorphism of CYP2D6. Another important enzyme example of genetic polymorphism of drug oxidation is that of the 4'-hydroxylation of the S-enantiomer of the antiepileptic drug mephenytoin, which is the subject of a review by Daniel and Edeki [8].

Cross Cultural Psychiatry. Edited by John M. Herrera, William B. Lawson and John J. Sramek.
© 1999 John Wiley & Sons Ltd.

HISTORICAL PERSPECTIVE

An early study on the metabolic fate of debrisoquine at St Mary's Hospital in London revealed the failure of a subject, unlike his colleagues, to oxidize the drug to its major 4-hydroxydebrisoquine metabolite [9]. Years later, this same subject developed severe orthostatic hypotension within 2 h of taking debrisoquine 32 mg base, a response that was not found with other subjects who ingested a similar dose [9]. Subsequent urine analysis revealed that non-responders to this dose excreted the drug as its major metabolite (4-hydroxydebrisoquine), whereas the sensitive responder excreted it unchanged. These observations were followed up with a population study which led to the subsequent description of genetic polymorphism of debrisoquine metabolism [5].

At about the same time in Bonn, Germany, independent studies on sparteine showed unusual responses in some subjects. During kinetic studies with a slow-release preparation of sparteine [10, 11] two subjects developed adverse effects including diplopia, blurred vision, dizziness and headache. These subjects had plasma levels of the sparteine 3–4 times higher than the others, although all the subjects had been given the same dose. Further observations in these two subjects revealed that:

1. Neither subject possessed the two metabolites of sparteine, 2-dehydrosparteine and 5-dehydrosparteine, which are normally present in plasma and urine.
2. Nearly 100% of either an intravenous or oral dose of the drug was recovered in urine as sparteine.

These initial observations and studies led to a population study and the subsequent description of another genetic drug polymorphism involving sparteine [6].

METHODS EMPLOYED IN THE STUDY OF DRUG POLYMORPHISMS

A number of study methods are employed in the identification of genetic polymorphism of drug metabolism to distinguish between hereditary and environmental factors contributing to variability in drug metabolism [12, 13]. These approaches are based on the use of carefully selected subjects under uniform and near basal environmental conditions.

Metabolic Phenotype

The first approach is to use a specific probe drug to determine the metabolic phenotype of an individual. Pharmacokinetic parameters such as half-life, clearance or metabolites of the drug might be measured in a large number of subjects. Based on the findings in these pharmacokinetic parameters, individuals are classified as either poor or extensive metabolizers [14, 15]. An intermediate heterozygous group may also be evident.

Population Study

This allows an estimate of the frequency of a particular deficiency trait (for example, metabolic capacity), and involves phenotyping a sufficient number of unrelated subjects from a homogenous population group [16]. The frequency distribution of this deficiency may indicate whether the inheritance of the defect is monogenic (mendelian) or polygenic. The frequency distribution of a monogenic trait may be either bimodal or trimodal, whereas it is usually unimodal if the trait is polygenic. The contribution of environmental factors in the polygenic traits is often difficult to differentiate. Studies in different ethnic groups demonstrate the variation in the frequencies of the different phenotypes of drug oxidation in various populations (Table 2.1).

Twin Study

The relative contribution of genetic and environmental factors to drug metabolism is determined by investigations in groups of monozygotic (identical) and dizygotic (fraternal) twins, under controlled clinical conditions. The contribution of heredity is calculated from a formula in which heritability ($H2$) is the variance within pairs of dizygotic twins (V_{Dz}) minus variance within pairs of monozygotic twins (V_{Mz}), divided by the variance between pairs of dizygotic twins [17, 18]:

$$H2 = (V_{Dz} - V_{Mz})/V_{Dz}$$

Variance (V) is calculated as:

sum of (difference between twins)$^2/2N$

where N is the number of twin pairs of same zygosity. A value ranging from 0 (negligible genetic contribution) to 1 (virtually complete genetic influence), is possible. The twin study offers a convenient initial step, although family studies are ultimately required.

Family/Pedigree Studies

The mode of inheritance is revealed by studying the transmission in families and generations of assigned phenotypes [19]. If the mode of inheritance follows a

TABLE 2.1 Frequency of CYP2D6 deficiency in different populations

Ethnicity (country)	Probe drug	% (PMs/total)		Reference
AFRICA				
American (USA, children)	DB	1.9	(2/106)	[94]
Ghanaian (Ghana)	SP	0	(0/154)	[95]
Ghanaian (Ghana)	DB	7	(10/141)	[88]
Ghanaian (Ghana)	DB	6.3	(5/80)	[96]
Nigerian (Nigeria)	SP	4	(7/165)	[97]
Nigerian (Nigeria)	SP	8	(10/123)	[98]
Nigerian (Nigeria)	DB	0	(0/138)	[89]
San Bushmen (South Africa)	DB	19	(18/96)	[99]
Zambian (Zambia)	DB	2	(2/102)	[100]
AMERICAN INDIANS				
Cuna (Panama)	SP	0	(0/170)	[101]
Cuna (Panama)	DB	0	(0/89)	[102]
Ngawbe' Guayme' (Panama)	SP	5.2	(5/121)	[103]
Canadian	DX	1.1	(1/95)	[104]
ASIA				
Chinese (China)	M	0	(0/98)	[105]
Chinese (China)	DB	1	(7/695)	[106]
Filipino (Saudi Arabia)	DX	0	(0/55)	[107]
Japanese (Japan)	DB	0	(0/100)	[108]
Japanese (Japan)	SP	2	(2/84)	[109]
Japanese (Japan)	M	0.5	(1/200)	[105]
Korean	DB	0	(0/152)	[110]
Maori (New Zealand)	DB	5	(5/101)	[111]
Sinhalese (Sri Lanka)	DB	1.8	(2/111)	[112]
Thai (Thailand)	DB	1.2	(2/173)	[113]
CAUCASIANS				
American (USA)	DX	6.7	(35/519)	[114]
American (USA)	DB	8.7	(16/183)	[108]
American (USA, children)	DB	7.7	(37/480)	[91]
Australian (Australia)	DB	6	(6/100)	[115]
Belgian (Belgium)	DB	7.2	(12/167)	[116]
Canadian (Canada)	SP	8.3	(4/48)	[117]
Danish (Denmark)	SP	7.3	(22/301)	[118]
Danish (Denmark)	SP	9.2	(33/358)	[119]
English (England)	DB	3	(3/94)	[5]
Estonian (Estonia)	DB	5.1	(4/78)	[120]
Estonian (Estonia)	DX	3.8	(3/78)	[120]
Finnish (Finland)	DB	3.2	(5/155)	[121]
Lapp (Finland)	DB	8.6	(6/70)	[121]
French (France)	DX	7.4	(45/610)	[122]
French (France)	DX	3.9	(4/103)	[123]
French (France)	DX	3	(4/132)	[124]
French (France)	DX(ELISA)	5.1	(216)	[125]
German (Germany)	DX	10	(46/450)	[126]
German (Germany)	SP	7.7	(15/194)	[127]

TABLE 2.1 *(continued)*

Ethnicity (country)	Probe drug	% (PMs/total)		Reference
Greenlander (Greenland)	SP	3.2	(6/185)	[128]
W. Greenlander (Greenland)	SP	2.3	(4/171)	[129]
E. Greenlander (Greenland)	SP	3.3	(10/300)	[129]
Italian (Italy)	DX	4.5	(11/246)	[130]
Spanish (Spain)	DB	6.6	(25/377)	[131]
Spanish (Spain)	DB	11	(14/127)	[132]
Spanish (Spain)	DX	10	(15/146)	[132]
Swedish (Sweden)	DB	6.82	(69/1011)	[106]
Swedish (Sweden)	DB	5.4	(41/757)	[133]
Swedish (Sweden)	DB	8.8	(18/205)	[134]
MIDDLE EASTERN				
Jordanian (Jordan)	DB	7.1	(14/195)	[135]
Jordanian (Jordan)	DB	7.7	(3/39)	[136]
Jordanian (Jordan)	DX	2.9	(7/241)	[137]
Saudi (Saudi Arabia)	DX	2	(2/102)	[107]
Saudi (Saudi Arabia)	DB	1	(1/102)	[138]
Turkish (Turkey)	DB	3.4	(11/326)	[139]

Abbreviations: DB debrisoquine; SP sparteine; DX dextromethorphan; M metoprolol

classical mendelian pattern, the trait can be classified as autosomal dominant, autosomal recessive or X-linked.

Panel Approach

Subjects who have been phenotyped with respect to a particular metabolic defect are given a single dose of the drug to be investigated and its pharmacokinetics and metabolism are studied [15]. These parameters are usually compared in two panels of subjects at both ends of the phenotype spectrum; for example, poor and extensive metabolizers. With this method, drugs with metabolic patterns that are affected by the genetic defect or polymorphism under investigation are detected.

In-vitro and Enzyme Studies

In-vitro techniques and enzyme studies are extensively employed as tools in the identification and study of genetic polymorphism of drug metabolism [20]. Some of these techniques involve the use of not only liver microsomes but also of isolated and purified enzymes and isoenzymes [21]. In-vitro techniques are useful in identifying the various forms of CYP enzymes involved in the oxidative metabolism of a particular drug [22] and also in determining the potential for drug interactions [23].

Genetic Studies

The principal studies of molecular biology, such as polymerase-chain reaction (PCR) and restriction fragment-length polymorphism (RFLP), are increasingly being used in the study of genetic drug polymorphism [24]. Poor metabolizers of debrisoquine have negligible amounts of the CYP enzyme that metabolizes this drug [25]. Poor metabolizers have mutant alleles that give rise to variant messenger RNA which produces a defective protein. DNA analysis of poor and extensive metabolizers has shown that different mutant alleles of varying combinations lead to different genotypes associated with both poor and extensive metabolizer pheno-types [26]. Thus it is now possible to genotype individuals to determine if they have metabolic deficiency traits by collection of a single blood sample [27].

GENETIC POLYMORPHISM OF DEBRISOQUINE/ SPARTEINE/DEXTROMETHORPHAN METABOLISM

Polymorphic hydroxylation of debrisoquine, an antihypertensive drug, was first described by Mahgoub et al. [5], and the polymorphic N-oxidation of sparteine was first described by Eichelbaum et al. [6]. The metabolism of these two drugs was later shown to be mediated by the same enzyme [28–31]; thus a poor metabolizer (PM) of debrisoquine will also be a PM of sparteine. Another drug that has been used extensively in phenotyping individuals with respect to their hepatic drug oxidizing capacity is dextromethorphan, an over-the-counter cough medication [32]. It is metabolized to dextro-orphan by cytochrome P4502D6 (CYP2D6). This enzyme is polymorphically distributed in different populations (see Table 2.1) and is involved in the metabolism of debrisoquine and sparteine (which are also used as probe drugs) and more than 30 other clinically important drugs [33, 34]. Based on their abilities to metabolize these drugs, individuals are classified as poor meta-bolizers (PMs) or extensive metabolizers (EMs). The metabolic phenotype of a subject is assigned based on the metabolic ratio (MR) of the probe drug in that individual, which is determined as follows:

- MR = amount of debrisoquine (moles)/amount of 4-hydroxydebrisoquine (moles) excreted in urine over 8 h;
- MR = amount of sparteine (moles)/amounts of 2- and 5-dehydrosparteine (moles) excreted in urine over 12 h;
- MR = amount of dextromethorphan (moles)/amount of dextrorphan (in moles) excreted in urine over 8 h.

Poor metabolizers are defined as having an MR greater than 12.6 (debrisoquine), 20 (sparteine), or 0.3 (dextromethorphan) [30–32].

The genetic polymorphism of the metabolism of debrisoquine, sparteine, and dextromethorphan is not affected by age, sex, or smoking; it is transmitted in a mendelian fashion and PM subjects are homozygous for an autosomal recessive gene [6, 31, 35–37]. The frequency in the European population of the allele controlling poor metabolism is 0.2321 and that for extensive metabolism is 0.7679 [37]. A study undertaken to find out if there is linkage of the polymorphic sparteine oxidation to various polymorphic marker systems showed a positive linkage to the P1 blood group [38]. The P1 blood group has been mapped to the long arm of chromosome 22, and thus it was concluded that the gene controlling debrisoquine/ sparteine metabolism polymorphism is situated on the long arm of chromosome 22 in close vicinity to P1. No relationship has been found between debrisoquine/ sparteine metabolism and drug acetylation, the excretion of bile acid and bile alcohol [39, 40], or 6-beta hydroxycortisol excretion [41]. Furthermore, the phenotype of a subject is not affected by viral or pneumococcal vaccination [42] and it is stable following repeated phenotyping in patients with insulin-dependent diabetes mellitus [43].

Pharmacokinetics and Phenotype

The plasma concentrations of debrisoquine are significantly higher in PMs than in EMs [15]. The 4-hydroxylation of debrisoquine by PMs following a 10 mg oral dose was capacity limited and dose dependent in the range of 1–20 mg; in EMs this oxidation did not deviate from first-order kinetics over a dose of 10–40 mg [44]. PM subjects also tend to have an increased pharmacodynamic response to drugs that are substrates of CYP2D6 [14].

Effect of Inducing Substances

A study was carried out to examine the influence of various enzyme inducers (1200 mg antipyrine, 100 mg phenobarbitone, 600 mg or 1200 mg rifampin daily for 7 days) on sparteine metabolism and 6-beta hydrocortisol excretion in panels of EM and PM subjects [45]. Drug metabolism was induced in both groups, as shown by increased 6-beta hydrocortisol excretion, although the increase caused by phenobarbitone was not significant—probably due to the low dose. Significant changes in elimination half-life and metabolic clearance were observed only in EMs following antipyrine and rifampin administration, with greater effect seen with 1200 mg/day rifampin. It was concluded that the regulation of the CYP isozyme involved in debrisoquine/sparteine polymorphism is predominantly under genetic control, with only a marginal effect from enzyme induction.

Enantioselectivity and Debrisoquine 4-Hydroxylation

Two early reports have focused attention on the interesting phenomenon of enantioselectivity by debrisoquine 4-hydroxylation [46, 47]. Debrisoquine has no

TABLE 2.2   Drugs metabolized by CYP2D6

Drug	Metabolic route/metabolite	Reference
Antidepressants		
Amitriptyline	Hydroxylation (nortriptyline)	[77]
Clomipramine	2-,8-hydroxylation (hydroxyclomipramine)	[140, 141]
Desmethylclomipramine	8-hydroxylation (hydroxydesmethylclomipramine)	[140]
Desipramine	2-hydroxylation (hydroxydesipramine)	[142]
Imipramine	2-hydroxylation (hydroxyimipramine; hydroxydesmethylimipramine)	[143, 144]
Desmethylimipramine	2-hydroxylation	[74, 145]
Risperidone	9-hydroxylation (hydroxyrisperidone)	[146]
Neuroleptics		
Reduced haloperidol	Oxidation (haloperidol)	[147]
Thioridazine	Side-chain oxidation (thioridazine-2-sulfoxide; thioridazine-2-sulfone)	[77, 148]
Selective serotonin reuptake inhibitors		
Citalopram	Demethylation (desmethylcitalopram)	[149]
Desmethylcitalopram	Demethylation (didesmethylcitalopram)	[149]
Fluvoxamine	Hydroxylation	[48]
Paroxetine	Oxidation	[48, 150]
Fluoxetine	Norfluoxetine	[142]
Sertraline	Demethylation (desmethylsertraline)	[142]
Nortriptyline	10-hydroxylation (hydroxynortriptyline)	[151]
Chlorpropamide	2-,3-hydroxylation (hydroxychlorpropamide)	[152]

chiral center; however hydroxylation in position 4 leads to the formation of an asymmetric carbon center with two possible enantiomers of absolute configurations: $R(-)$ and $S(+)$ 4-hydroxydebrisoquine. Extensive metabolizers exhibited pronounced enantioselectivity in debrisoquine 4-hydoxylation, with more than 99% of 4-hydroxydebrisoquine excreted as the $S(+)$ enantiomer. The PMs on the other end are characterized not only by reduced metabolite formation but also by loss of enantioselectivity, with 5–36% of the total 4-hydroxydebrisoquine being excreted as the $R(-)$ enantiomer. It was the view of the authors that 4-hydroxydebrisoquine enantiomer formation might provide an additional phenotyping criterion, especially in those subjects with metabolic ratios close to the antimode.

Substrates of CYP2D6

CYP2D6 is involved in the metabolism of more than 30 drugs that are very important in the clinical arena [33, 34]. Major classes include beta-adrenoceptor blockers, antiarrhythmics, tricyclic antidepressants, neuroleptics, and serotonin reuptake inhibitors [23, 48] (Table 2.2).

CLINICAL AND THERAPEUTIC IMPLICATIONS

There are a number of important clinical, therapeutic and toxicological implications in the deficiency of CYP2D6.

Increased Adverse Effects

As a result of impaired metabolic capacity, PMs, even at normal doses, usually have higher plasma concentrations of drugs that are substrates of CYP2D6. This has been demonstrated for several drugs—indoramin [49], amitriptyline, nortriptyline [50], timolol [15], and others [34]. Thus, PM subjects may simply be prone to the development of adverse effects during the course of a normal therapeutic use of a drug. It is noteworthy that adverse effects in two PM subjects during the course of an initial investigation led to the discovery of the genetic polymorphism of sparteine metabolism [6]. Therefore, in order to avoid increased adverse effects such patients will require a lower than usual dose [51], as deficient metabolism may lead to increased response [9, 14]. The administration of perhexiline is associated with peripheral neuropathy in subjects who poorly hydroxylate debrisoquine [52]. Phenformin 4-hydroxylation co-segregates with debrisoquine hydroxylation [53], and this might be an important factor in the development of lactic acidosis, when PM patients take phenformin [54, 55]. The metabolism of some beta-adrenoceptor blockers (such as bufuralol, timolol, propranolol, and metoprolol) is controlled by the debrisoquine gene locus, although that of atenolol is not; thus PMs have increased plasma concentrations and may have increased beta-adrenoceptor blockade and be prone to more adverse effects than EMs when on these drugs [56–63]. Failure to consider the pharmacogenetic phenotype of a subject could lead to overtreatment of PMs and undertreatment of EMs.

Drug Interactions

Certain drugs have very high affinity for CYP2D6, bind strongly to it and prevent it from metabolizing other drugs, including such CYP2D6 substrates as propafenone, fluoxetine and norfluoxetine (its main metabolite) [23], and other drugs like quinidine which, although it has high affinity for CYP2D6 [64], is not metabolized by it [65]. This inhibitory effect of quinidine has been demonstrated not only in vitro [64, 66] but also in vivo. Quinidine inhibits 2-hydroxylation of desipramine in both PMs and EMs, whereas its diastereoisomer quinine inhibits this metabolism only in EMs, indicating a possible stereoselective mechanism [67]. The high inhibitory potency of quinidine was recently demonstrated by the fact that even low doses inhibited the metabolism of ophthalmic timolol, leading to significant increases in plasma timolol concentrations and pharmacodynamic response [15].

In-vitro studies have shown that the selective serotonin reuptake inhibitors (SSRIs) paroxetine and fluvoxamine inhibit desipramine hydroxylation, albeit to different extents [48]. Fluoxetine has been shown to reduce the oral clearance of tricyclic antidepressants [68, 69]. Some clinical case reports have also provided evidence to suggest that fluoxetine interacts with tricyclic antidepressants and antipsychotics [70]. The drug interactions between neuroleptics and tricyclic antidepressants [71] could also be explained on the basis of the involvement of CYP2D6. The potential for drug interaction is much greater in EMs than in PMs.

It is also of interest that the metabolism of desipramine, a drug which cosegregates with debrisoquine metabolism [72–74], was inhibited by cimetidine in EMs but not in PMs [75]. Because several drug types used in psychiatry are substrates of CYP2D6, pharmacogenetic evaluation is an important factor that needs to be considered in clinical situations when psychotropic medications are administered. Studies have indicated that psychiatric drug treatment is capable of increasing the metabolic ratios and changing the pharmacogenetic status of patients [76–78].

Shift to a More Toxic Metabolite

Another important consequence of impaired drug metabolism is a shift in the metabolic pathway leading to the formation of a toxic metabolite, when the main pathway of detoxification is impaired while that of the toxic metabolite is not. This is exemplified by phenacetin, impaired o-de-ethylation of which leads to increased formation of 2-hydroxyphenetidin, a metabolite implicated in the development of methemoglobinemia following phenacetin administration. This has been confirmed by observations of more cases of methemoglobinemia in PMs than in EMs receiving the same dose of phenacetin [79, 80].

Therapeutic Failure

Defective drug metabolism could also lead to therapeutic failure if formation of an active metabolite responsible for therapeutic activity is impaired. An example is the antiarrhythmic drug encainide; the o-demethylated metabolites have antiarrhythmic activity and their formation is under genetic control similar to that of debrisoquine [81, 82]. However, it seems that the possible failure in the PM is offset by the antiarrhythmic activity of the very high concentration of the parent drug [82].

Another example of therapeutic failure in PMs occurs with codeine, which is o-demethylated to morphine by CYP2D6 [83]. The role of the genetic phenotype of a subject in the analgesic efficacy of codeine is supported by a study in which codeine increased the pain threshold in EMs but not in PMs [84], thus providing evidence that morphine formation is essential for analgesia during treatment with codeine. PMs may therefore not benefit as much as EMs from the analgesic effect of codeine.

Rapid Metabolism Leading to Therapeutic Failure

The phenomenon of 'ultra-rapid metabolism' of debrisoquine was first brought to light by the case of a depressed patient taking nortriptyline who failed to attain adequate therapeutic plasma concentrations because the drug was very rapidly metabolized [85]. As a result of RFLP analysis of the CYP2D locus in two families, the basis of the very rapid metabolism of debrisoquine was identified as being due to a variant CYP2D6 gene, CYP2D6L [86]: the members of these families had inherited amplification of the CYP2D6L. The prevalence of subjects with duplication of CYP2D6L in a Spanish population was about 7% [87], similar to that of PMs. Ultra rapid metabolism is therefore another important factor that should be considered in order to avoid therapeutic failure of CYP2D6 substrates.

Interethnic Differences

The frequency of the PM phenotypes varies with ethnic origin (see Table 2.1). Most of the studies on deficient metabolism of drugs by PMs have been carried out in Caucasian populations, and these findings may not always be applicable to other populations. This is supported by a study in Ghanaians, which failed to show that poor metabolizers of sparteine are also poor metabolizers of debrisoquine, quite unlike the findings in Caucasian populations [88]. A study in a Nigerian population did not identify PMs of metoprolol or debrisoquine [89].

Differences in gene frequencies have also been demonstrated in various populations. For example, Spaniards had lower frequency of the CYP2D6(B) allele and a higher frequency of the wild-type allele than other Caucasian populations [90]. The CYP2D6Ch alleles were very frequent in Orientals, whereas CYP2D6A or CYP2D6B were not identified [91]. Also, the lower prevalence of debrisoquine PMs has been said to be due to reduced frequency of the CYP2D6(B) mutation [92].

Implications for Drug Development

Genetic polymorphism of drug oxidation has implications in the development of new drugs [12, 93]. Subjects should be enlisted for the initial Phase 1 and 2 studies of new drugs based on their phenotypes with already established probe drugs. This will avoid the use of subjects from extremes of the phenotype spectrum. Secondly, the varying incidence of polymorphisms in different ethnic groups raises doubts on the reliability of extrapolating findings from one population group to others. In order to give reliable dosage recommendations in a population, studies are needed using representative subjects of that particular population. Extensive applications of in-vitro drug-metabolism studies have provided early information on the types of various CYP enzymes involved in the metabolism of a particular drug and on potential drug interactions and have enabled more meaningful clinical studies to be conducted.

CONCLUSION

The recent advances in the field of genetic polymorphism of drug oxidation has brought to light the important concept that pharmacogenetic evaluation should be considered in drug therapy. This will not only allow for optimization of drug therapy but will also avoid unnecessary adverse effects. These considerations are especially relevant in the use of cardiovascular drugs and in the drug treatment of psychiatric disorders.

REFERENCES

1. Chapman CJ. 1977. Drugs and genes. Therapeutic implications. *Drugs* **14**: 120–7.
2. Kutt H, Wolk M, Scherman R, McDowell F. 1964. Insufficient parahydroxylation as a cause of diphenylhydantoin toxicity. *Neurology* **14**: 542–8.
3. Edeki T, Brase D. 1995. Phenytoin disposition and toxicity: Role of Pharmacogenetic and Interethnic Factors. *Drug Metab Rev* **27**(3): 449–69.
4. Shahidi NT. 1968. Acetophenetidin-induced methemoglobinemia. *Ann NY Acad Sci* **151**(2): 822–32.
5. Mahgoub A, Dring LG, Idle JR, Lancaster R, Smith RL. 1977. Polymorphic hydroxylation of debrisoquine in man. *Lancet* **2**: 584–6.
6. Eichelbaum M, Spannbrucker N, Steincker B, Dengler HJ. 1979. Defective *N*-oxidation of sparteine in man: A new pharmacogenetic defect. *Eur J Clin Pharmacol* **16**: 183–7.
7. Guengerich FP. 1992. Human cytochrome P-450 enzymes. *Life Sci* **50**: 1471–8.
8. Daniel H, Edeki T. 1996. Genetic Polymorphism of S-Mephenytoin 4'-hydroxylation. *Psychopharmacol Bull* **32**(2): 219–30.
9. Smith RL. 1986. Discovery of the genetic polymorphism of drug oxidation. *Xenobiotica* **16**: 361–5.
10. Eichelbaum M, Spannbrucker N, Dengler HJ. 1975. *N*-oxidation of sparteine in man and its interindividual differences. *Arch Pharmacol* **287**: R94.
11. Eichelbaum M, Spannbrucker N, Dengler HJ. 1975. Lack of *N*-oxidation of sparteine in certain healthy subjects. Sixth International Congress of Pharmacology, Helsinki, July 20–25, 1071.
12. Eichelbaum M. 1981. Polymorphism of drug oxidation in man: novel findings. *Trends in Pharmacological Sciences*. New York: Elsevier/North Holland Biochemical Press.
13. Edeki T. 1989. Antipyrine and debrisoquine as pharmacologic probe drugs in assessing drug therapy and disease states. PhD dissertation, University of London, England.
14. Al-Sereiti MD, Edeki T, Lledo P, Turner P. 1990. The effects of timolol on intraocular pressure and exercise heart rate in poor and extensive debrisoquine metabolizers. *Int J Clin Pharmacol Res* **6**: 339–45.
15. Edeki TI, He H, Wood AJJ. 1995. Pharmacogenetic explanation for excessive β-blockade following timolol eye drops. Potential for oral–ophthalmic drug interaction. *JAMA* **274**: 1611–13.
16. He N, Edeki T. 1995. Polymorphism of Dextromethorphan Oxidation in African Americans [abstract]. *J Invest Med* **43**: 256A.
17. Vesell ES, Page JG. 1968. Genetic control of drug levels in man: Antipyrine. *Science* **161**: 72–3.
18. Penno MB, Dvorchik BH, Vesell ES. 1981. Genetic variation in rates of antipyrine metabolism formation: A study in uninduced twins. *Proc Natl Acad Sci USA* **78**: 5193–6.

19. Evans DAP, Mahgoub A, Sloan TP, Idle JR, Smith RL. 1983. A family and population study of the genetic polymorphism of debrisoquine oxidation in a white British population. *J Med Genet* **17**: 102–5.

20. Newton DJ, Wang RW, Lu AYH. 1995. Cytochrome P450 inhibitors—evaluation of specificities in the in vitro metabolism of therapeutic agents by human liver microsomes. *Drug Metab Dispos* **23**: 154–8.

21. Distlerath LM, Reilly PEB, Martin AV, Davis GG, Wilkinson GR, Guengerich FP. 1985. Purification and characterization of the human liver cytochromes P-450 involved in debrisoquine 4-hydroxylation and phenacetin *o*-deethylation, two prototypes for genetic polymorphism in oxidative drug metabolism. *J Biol Chem* **260**: 9057–67.

22. Masabuchi Y, Hosokawa S, Horie T, Suzuki T, Ohmori S, Kitada M, Narimatsu S. 1994. Cytochrome P450 isozymes involved in propranolol metabolism in human liver microsomes: The role of CYP2D6 as ring-hydroxylase and CYP1A2 as *N*-desisopropylase. *Drug Metab Dispos* **22**: 909–15.

23. Otton SV, Wu D, Joffe RT, Cheung SW, Sellers EM. 1993. Inhibition by fluoxetine of cytochrome P450 2D6 activity. *Clin Pharmacol Ther* **53**: 401–9.

24. Steen VM, Andreassen OA, Daly AK, Tefre T, Borresen AL, Idle JR, Gulbrandsen AK. 1995. Detection of the metabolizer-associated CYP2D6(D) gene deletion allele by long-PCR technology. *Pharmacogenetics* **5**: 215–23.

25. Gonzalez FJ, Skoda CR, Kimura SM, Umeno M, Zanger UM, Nebert DW *et al.* 1988. Characterization of the common genetic defect in humans deficient in debrisoquine metabolism. *Nature* **331**: 442–6.

26. Skoda CK, Gonzalez FJ, Demierre A, Meyer UA. 1988. Two mutant alleles of the human cytochrome P-450 db1 gene (P450C2D1) associated with genetically deficient metabolism of debrisoquine and other drugs. *Proc Natl Acad Sci USA* **85**: 5240–3.

27. Broly F, Gaedigk A, Heim M, Eichelbaum M, Morike K, Meyer UA. 1991. Debrisoquine/sparteine hydroxylation genotype and phenotype: Analysis of common mutations and alleles of CYP2D6 in a European population. *DNA Cell Biol* **10**: 545–58.

28. Inaba T, Otton SV, Kalow W. 1980. Deficient metabolism of debrisoquine and sparteine. *Clin Pharmacol Ther* **27**: 547–9.

29. Inaba T, Vinks A, Otton SV, Kalow W. 1983. Comparative pharmacogenetics of sparteine and debrisoquine. *Clin Pharmacol Ther* **33**: 394–9.

30. Eichelbaum M, Bertilsoon L, Sawe J, Zekorn C. 1982. Polymorphic oxidation of sparteine and debrisoquine related pharmacogenetic entities. *Clin Pharmacol Ther* **31**: 184–6.

31. Evans DAP, Harmer D, Downham DY, Whibley EJ, Idle JR, Ritchie, Smiths RL. 1983. The genetic control of sparteine and debrisoquine metabolism in man with new methods of analyzing bimodal distributions. *J Med Genet* **20**: 321–9.

32. Schmid B, Bircher J, Preisig R, Kupfer A. 1985. Polymorphic dextromethorphan metabolism: Co-segregation of oxidative *o*-demethylation with debrisoquin hydroxylation. *Clin Pharmacol Ther* **38**(6): 618–24.

33. Jacqz E, Hall SD, Branch RA. 1986. Genetically determined polymorphisms in drug oxidation. *Hepatology* **6**: 1020–32.

34. Eichelbaum M, Gross AS. 1990. The genetic polymorphism of debrisoquine/sparteine metabolism—clinical aspects. *Pharmacol Ther* **46**: 377–94.

35. Idle J, Smith RL. 1984. The debrisoquine hydroxylation gene. A gene of multiple consequence. In: Lemberger L, Reidenberg M eds, Proceedings of the Second World Conference on Clinical Pharmacology and Therapeutics. Bethesda, MD: American Society for Pharmacology Experimental Therapeutics, pp. 148–64.

36. Brosen K, Klysner R, Gram LF, Otton SV, Bech P, Bertilsson L. 1986. Steady-state concentrations of imipramine and its metabolites in relation to the sparteine/debrisoquine polymorphism. *Eur J Clin Pharmacol* **30**: 679–84.

37. Eichelbaum M, Reetz KP, Schmidt EK, Zekorn C. 1986. The genetic polymorphism of sparteine metabolism. *Xenobiotica* **16**: 405–81.
38. Eichelbaum M, Baur MP, Dengler HJ, Osikowska-Evers BO, Tieves G, Zekron C, Rittner C. 1987. Chromosome assignment of human cytochrome P-450 (debrisoquine/sparteine type) to chromosome 22. *Br J Clin Pharmacol* **23**: 455–8.
39. Karlaganis G, Küpfer A, Preisig R. 1984. Urinary bile alcohol excretion does not reflect the genetic polymorphism of debrisoquine hydroxylation. *Br J Clin Pharmacol* **17**: 470–3.
40. Harmer D, Pevans DA, Eze LC, Jolly M, Whibley EJ. 1986. The relationship between the acetylator and the sparteine hydroxylation polymorphisms. *J Med Genet* **23**: 155–6.
41. Park BK, Eichelbaum M, Ohnhaus EE. 1982. 6-beta hydroxycortisol excretion in relation to polymorphic *N*-oxidation of sparteine [letter]. *Br J Clin Pharmacol* **13**: 737–40.
42. Ayesh R, Scandding G, Brostoff J, Idle JR, Smith RL. 1988. Stability of the debrisoquine metabolic ratio to immunoperturbation by influenza and pneumococcus vaccines [abstract]. *Br J Clin Pharmacol* **25**: 141P.
43. Bechtel YC, Joanne C, Grandmottet M, Bechtel PR. 1988. The influence of insulin-dependent diabetes on the metabolism of caffeine and the expression of debrisoquine. *Clin Pharmacol Ther* **44**: 408–17.
44. Sloan TP, Lancaster R, Shann RR, Idle JR, Smith RL. 1983. Genetically determined oxidation capacity and the disposition of debrisoquine. *Br J Clin Pharmacol* **15**: 443–50.
45. Eichelbaum M, Mineshita S, Ohnhaus EE, Zekorn C. 1986. The influence of enzyme induction on polymorphic sparteine oxidation. *Br J Clin Pharmacol* **22**: 49–53.
46. Meese CO, Bertilsson L, Fisher C, Küpfer A, Steiner E, Eichelbaum M. Stereoselectivity of 4-hydroxydeberisoquine enantiomer formation in relation to debrisoquine phenotype. Third World Conference on Clinical Pharmacology and Therapeutics, July–August 1986.
47. Eichelbaum M, Bertilsson L, Küpfer A, Steiner E, Meese CO. 1988. Enantioselectivity of 4-hydroxylation in extensive and poor metabolisers of debrisoquine. *Br J Clin Pharmacol* **25**: 505–8.
48. von Molte L, Greenblatt D, Court M, Duan S, Harmatz J, Shader R. 1995. Inhibition of alprazolam and desipramine hydroxylation in vitro by paroxetine and fluvoxamine: Comparison with other selective serotonin reuptake inhibitor antidepressants. *J Clin Psychopharmacol* **15**: 125–31.
49. Pierce DM, Smith SE, Franklin RA. 1987. The pharmacokinetics of Indoramin and 6-hydroxyindoramin on poor and extensive hydroxylators of debrisoquine. *Eur J Clin Pharmacol* **33**: 59–65.
50. Baumann P, Jonzier-Perey M, Koeb L, Küpfer A, Tinguely D, Schopf J. 1986. Amitriptyline pharmacokinetics and clinical response: 11. Metabolic polymorphism assessed by hydroxylation of debrisoquine and mephenytoin. *Int J Clin Psychopharmacol* **1**: 102–12.
51. Silas JH, Lennard MS, Tucker GT, Smith AJ, Malcolm SL, Marten TR. 1977. Why hypertensive patients vary their response to oral debrisoquine. *BMJ* **1**: 422–5.
52. Shah RR, Oates NS, Idle JR, Smith RL, Lockhart JDF. 1988. Prediction of subclinical perhexiline neuropathy in a patient with inborn error of debrisoquine hydroxylation. *Am Heart J* **105**: 159–61.
53. Oates NS, Shah RR, Idle JR, Smith RL. 1982. Genetic polymorphism of phenformin 4-hydroxylation. *Clin Pharmacol Ther* **32**: 81–9.
54. Shah RR, Oates NS, Idle JR, Smith RL. 1980. Genetic impairment of phenformin metabolism. *Lancet* **1**: 1147.
55. Wiholm B, Alvan G, Bertilsson L, Sawe J, Sjöqvist F. 1981. Hydroxylation of debrisoquine in patients with lactic acidosis after phenformin: *Lancet* **1**(8229): 1098–9.

56. Lennard MS, Silas JH, Freestone S, Ramsay LE, Tucker GT, Woods HF. 1982. Oxidation phenotype—a major determinant of metoprolol metabolism and response. *N Engl J Med* **307**: 1558–60.
57. Lennard MS, Jackson PR, Freestone S, Tucker GT, Ramsay LE, Woods HF. 1982. The relationship between debrisoquine oxidation phenotype and the pharmacokinetics and pharmacodynamics of propranolol. *Br J Clin Pharmacol* **17**: 679–85.
58. Lennard MS, Tucker GT, Silas JH, Woods HF. 1986. Debrisoquine polymorphism and the metabolism and action of metoprolol, timolol, propranolol, and atenolol. *Xenobiotica* **16**: 435–47.
59. Dayer P, Kubli A, Küpfer A, Courvoisier F, Balant L, Fabre J. 1982. Defective hydroxylation of bufuralol associated with side-effects of the drug in poor metabolisers. *Br J Clin Pharmacol* **13**: 750–1.
60. Dayer P, Balant L, Küpfer A, Courvoisier F, Fabre J. 1983. Contribution of the genetic status of oxidative metabolism to variability in the plasma concentrations of beta-adrenoceptor blocking agents. *Eur J Clin Pharmacol* **24**: 797–9.
61. Raghuram TC, Koshakji RP, Wilkinson GR, Wood AJJ. 1984. Polymorphic ability to metabolize propranolol alters 4-hydroxypropranolol levels but not beta blockade. *Clin Pharmacol Ther* **36**: 51–6.
62. McGourty JC, Silas JH. 1985. Metoprolol metabolism and debrisoquine oxidation polymorphism—population and family studies. *Br J Clin Pharmacol* **20**: 555–6.
63. McGourty JC, Silas JH, Fleming JJ, McBurney A, Ward JW. 1985. Pharmacokinetics and beta-blocking effects of timolol in poor and extensive metabolisers of debrisoquin. *Clin Pharmacol Ther* **38**: 409–13.
64. Otton SV, Inaba T, Kalow W. 1984. Competitive inhibition of sparteine oxidation in human liver by β-adrenoceptor antagonists and other cardiovascular drugs. *Life Sci* **34**: 73–80.
65. Mikus G, Ha HR, Vozen S, Zekorm C, Follath F, Eichelbaum M. 1986. Pharmacokinetics and metabolism of quinidine in extensive and poor metabolisers of sparteine. *Eur J Clin Pharmacol* **31**: 69–72.
66. Brosen K, Gram L. 1987. Quinidine inhibits the 2-hydroxylation of imipramine and desipramine but not the demethylation of imipramine. *Eur J Clin Pharmacol* **37**: 155–60.
67. Steiner E, Dumont E, Spina E, Dahlqvist R. 1988. Inhibition of desipramine 2-hydroxylation by quinidine and quinine. *Clin Pharmacol Ther* **43**: 577–81.
68. Bergstrom RF, Peyton AL, Lemberger L. 1992. Quantification and mechanism of the fluoxetine and tricyclic antidepressant interaction. *Clin Pharmacol Ther* **51**: 239–48.
69. Preskorn SH, Alderman J, Chung M, Harrison W, Messig M, Harris S. 1994. Pharmacokinetics of desipramine coadministered with sertraline or fluoxetine. *J Clin Psychopharmacol* **14**: 90–8.
70. Ciraulo DA, Shader RI. 1990. Fluoxetine drug–drug interactions: I. Antidepressants and antipsychotics. *J Clin Psychopharmacol* **10**: 48–50.
71. Gram LF, Overo KF. 1972. Drug interaction. Inhibitory effect of neuroleptics on metabolism of tricyclic antidepressants in man. *BMJ* **1**: 463–5.
72. Bertilsson L, Aberg-Wistedt A. 1983. The debrisoquine hydroxylation test predicts steady-state plasma levels of desipramine. *Br J Clin Pharmacol* **15**: 388–90.
73. Spina E, Birgersson C, von Bahr C, Ericsson O, Mellström B, Steiner E, Sjöqvist F. 1984. Phenotypic consistency in hydroxylation of desmethylimipramine and debrisoquine in healthy subjects and in human liver microsomes. *Clin Pharmacol Ther* **36**: 677–82.
74. Spina E, Steiner E, Ericsson O, Sjoqvist F. 1987. Hydroxylation of desmethylimipramine: Dependence on debrisoquine hydroxylation phenotype. *Clin Pharmacol Ther* **41**: 314–19.
75. Steiner E, Spina E. 1987. Differences in the inhibitory effect of cimetidine on desipra-

mine metabolism between rapid and slow debrisoquin hydroxylators. *Clin Pharmacol Ther* **42**: 278–82.

76. Derenne F, Joanne C, Vandel S, Bertschy G, Volmat, Bechtel P. 1989. Debrisoquine oxidative phenotyping and psychiatric drug treatment. *Eur J Clin Pharmacol* **36**: 53–8.

77. Baumann P, Meyer JW, Amey M, Baettig D, Bryois C, Perey MJ *et al.* 1992. Dextromethorphan and mephenytoin phenotyping of patients treated with thioridazine or amitriptyline. *Ther Drug Monit* **14**: 1–8.

78. Llerena A, Herraiz AG, Cobaleda J, Johansson I, Dahl ML. 1993. Debrisoquin and mephenytoin hydroxylation phenotypes and CYP2D6 genotype in patients treated with neuroleptic and antidepressant agents. *Clin Pharmacol Ther* **54**: 606–11.

79. Sloan TP, Mahoub A, Lancaster R, Idle JR, Smith RL. 1978. Polymorphism of carbon oxidation of drugs and clinical implications. *BMJ* **2**: 655–7.

80. Ritchie JC, Sloan TP, Idle JP, Smith RL. 1980. Toxicological implications of polymorphic drug metabolism. *Ciba Found Symp* **76**: 219–44.

81. Woosely RL, Roden DM, Duff HJ, Carey EL, Wood AJJ, Wilkinson GR. 1981. Coinheritance of deficient oxidative metabolism of encainide and debrisoquine. *Clin Res* **29**: 501A.

82. McAllister CB, Wolfenden HT, Aslanian WS, Woosley RL, Wilkinson GR. 1986. Oxidative metabolism of encainide: polymorphism, pharmacokinetics and clinical considerations. *Xenobiotica* **16**: 483–90.

83. Yue QY, Svensson JO, Alm C, Sjoqvist F, Sawe J. 1989. Codeine O-demethylation co-segregates with polymorphic debrisoquine hydroxylation. *Br J Clin Pharmacol* **28**: 639–45.

84. Sindrup S, Brosen K, Bjerring P, Nielson L, Larsen U, Angelo H, Gram L. 1991. Codeine increases pain thresholds to copper vapor laser stimuli in extensive but not poor metabolizers of sparteine. *Clin Pharmacol Ther* **49**: 686–93.

85. Bertilsson L, Aberg-Wistedt A, Gustafsson LL, Nordin C. 1985. Extremely rapid hydroxylation of debrisoquine. A case report with implication for treatment with nortriptyline and other tricyclic antidepressants. *Ther Drug Monit* **7**: 478–80.

86. Johansson I, Ludqvist E, Bertilsson L, Dahl ML, Sjoqvist F, Sundberg M. 1993. Inherited amplification of an active gene in the cytochrome P450 CYP2D locus as a cause of ultrarapid metabolism of debrisoquine. *Proc Natl Acad Sci USA* **90**: 11825–9.

87. Agundez J, Ledesma MC, Ladero JM, Benitez J. 1995. Prevalence of CYP2D6 gene duplication and its repercussion on the oxidative phenotype in a white population. *Clin Pharmacol Ther* **57**: 265–9.

88. Woolhouse NM, Eichelbaum M, Oates NS, Idle JR, Smith RL. 1985. Dissociation of co-regulatory control of debrisoquin/phenformin and sparteine oxidation in Ghanaians. *Clin Pharmacol Ther* **37**: 512–21.

89. Iyun AO, Lennard MS, Tucker GT, Woods HF. 1986. Metoprolol and debrisoquin metabolism in Nigerians: Lack of evidence for polymorphic oxidation. *Clin Pharmacol Ther* **40**: 387–94.

90. Agundez J, Martinez C, Ledesma MC, Ladona M, Ladero J, Benitez J. 1994. Genetic basis for differences in debrisoquin polymorphism between a Spanish and other white populations. *Clin Pharmacol Ther* **55**: 412–17.

91. Dahl ML, Yue QY, Roh HK, Johansso I, Sawe J, Sjoqvist F, Bertilsson L. 1995. Genetic analysis of the CYP2D locus in relation to debrisoquine hydroxylation capacity in Korean, Japanese, and Chinese subjects. *Pharmacogenetics* **5**: 159–64.

92. Evans WE, Relling MV, Rahman A, McLeod HL, Scott EP, Lin JS. 1993. Genetic basis for a lower prevalence of deficient CYP2D6 oxidative drug metabolism phenotypes in Black Americans. *J Clin Invest* **91**: 150–4.

93. Eichelbaum M. 1982. Defective oxidation of drugs: Pharmacokinetic and therapeutic implications. *Clin Pharmacokinet* **7**: 1–22.

94. Relling MV, Cherrie J, Schell MJ, Petros WP, Meyer WH, Evans WE. 1991. Lower prevalence of the debrisoquin oxidative poor metabolizer phenotype in American black versus white subjects. *Clin Pharmacol Ther* **50**: 308–13.

95. Eichelbaum M, Woolhouse NM. 1985. Inter-ethnic difference in sparteine oxidation among Ghanaians and Germans. *Eur J Clin Pharmacol* **28**: 79–83.

96. Woolhouse NM, Andoh B, Mahgoub A, Sloan TP, Idle JR, Smith RL. 1979. Debrisoquin hydroxylation polymorphism among Ghanaians and Caucasians. *Clin Pharmacol Ther* **26**: 584–91.

97. Lennard MS, Iyun AO, Jackson PR, Tucker GT, Woods HF. 1992. Evidence for a dissociation in the control of sparteine, debrisoquine and metoprolol metabolism in Nigerians. *Pharmacogenetics* **2**: 89–92.

98. Mbanefo C, Bababunmi EA, Mahgoub A, Sloan TP, Idle JR, Smith RL. 1980. A study of the debrisoquine hydroxylation polymorphism in a Nigerian population. *Xenobiotica* **10**: 811–18.

99. Sommers DK, Moncrieff J, Avenant J. 1988. Polymorphism of the 4-hydroxylation of debrisoquine in the San Bushmen of Southern Africa. *Human Toxicol* **7**: 273–6.

100. Simooya O, Njunju E, Hodjegan AR, Lennard MS, Tucker GT. 1993. Debrisoquine and metoprolol oxidation in Zambians: a population study. *Pharmacogenetics* **3**: 205–8.

101. Arias TD, Jorge LF, Lee D, Barrantes R, Inaba T. 1988. The oxidative metabolism of sparteine in the Cuna Amerindians of Panama. Absence of evidence for deficient metabolizers. *Clin Pharmacol Ther* **43**: 456–65.

102. Jorge LF, Arias TD, Inaba T, Jackson, PR. 1990. Unimodal distribution of the metabolic ratio for debrisoquine in Cuna Amerindians of Panama. *Br J Clin Pharmacol* **30**: 281–5.

103. Arias TD, Inaba T, Cooke RG, Jorge LF. 1988. A preliminary note on the transient polymorphic oxidation of sparteine in the Ngawbe Guaymi Amerindians. A case of genetic divergence with tentative phylogenetic time for the pathway. *Clin Pharmacol Ther* **44**: 343–52.

104. Nowak MP, Tyndale RF, Sellers EM. 1997. CYP2D6 phenotype and genotype in a Canadian native Indian population. *Pharmacogenetics* **7**: 145–8.

105. Horai Y, Nakano M, Ishizaki T, Ishikawa K, Zhou HH, Zhou BJ *et al.* 1989. Metoprolol and mephenytoin oxidation polymorphisms in Far Eastern Oriental subjects: Japanese versus mainland Chinese. *Clin Pharmacol Ther* **46**: 198–207.

106. Bertilsson L, Lou, YQ, Yun-Long D, Uin L, Tang-Yun K, Xia-Mau L *et al.* 1992. Pronounced differences between native Chinese and Swedish populations in the polymorphic hydroxylations of derisoquin and *S*-mephenytoin. *Clin Pharmacol Ther* **51**(4): 388–97.

107. Evans DA, Krahn P, Narayanan N. 1995. The mephenytoin (cytochrome P450 2C19) and dextromethorphan (cytochrome P450 2D6) polymorphisms in Saudi Arabians and Filipinos. *Pharmacogenetics* **5**: 64–71.

108. Nakamura K, Goto F, Ray WA, McAllister CB, Jacqz E, Wilkinson GR, Branch RA. 1985. Interethnic differences in genetic polymorphism of debrisoquin and mephenytoin hydroxylation between Japanese and Caucasian populations. *Clin Pharmacol Ther* **38**: 402–8.

109. Ishizaki T, Eichelbaum M, Horai Y, Hashimoto K, Chiba K, Dengler HJ. 1987. Evidence for polymorphic oxidation of sparteine in Japanese subjects. *Br J Clin Pharmacol* **23**: 482–5.

110. Roh HK, Dahl MI, Johansson I, Sundberg MI, Cha YN, Bertilsson L. 1996. Debrisoquine and *S*-mephenytoin hydroxylation phenotypes and genotypes in a Korean population. *Pharmacogenetics* **6**: 441–7.

111. Wanwimolruk S, Pratt EL, Denton JR, Charcroft SCW, Barron PA, Broughton JR.

1995. Evidence for the polymorphic oxidation of debrisoquine and proguanil in a New Zealand Maori population. *Pharmacokinetics* **5**: 193–8.

112. Weerasuriya K, Jayakody RL, Smith AD, Wolf CR, Tucker GT, Lennard MS. 1994. Debrisoquine and mephenytoin oxidation in Sinhalese: a population study. *Br J Clin Pharmacol* **38**: 466–70.

113. Wanwimolruk S, Patamasucon P, Lee EJD. 1990. Evidence for the polymorphic oxidation of debrisoquine in the Thai population. *Br J Clin Pharmacol* **29**: 244–7.

114. Guttendorf RJ, Britto M, Blouin RA, Foster TS, John W, Pittman KA, Wedlund PJ. 1990. Rapid screening for polymorphisms in dextromethorphan and mephenytoin metabolism. *Br J Clin Pharmacol* **29**: 373–80.

115. Peart GF, Boutagy J, Shenfield GM. 1986. Debrisoquine oxidation in an Australian population. *Br J Clin Pharmacol* **21**: 465–71.

116. Leclercq V, Desager JP, Nieuwenhuyze YV, Harvengt C. 1987. Prevalence of drug hydroxylator phenotypes in Belgium. *Eur J Clin Pharmacol* **33**: 439–40.

117. Vinks A, Inaba T, Otton SV, Kalow W. 1982. Sparteine metabolism in Canadian Caucasians. *Clin Pharmacol Ther* **31**: 23–9.

118. Brosen K, Otton SV, Gram LF. 1985. Sparteine oxidation polymorphism in Denmark. *Acta Pharmacol Toxicol* **57**: 357–60.

119. Drohse A, Bathum L, Brosen K, Gram LF. 1989. Mephenytoin and sparteine oxidation: genetic polymorphisms in Denmark. *Br J Clin Pharmacol* **27**: 620–5.

120. Kiivet RA, Svenson JO, Bertilsson L, Sjoqvist. 1993. Polymorphism of debrisoquine and mephenytoin hydroxylation among Estonians. *Pharmacol Toxicol* **72**: 113–15.

121. Arvela P, Kirjarinta M, Kirjarinta M, Karki N, Pelkonen O. 1988. Polymorphism of debrisoquine hydroxylation among Finns and Lapps. *Br J Clin Pharmacol* **26**: 601–3.

122. Viry MV, Fournier B, Siest G, Galteau MM. 1992. Dextromethorphan o-demethylation in a large number of French Caucasian families. *Pharmacogenetics* **2**: 135–8.

123. Larrey D, Amouyal G, Tinel M, Letteron P, Berson A, Lagge G, Pessayre D. 1987. Polymorphism of dextromethorphan oxidation in a French population. *Br J Clin Pharmacol* **24**: 676–9.

124. Jacqz E, Dulac H, Mathieu H. 1988. Phenotyping polymorphic drug metabolism in the French Caucasian population. *Eur J Clin Pharmacol* **35**: 167–71.

125. Freche JP, Dragacci SM, Petit AM, Siest JP, Galteau MM, Siest G. 1990. Development of an ELISA to study the polymorphism of dextromethorphan oxidation in a French population. *Eur J Clin Pharmacol* **39**: 481–5.

126. Hildebrand M, Seifert W, Reichenberger. 1989. Determination of dextromethorphan metabolizer phenotype in healthy volunteers. *Eur J Clin Pharmacol* **36**: 315–18.

127. Bock KW, Schrenk D, Forster A, Griese EU, Morike K, Brockmeier D, Eichelbaum M. 1994. The influence of environmental and genetic factors on CYP2D6, CYP1A2 and UDP-glucuronosytransferases in man using sparteine, caffeine, and paracetamol as probes. *Pharmacogenetics* **4**: 209–18.

128. Brosen K. 1986. Sparteine oxidation polymorphism in Greenlanders living in Denmark. *Br J Clin. Pharmacol* **22**: 415–19.

129. Clasen K, Madsen L, Brosen K, Alboge K, Misfeldt S, Gram L. 1991. Sparteine and mephenytoin oxidation: Genetic polymorphisms in East and West Greenland. *Clin Pharmacol Ther* **49**: 624–31.

130. Spina E, Campo GM, Avenoso A, Caputi AP, Zuccaro P, Pacifici R *et al.* 1994. CYP2D6-Related oxidation polymorphism in Italy. *Pharmacol Res* **29**: 281–9.

131. Benitez J, Llerena A, Cobaleda J. 1988. Debrisoquin oxidation polymorphism in a Spanish population. *Clin Pharmacol Ther* **44**: 74–7.

132. Henthorn TK, Benitez J, Avram MJ, Martinez C, Llerena A, Cobaleda J *et al.* 1989. Assessment of the debrisoquin and dextromethorphan phenotyping tests by gaussian mixture distributions analysis. *Clin Pharmacol Ther* **45**: 328–33.

133. Steiner E, Bertilsson L, Sawe J, Bertling I, Sjoqvist F. 1988. Polymorphic debrisoquin hydroxylation in 757 Swedish subjects. *Clin Pharmacol Ther* **44**: 431–5.
134. Sanz EJ, Villen T, Alm C, Bertilsson L. 1989. *S*-mephenytoin hydroxylation phenotypes in a Swedish population determined after coadministration with debrisoquin. *Clin Pharmacol Ther* **45**: 495–8.
135. Hadidi HF, Cholerton S, Monkman SC, Armstrong M, Irshaid YM, Rawashdeh NM *et al.* 1994. Debrisoquine 4-hydroxylation (CYP2D6) polymorphism in Jordanians. *Pharmacogenetics* **4**: 159–61.
136. Al-Hadidi HF, Irshaid YM, Rawashdeh NM. 1994. Metoprolok A-hydroxylation is a poor probe for debrisoquine oxidation (CYP2D6) polymorphism in Jordanians. *Eur J Clin Pharmacol* **47**: 311–14.
137. Irshaid YM, Al-Hadidi HF, Rawashdeh NM. 1993. Dextromethorphan *o*-demethylation polymorphism in Jordanians. *Eur J Clin Pharmacol* **45**: 271–3.
138. Islam SI, Idle JR, Smith RL. 1980. The polymorphic 4-hydroxylation of debrisoquine in a Saudi Arab population. *Xenobiotica* **10**: 819–25.
139. Bozkurt A, Basci N, Isimer A, Sayal A, Kayaalp O. 1994. Polymorphic debrisoquin metabolism in a Turkish population. *Clin. Pharmacol Ther* **55**: 399–401.
140. Gorgia AE, Balnt LP, Genet C, Dayer P, Aeschlimann JM, Garrone G. 1986. Importance of oxidative polymorphism and levomepromazine treatment on the steady-state blood concentrations of clomipramine and its major metabolites. *Eur J Clin Pharmacol* **31**: 449–55.
141. Nielson K, Brosen K, Hansen M, Gram L. 1994. Single-dose kinetics of clomipramine: Relationship to the sparteine and *S*-mephenytoin oxidation polymorphisms. *Clin Pharmacol Ther* **55**: 518–27.
142. von Molte L, Greenblatt D, Coteau-Bibbo M, Duan S, Harmatz J, Shader R. 1994. Inhibition of desipramine hydroxylation in vitro by serotonin reuptake inhibitor antidepressants, and by quinidine and ketoconazole: A model system to predict drug interacts in vivo. *J Pharmacol Exp Ther* **268**: 1278–83.
143. Brosen K, Gram LF. 1989. Quinidine inhibits the 2-hydroxylation of imipramine and desipramine but not the demethylation of imipramine. *Eur J Clin Pharmacol* **37**: 155–60.
144. Brosen K, Zeugin T, Meyer U. 1991. Role of P450IID6, the target of the sparteine-debrisoquin oxidation polymorphism, in the metabolism of imipramine. *Clin Pharmacol Ther* **49**: 609–17.
145. Spina E, Birgersson C, Bahr C, Ericsson O, Mellstrom B, Steiner E, Sjoqvist F. 1984. Phenotypic consistency in hydroxylation of desmethylimipramine and debrisoquine in healthy subjects and in human liver microsomes. *Clin Pharmacol Ther* **36**: 677–82.
146. Huang ML, Peer AV, Woestenborghs R, Coster R, Heykants J, Jansen AI *et al.* 1993. Pharmacokinetics of the novel antipsychotic agent risperidone and the prolactin response in healthy subjects. *Clin Pharmacol Ther* **54**: 257–68.
147. Llerena A, Dahl M, Ekqvist B, Bertilsson L. 1992. Haloperidol disposition is dependent on the debrisoquine hydroxylation phenotype: Increased plasma levels of the reduced metabolite in poor metabolizers. *Ther Drug Monit* **14**: 261–4.
148. Bahr C, Movin G, Nordin C, Liden A, Udenaes M, Hedberg A *et al.* 1991. Plasma levels of thioridazine and metabolites are influenced by the debrisoquin hydroxylation phenotype. *Clin Pharmacol Ther* **49**: 234–40.
149. Sindrup SH, Brosen K, Hansen MG, Jorgensen A, Overo K, Gram L. 1993. Pharmacokinetics of citalopram in relation to the sparteine and the mephenytoin oxidation polymorphisms. *Ther Drug Monit* **15**: 11–17.
150. Sindrup S, Brosen K, Gram L. 1992. Pharmacokinetics of the selective serotonin reuptake inhibitor paroxetine: Nonlinearity and relation to the sparteine oxidation polymorphism. *Clin Pharmacol Ther* **51**: 288–95.

151. Woolhouse N, Yamoah K, Mellstrom B, Hedman A, Bertilsson L, Sjoqvist F. 1984. Nortriptyline and debrisoquine hydroxylations in Ghanaian and Swedish subjects. *Clin Pharmacol Ther* **36**: 374–8.
152. Kallio J, Huupponeen R, Pyykko K. 1990. The relationship between debrisoquine oxidation phenotype and the pharmacokinetics of chlorpropamide. *Eur J Clin Pharmacol* **39**: 93–5.

3

Pharmacokinetic Analysis of Ethnic Groups Using Population Methods

Stanford S. Jhee and Neal R. Cutler

California Clinical Trials, Beverly Hills, CA, USA

INTRODUCTION

The influence of patient characteristics such as age, sex, hepatic/renal function and disease states on pharmacokinetics (PK) and pharmacodynamics (PD) have received much attention in past years [1–3]. Dosing guidelines for elderly people and hepatic/renal impaired patients are frequently found in product package inserts. It has been recognized that ethnicity also represents an important factor in determining the response of patients to a wide variety of medications, especially psychotropics [4–8]. Despite this, current information on the role ethnicity plays in drug dosage design is limited: exploration of ethnic factors is not part of the drug development process and thus this information is not available for the clinician upon release of new medications. Clinicians are often left without clear guidelines for the design of an initial, individualized optimum-dosage regimen or for subsequent dosage adjustments.

Ideally, these programs should be incorporated into each stage of the drug development process. Although many concerns for costs and logistical issues are involved with such endeavors, careful planning from the early stage can enable sponsors to incorporate the role of ethnicity into drug development. Until programs to incorporate ethnicity are implemented into the drug development process, advances in population PK modeling can enable characterization of a drug's PK in different populations with limited data obtained from routine clinical practice. In this chapter, we will explore population PK method as a tool for assessing the influence of patient characteristics on the PK of drugs.

POPULATION PHARMACOKINETICS

Definition and Purpose

Definition of population PK may vary. Owing to its popularity, the non-linear mixed-effects model (NONMEM) method has most often been used to describe

Cross Cultural Psychiatry. Edited by John M. Herrera, William B. Lawson and John J. Sramek.
© 1999 John Wiley & Sons Ltd.

population PK. Sometimes NONMEM and population PK are used interchangeably; however, population PK is a general term describing both the PK and PD in groups of patients with similar characteristics. Population PK attempts to discover factors, including ethnicity, that are causing changes in the dose–concentration relationship. Providing a quantitative guideline for drug dosage individualization is the ultimate purpose of population PK. One example of the use of population PK is identifying an antipsychotic dosage regimen for Asian schizophrenics that will yield the same plasma level as obtained in Caucasian schizophrenics.

Traditional Pharmacokinetic Modeling Approach

Mean PK parameter values have traditionally been obtained by studies involving numerous samplings in limited numbers of individuals. The PK parameters are estimated for each individual and the population parameters are represented by measures of central tendency (that is, mean, logarithmic mean, median). Estimates of parameters were calculated by unweighted or weighted least squares non-linear regression analysis using a compartmental or non-compartmental PK model. However, there are problems associated with this two-stage approach. Inter- and intraindividual variation may result in imprecise estimates of the true individual parameter as this method does not partition random variability: even as many as five samples per patient may yield poor individual PK estimates and have the potential to produce biased and/or suboptimal results [9]. This often leads to the selection of subjects with minimal variability, who seldom represent the patient population intended to receive the drug. Furthermore, for various reasons, it is difficult to obtain large numbers of samples per patients, which results in inaccurate estimates [10].

Population Approach

Perhaps the most important difference with the population approach is that the complete sample, rather than the individual, is considered as a unit of analysis. This unit is used to estimate the distribution of the parameters. It uses individual scores, simultaneously, to estimate parameters in a single stage of analysis. Unlike traditional methods, the population approach accounts for all sources of variability. Factors that contribute to the variability of the measured observation are known as 'effects' and are of two types: fixed and random. Fixed effects are known factors that are assumed to have no errors—such as patient age, weight, dose, and renal function. Random effects include any unexplainable variation between or within individuals.

Consideration of all this variability has led to the development of mixed-effects model methods, which are viewed as the optimal population modeling method: the individuality of each subject is maintained and accounted for even when the data are sparse and the data are collected under less stringent conditions in recognition of the practical problems in sample collection and patient recruitment. This population approach was proposed by Sheiner and coworkers [11].

The most well known program for applying mixed effects method is NONMEM. Further discussion in this chapter will involve this method.

EXECUTION OF POPULATION PHARMACOKINETICS MODEL

The Software

NONMEM software is readily available from the NONMEM project group [12]. A comprehensive list of related publication is also available from this group.

Prerequisites

Before conducting population PK studies, researchers should be familiar with the basic PK characteristics of the drug to be studied. For example, the major route of drug elimination should be identified and basic models describing the drug's behavior should be available, as should a validated sensitive and specific assay. This information must include not only the compound of interest but also known metabolites that may be clinically important.

A protocol should be written outlining the objectives of the population pharmacokinetic study: patient selection criteria, sampling procedures and method for data analysis should be stated. The data analysis plan should always be described in advance as specifically as possible. The difference between statistically significant and clinically relevant PK parameters should be distinguished. Special data collection forms that can easily be used by study staff or ward nurses should be designed. One of the most important factors in NONMEM analysis is accurate documentation of dosing and sampling information. The personnel involved in the study must be made to understand that accurate recording of the dose/sampling time is much more important than adherence to the scheduled times.

Practical Considerations

How Many Patients do I Need?

Perhaps the biggest advantage of using the population approach is the loose nature of patient selection. Data can be generated directly from routine patient monitoring. Heterogeneous patient distribution is encouraged in population analysis because the covariates can easily be incorporated into the analysis. The more patients included in the analysis, the better, but sufficient numbers from each ethnic group of interest are needed to see if ethnicity contributes to a significant pharmacokinetic variability. It is recommended that 10–20 patients from any ethnic group are included [13].

How Many Samples are Needed from Each Patient?

One of the advantages of using NONMEM is that a single data point from a single patient is still useful in the analysis. However, the data set should not be composed only of single data points. There is no minimum for the number of samples required but more samples will yield a more robust analysis. The goal should be to collect several (1–6) samples from each patient, giving several data points for each.

When Should the Samples be Collected?

In general, there are no sampling time restraints imposed on NONMEM. However, collection of just trough or peak samples should be avoided. Attention to the timing of the samples is more likely to yield useful information [14]. Samples collected near the trough will yield more information about clearances, peak samples may provide more information about the volume of distribution.

APPLICATION OF FINDINGS

Pharmacokinetic parameterization of a population such as that of Hispanic schizophrenics provides population 'priors,' parameters that may be used to develop dosing regimens for the compound of interest. Although these population 'priors' can, to an extent, help to define a dosage regimen, they should be used in combination with individual plasma concentration data (obtained during routine care) to provide the most reliable estimation of individual parameters—which would not be possible using either set of information alone [15, 16]. The mathematical derivation of this procedure is based on Bayes' theorem for conditional probabilities [17]. There are numerous computer software programs available to assist the clinician in individualizing dosage regimens—for example, the NONMEM package already mentioned.

SUMMARY

Incorporation of ethnicity into drug development programs will probably take some time and in the meantime clinicians (especially in psychiatry) inevitably face dosing questions with various ethnicities. Population variabilities can be more accurately modeled with population methods. NONMEM is a unique tool enabling clinicians to use routine clinical data to estimate all sources of variability, including ethnicity, for optimal drug therapy.

REFERENCES

1. Samara E, Granneman R. 1997. Role of population pharmacokinetics in drug development. A pharmaceutical industry perspective. *Clin Pharmacokinet* **32**: 294–312.
2. Vozeh S, Steimer JL, Rowland M, Morselli P, Mentre F, Balant LP, Aarons L. 1996. The use of population pharmacokinetics in drug development. *Clin Pharmacokinet* **30**: 81–93.
3. Troconiz IF. 1996. Population-based approach to the assessment of pharmacokinetic–pharmacodynamic data. *Methods Find Exp Clin Pharmacol* **18S**: C51–2.
4. Kalow W. 1989. Race and therapeutic drug response. *N Engl J Med* **320**: 588–9.
5. Kalow W, ed. 1992. *Pharmacogenetics of Drug Metabolism*. New York: Pergamon Press.
6. Lin KM, Poland RE, Nakasaki G, eds. 1993. *Psychopharmacology and Psychobiology of Ethnicity*. Washington DC: American Psychiatric Press.
7. Wood AJ, Zhou HH. 1991. Ethnic difference in drug disposition and responsiveness. *Clin Pharmacokinet* **20**: 1–24.
8. Zhou HH, Koshakji RP, Silberstein DJ, Wilkinson GR, Wood AJ. 1989. Altered sensitivity to and clearance of propranolol in men of Chinese descent as compared with American whites. *N Engl J Med* **320**: 565–70.
9. Kataria BK, Ved SA, Nicodemus HF, Hoy GR, Lea D, Dubois My, Mandama JW, Schafer SL. 1994. The pharmacokinetics of propofol in children using three different data analysis approaches. *Anesthesiology* **80**: 104–22.
10. Sheiner LB, Beal SL. 1983. Evaluation of methods for estimating population pharmacokinetic parameters. III. Monoexponential model: Routine clinical pharmacokinetic data. *J Pharmacokinet Biopharm* **11**: 303–19.
11. Sheiner LB, Rosenberg B, Marathe W. 1977. Estimation of population characteristics of pharmacokinetic parameters from routine clinical data. *J Pharmacokinet Biopharm* **5**: 445–79.
12. Boeckmann AJ, Sheiner LB, Beal SL, eds. 1992. *NONMEM User's Guide*. University of California at San Francisco: NONMEM Project Group.
13. Sheiner LB, Benet LZ. 1985. Premarketing observational studies of population pharmacokinetics of new drugs. *Clin Pharmacol Ther* **38**: 481–7.
14. D'Argenio DZ. 1981. Optimal sampling times for pharmacokinetic experiments. *J Pharmacokinet Biopharm* **9**: 739–55.
15. Shiener LB, Rosenburg B, Melmon KL. 1972. Modelling of individual pharmacokinetics for computer-aided drug dosage. *Comput Biomed Res* **5**: 411–59.
16. Bruno R, Iliadis MC, Lacarelle B, Cosson V, Mandema JW, Le Roux Y *et al.* 1992. Evaluation of Bayesian estimation in comparison to NONMEM for population pharmacokinetic data analysis: Application to perfloxacin in intensive care unit patients. *J Pharmacokinet Biopharm* **20**: 653–69.
17. Sheiner LB, Beal S, Rosenberg B, Marathe VV. 1979. Forecasting individual pharmacokinetics. *Clin Pharmacol Ther* **26**: 294–305.

Psychopharmacology

4

Psychopharmacology in Cross Cultural Psychiatry

Keh-Ming Lin, Michael W. Smith and Ricardo P. Mendoza

Department of Psychiatry, Harbor-UCLA Medical Center, Torrance, CA, USA

INTRODUCTION

Findings of substantial and clinically significant cross ethnic differences in psychotropic responses have been repeatedly reported since the early 1960s [1–5]. However, despite this body of literature, most clinicians and researchers have remained unaware of such a possibility and often suggestions of ethnic differences in drug responses were regarded as either unlikely or unimportant. Reflecting this general attitude, very few well-designed research efforts have been made to examine the validity and clinical relevance of these observations, as well as the mechanisms responsible for them. This is ironic and regrettable, especially in light of the potency of modern psychopharmacology, with its promise of miraculous cure, as well as the danger of substantive harmful effects when administered inappropriately. Since the 1950s, these modern psychotropics have revolutionized psychiatric care world wide; their widespread use attests to their efficacy and utility. At the same time, however, it is disconcerting to realize that, despite the remarkable success in the practice of psychopharmacology across cultural and ethnic lines, so little is currently known regarding the potential contribution of cultural and ethnic factors in determining whether a particular patient would benefit from a particular treatment regimen, or if he or she is at a particular risk for certain potentially dangerous or devastating adverse effects.

THE NEGLECT OF ETHNICITY AND CULTURE IN PSYCHOPHARMACOLOGICAL RESEARCH

Many factors possibly contributed towards such neglect. First of all, contrary to clear evidence indicating otherwise [5], there is a pervasive belief in psychiatry that equates biology with universality, and attributes cross cultural/cross ethnic diversity

Cross Cultural Psychiatry. Edited by John M. Herrera, William B. Lawson and John J. Sramek.
© 1999 John Wiley & Sons Ltd.

only to psychosocial factors [6]. Such a belief leads to the neglect of remarkable biological diversities that exist in all living organisms, including the human species, both within and between ethnic groups, and has been at least partially responsible for the slow progress of cross cultural research on biologically related issues.

Similarly, because of the long history of the racist misinterpretation and distortion of scientific data [7], researchers and clinicians are often uncomfortable with the idea that people with divergent ethnic and ancestral backgrounds might differ significantly in their biological endowments, including pharmacological responses. This 'color-blind' approach, 'politically correct' and innocuous in appearance, probably results in the neglect of issues that may be of pressing importance for ethnic minority populations. Further, because of past incidents of the flagrant abuse of minority patients in biomedical research [7], there is a pervasive sense of distrust in many minority communities towards the 'mainstream' biomedical establishment in general and research endeavors in particular. These forces, as well as other more general factors related to the accessibility of healthcare, combined to make it difficult for patients and volunteers of ethnic minority to participate in biomedical research in general, and research in psychopharmacology in particular. As a result, until most recently, most studies drew their conclusions from subjects that were almost exclusively 'white males.' Ironically, once published, such findings are typically applied to the populations that have been largely excluded from research. Further, the absence of data indicating ethnic variation in responses is then taken to mean that ethnicity and culture do not represent significant factors in determining treatment effects. This leads to a vicious cycle, preventing the serious consideration of issues that may be of central relevance to the majority of our patients, who are increasingly culturally and ethnically diversified.

THE EMERGENCE OF PHARMACOGENETICS

The need to include ethnically diverse populations in psychiatric research, including psychopharmacological research, takes on a renewed sense of significance and urgency along with the emergence and rapid progress of molecular biology. As the field enfolds, it becomes increasingly clear that gene polymorphism exists widely in most, if not all, human genes, including those involved in the mediation of drug metabolism and/or responses. At the same time, for almost all of the genes demonstrating polymorphism, ethnic variation is the rule rather than the exception. For example, the activity of most extensively studied cytochrome P-450 (CYP) enzymes, such as the CYP2D6 and CYP2C19, is significantly influenced by a number of distinctive mutations, some of which are to a large extent ethnically specific. Receptor polymorphisms that have been identified thus far, such as those involving D_2 and D_4, also show remarkable ethnic variations in their mutation patterns [8–10]. Although the meaning and clinical relevance of these variations remain to be further examined, there is every reason to believe that such differences are far from trivial, both for clinical and for research purposes (for example, the controversy regarding the association between D_2 polymorphism and alcoholism was partially generated by the neglect of ethnic difference in the former [11]). With the expectation that new developments in phenotyping (the measurement of enzyme activities) and genotyping (the detection of mutations using molecular biology methods) procedures will soon lead to the establishment of pharmacogenetic probes that could be applied widely in clinical settings, it is even more important that the role of ethnicity is not neglected. Otherwise, there may be situations where the probes are developed based on norms of one ethnic group, yet applied on other ethnic groups where they would yield little clinically useful information.

The progress of pharmacogenetics and molecular biology also makes it increasingly clear that the expression of genes is typically remarkably responsive to environmental, and thus cultural, influences. This is very clearly seen in the case of pharmacogenetics: major CYP enzymes, such as CYP1A2, CYP3A4 and CYP1E2, have been demonstrated to be particularly sensitive to the influences of environmental factors [12–17]. A large number of natural substances, including constituents of tobacco, micronutrients, macronutrients, herbs, industrial toxins and even environmental pollution, could either induce or inhibit the expression of these enzymes in a significant manner [12–17]. For example, the activity of CYP3A4 is significantly lower in Mexican Americans and Asian Indians than in other groups [18]. Although the reason for such a difference is not completely clear, it is assumed that it is most probably caused by ethnic differences in dietary practices, especially the intake of certain vegetables that may inhibit the enzyme. Similar explanations may be applicable to earlier observations of lower clearance rates in Asian Indians and Sudanese people for substances such as antipyrine [19–20] and clomipramine [21] than seen in their British White counterparts. This hypothesis was further strengthened by the fact that those who switched from their traditional (mostly vegetarian) diet to a British diet (which included meat) developed a metabolic pattern similar to that of the Whites. Other factors might also be responsible for changes in the metabolic profiles in migrants who moved from rural to urban settings. As an example, a recent study reported the rate of metabolism of CYP1A2 to be higher in a group of Koreans living in urban areas than in their compatriots residing in rural Korea [22]. Since both groups were non-smokers and had similar dietary intake, the authors suggested that exposure to a higher level of air pollution might be responsible for the induction of the drug-metabolizing enzyme in the urban group.

While the Western world is going through a resurgence or revival for the medicinal use of herbs [23], such practices have always been extremely common among ethnic minorities in the USA, and among non-Westerners around the world [24]. Herbs as well as other natural substances are the natural substrates for the 'drug-metabolizing' [1], and are thus likely to modify the activity of these enzymes through induction or inhibition [25]. Because many of these herbs are taken concurrently with psychotropic medications, drug–herb interactions are most likely to occur, but have rarely been reported because such a possibility is rarely considered.

Thus, for a number of important reasons, advances in pharmacogenetics have contributed greatly to our understanding of the mechanisms underlying cross ethnic as well as interindividual variations in drug responses. The incorporation of these research tools and concepts in future studies is crucial, not only for the further clarification of the extent, of and mechanisms responsible for, such variations but also for the establishment of guidelines for rational psychopharmacotherapy that are ethnically and culturally appropriate and useful.

DANGER OF STEREOTYPING AND OVERGENERALIZATION

As amply demonstrated throughout this volume, cross ethnic differences in pharmacological responses are often substantial and of clinical significance. However, unless these findings are understood in the context of interindividual variability in drug responses that exist in any given ethnic group, they are likely to be interpreted stereotypically and simplistically. Such a misunderstanding might lead to the indiscriminate treatment of all patients from a particular group with a set dose range, thereby neglecting the need for individual tailoring of any treatment regimen in the clinical settings. Figure 4.1 shows that in one of our earlier studies of the metabolism of haloperidol, cross ethnic and interindividual variations are both substantial, and superimposed [26].

Largely for political reasons, populations in the USA are customarily divided into several major ethnic groups, including African Americans, Asians, Caucasians, Hispanics and Native Americans. Included in each of these major groupings are a large number of distinct cultural or 'nationality' groups. Although these 'subgroups' often share important historical and cultural roots, as well as biological traits, each is unique in many aspects, rendering indiscriminate generalization a precarious business. For example, although the CYP2D6*4 (B mutation) may be regarded as a Caucasian-specific mutation because it is extremely rare in Asians and African Blacks but is commonly seen in all Caucasian groups ranging from Latvian to Spanish, studies conducted in Spain have consistently shown a lower rate relative to the other Caucasian groups (but still substantially higher than any non-Caucasian groups studied thus far) [27]. Another prominent example is the enzymes involved in the metabolism of alcohol and acetaldehyde (alcohol dehydrogenase and aldehyde dehydrogenase, respectively) [28]. Although high rates of specific mutations involving these enzymes render close to half of any given East Asian populations (e.g. Chinese, Japanese and Koreans) extremely sensitive to the effect of alcohol [29–30], this is not the case with Asians with Malay origin, such as Filipinos, Filipino Americans and Taiwanese aborigines [31].

Similar danger exists in the indiscriminate lumping together of different Hispanic groups. Although Puerto Ricans and Mexican Americans share important biological and cultural roots, there are also distinct differences in the history of

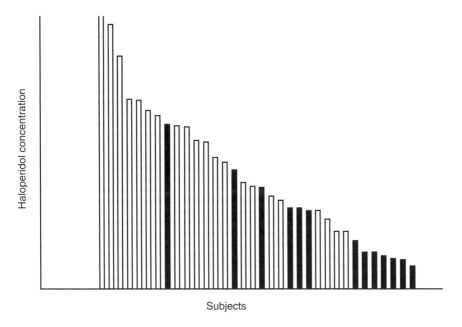

FIGURE 4.1   Variability of haloperidol concentrations in normal Asian (□) and Caucasian (■) volunteers after the administration of haloperidol (1.0 mg, orally). The graph shows: (1) substantial interindividual variability within each of the ethnic groups; (2) dramatic differences in the pharmacokinetics of haloperidol between the two ethnic groups; and (3) overlap of the pharmacokinetics between the two groups

migration and the intermixture of various racial groups leading to significant variations in behavioral patterns and possibly pharmacological responses. This may be a reason for the discrepancy previously observed in Hispanics' responses to tricyclic antidepressants: while a clinical study conducted in New York showed that Puerto Ricans were extremely sensitive to the medication [32], research conducted by Gaviria *et al.* [33] and by our group showed little difference between Mexican Americans and their Caucasian counterparts in the metabolism of these medications [33].

THE IMPORTANCE OF 'NON-PHARMACOLOGICAL' FACTORS

Lastly, it should be emphasized that, irrespective of specificity and potency of any given pharmacological intervention, treatment effects are invariably even more powerfully determined by factors that are primarily 'non-biological' in nature [34]. These include issues related to expectations, adherence (compliance), placebo response and clinician–patient relationships [32]. As these responses are all largely mediated through processes that are symbolic and interactive in nature, there is little question that culture should play an extremely important role in shaping them, and in turn powerfully determine whether any given patient will respond to a particular treatment regimen.

As important as these issues are, unfortunately they have thus far rarely been the focus of systematic research attention, and the literature covering this important area is meager or next to non-existent. However, data derived from a large variety of sources, including clinical reports, anthropological observations and utilization studies, converge to support the hypothesis that cultural factors are indeed extremely important in influencing patients' attitudes, adherence and ultimately responses to pharmacological treatment [34–38]. As an example, among Asians and Asian Americans there is a widespread belief in the danger of the long-term use of 'Western' medications, which may contribute significantly to problems of non-compliance [34]. However, without systematic research data the extent to which this may be the case remains unclear.

The therapeutic relationship is a two-way process, and the outcome of the therapeutic interaction is influenced not only by the patient but also by the clinician. In the cross cultural situation, the clinician's ability to accurately assess a patient's symptoms as well as his or her responses to treatment may be hampered by lack of an adequate understanding of the patient's cultural norms [34], as well as misperceptions. This is probably the reason for higher doses of neuroleptics being prescribed for African American patients than to their Caucasian counterparts [39]. In several studies, African Americans have also been shown to suffer from a higher rate of tardive dyskinesia [40–42], which is probably related to their exposure to higher doses of neuroleptics over time. This is thus not an innocuous condition and deserves more careful and systematic exploration.

SUMMARY AND CONCLUSION

In this short chapter we focused on some of the conceptual issues that may be of particular relevance for research and practice of psychopharmacotherapy in the cross cultural setting. Although observations suggesting the existence of ethnic differences in psychotropic responses appeared soon after the introduction of these powerful therapeutic drugs in the 1950s, objective data documenting such differences started to emerge only in the last two decades. Progress of the field in recent years has accelerated. Together with the phenomenal growth of pharmacogenetics and the maturation of research methodology in other relevant areas, it is expected that our knowledge in the application of psychopharmacology in cross cultural psychiatric practices will continue to expand, such that the use of these powerful agents will become increasingly targeted, rational and effective irrespective of a patient's ethnic and cultural backgrounds.

ACKNOWLEDGMENTS

This study was undertaken by the Research Center on the Psychobiology of Ethnicity and the Department of Psychiatry, Harbor-UCLA Medical Center. It was supported in part by NIMH Research Center on the Psychobiology of Ethnicity MH47193.

REFERENCES

1. Kalow, W. ed. 1992. *Pharmacogenetics of Drug Metabolism.* New York: Pergamon Press.
2. Nebert DW, Weber WW. 1989. Pharmacogenetics. In: *Pharmacogenetics. Principles of Drug Action,* 3rd ed. Churchill Livingstone, pp. 469–531.
3. Mendoza R, Smith M, Poland R, Lin K, Strickland, T. 1991. Ethnic psychopharmacology: the Hispanic and Native American perspective. *Psychopharmacol Bull* **27**: 449–61.
4. Goedde HW, Agarwal DP, eds. 1986. *Ethnic Differences in Reactions to Drugs and Xenobiotics.* New York: Liss.
5. Lin KM, Poland RE, Nakasaki G. 1993. *Psychopharmacology and Psychobiology of Ethnicity.* Washington, DC: American Psychiatric Press.
6. Kleinman A. 1988. *Rethinking Psychiatry.* New York: Free Press.
7. Lawson W. 1986. Racial and ethnic factors in psychiatric research. *Hosp Community Psychiatry* **37**: 50–4.
8. Lee MS, Lee KJ, Kwak DI. 1997. No association between the dopamine D2 receptor gene and Korean alcoholism. *Psychiatr Genet* **7**: 93–5.
9. Blum K, Noble EP, Sheridan PJ, Finley O, Montgomery A, Ritchie T *et al.* 1991. Association of the A1 allele of the D2 dopamine receptor gene with severe alcoholism. *Alcohol* **8**: 409–16.
10. Dobashi I, Inada T, Hadano K. 1997. Alcoholism and gene polymorphisms related to central dopaminergic transmission in the Japanese population. *Psychiatr Genet* **7**: 87–91.
11. Chen CH, Chien SH, Hwu HG. 1996. Lack of association between TaqI A1 allele of dopamine D2 receptor gene and alcohol-use disorders in atayal natives of Taiwan. *Am J Med Genet* **67**: 488–90.
12. Dollery C, Fraser H, Mucklow J. 1979. Contribution of environmental factors to variability in human drug metabolism. *Drug Metab Rev* **9**: 207–20.
13. Shils ME, Young VR, eds. 1988. Diet, nutrition and drug reactions. In: *Modern Nutrition in Health and Disease,* 7th ed. Philadelphia: Lea & Febiger.
14. Conney AH, Pantuck EJ, Hsiao KC, Kuntzman R, Alvares AP, Kappas A. 1977. Regulation of drug metabolism in man by environmental chemicals and diet. *Fed Proc* **36**(5): 1647–52.
15. Ereshefsky L. 1996. Pharmacokinetics and drug interactions: update for new antipsychotics. *J Clin Psychiatry* **57** (Suppl 11): 12–25.
16. Murray M, Reidy G. 1990. Selectivity in the inhibition of mammalian cytochromes P-450 by chemical agents. *Pharmacol Rev* **42**: 2–101.
17. Anderson KE, Conney AH, Kappas A. 1986. Nutrition as an environmental influence on chemical metabolism in man. Ethnic differences in reactions to drugs and xenobiotics. *Progr Clin Biol Res* **214**: 39–54.
18. Ahsan C, Renwick A, Waller D, Challenor V, George C, Amanullah M. 1993. The influences of dose and ethnic origins on the pharmacokinetics of nifedipine. *Clin Pharmacol Ther* **54**: 329–38.
19. Desai NK, Sheth UK, Mucklow JC. 1980. Antipyrine clearance in Indian villagers. *Br J Clin Pharmacol* **9**: 387–94.

20. Branch R, Salih S, Homeida M. 1978. Racial differences in drug metabolizing ability: a study with antipyrine in the Sudan. *Clin Pharmacol Ther* **24**: 283–6.
21. Shimoda K, Minowada T, Noguchi T, Takahashi S. 1993. Interindividual variations of desmethylation and hydroxylation of clomipramine in an Oriental psychiatric population. *J Clin Psychopharmacol* **13**(3): 181–8.
22. Chung WG, Kang JH, Lee KH, Roh HK, Cha YN. Differences of CYP1A2 activity between urban and rural people. *Clin Pharmacol Ther* **63**: 216.
23. Eisenberg DM, Kessler RC, Foster C, Norlock FE, Calkins DR, Delbanco TL. 1993. Unconventional medicine in the United States. Prevalence, costs, and patterns of use. *N Engl J Med* **328**(4): 246–52.
24. Lam CL, Catarivas MG, Munro C, Lauder IJ. 1994. Self-medication among Hong Kong Chinese. *Soc Sci Med* **39**(12): 1641–7.
25. Liu G. 1991. Effects of some compounds isolated from Chinese medicinal herbs on hepatic microsomal cytochrome P-450 and their potential biological consequences. *Drug Metab Rev* **23**: 439–65.
26. Lin KM, Finder E. 1983. Neuroleptic dosage in Asians. *Am J Psychiatry* **140**: 490–1.
27. Agundez JAG, Martinez C, Ledesma MC, Ladona MG, Ladero JM, Benitez J. 1994. Genetic basis for differences in debrisoquin polymorphism between a Spanish and other white populations. *Clin Pharmacol Ther* **55**: 412–17.
28. Agarwal D, Goedde H. 1990. *Alcohol Metabolism, Alcohol Intolerance and Alcoholism: Biochemical and Pharmacogenetic Approaches*. Berlin: Springer-Verlag.
29. Shibuya A, Yoshida A. 1988. Frequency of the atypical aldehyde dehydrogenase-2 gene (ALDH2/2) in Japanese and Caucasians. *Am J Hum Genet* **43**: 744–8.
30. Yoshida A. 1983. *Differences in the Isozymes Involved in Alcohol Metabolism Between Caucasians and Orientals*. New York: Alan R. Liss.
31. Lubben JE, Chi I, Kitano HH. 1988. Exploring Filipino American drinking behavior. *J Stud Alcohol* **49**: 26–9.
32. Marcos LR, Cancro R. 1982. Pharmacotherapy of Hispanic depressed patients: clinical observations. *Am J Psychother* **36**(4): 505–13.
33. Gaviria M, Gil AA, Javaid JI. 1986. Nortriptyline kinetics in Hispanic and Anglo subjects. *J Clin Psychopharmacol* **6**: 227–31.
34. Smith M, Lin KM, Poland RE, Nuccio I, Zheng Y, McGeoy S, Lesser I. 1998. Ethnicity and imipramine response: I. Pharmacokinetic comparisons (submitted for publication).
35. Smith M, Lin K, Mendoza R. 1993. 'Non-Biological' issues affecting psychopharmacotherapy: Cultural considerations. In: Lin K, Poland R, Nakasaki G, eds. *Psychopharmacology and Psychobiology of Ethnicity*. Washington: American Psychiatric Press.
36. Smith M, Lin KM. 1996. Biological Implications for Ethnic Differences in Treatment. In: Kato PM, Mann T, eds. *Health Psychology of Special Populations: Issues of Age, Gender, and Ethnicity*. New York: Plenum.
37. Moerman D. 1979. Anthropology of symbolic healing. *Curr Anthropol* **20**: 59–80.
38. Jenkins JH. 1988. Conceptions of schizophrenia as a problem of nerves: a cross-cultural comparison of Mexican-Americans and Anglo-Americans. *Soc Sci Med* **26**: 1233–43.
39. Strickland T, Ranganath V, Lin K, Poland R, Mendoza R, Smith M. 1991. Psychopharmacologic considerations in the treatment of Black American populations. *Psychopharmacol Bull* **27**: 441–8.
40. Jeste DV, Lindamer LA, Evans J, Lacro JP. 1996. Relationship of ethnicity and gender to schizophrenia and pharmacology of neuroleptics. *Psychopharmacol Bull* **32**(2): 243–51.
41. Glazer WM, Morgenstern H, Doucette J. 1994. Race and tardive dyskinesia among outpatients at a CMHC. *Hosp Community Psychiatry* **45**(1): 38–42.
42. Lawson WB. 1996. Clinical issues in the pharmacotherapy of African-Americans. *Psychopharmacol Bull* **32**(2): 275–81.

5

Prescribing for Africans: Some Transcultural Guidelines

Samuel O. Okpaku

Vanderbilt University School of Medicine, Nashville, TN, USA

INTRODUCTION

Historically, the number of Africans who study abroad is considerable. This has to do with the colonial past of that continent as well as an almost insatiable appetite for educational advancement and a search for self-enhancement. Three or four decades ago, most Africans who studied abroad generally planned to return home. However, with political unrest and economic deterioration, many Africans abroad have become self-exiled in their host countries. Civil and intergroup wars have led to a cadre of African refugees and immigrants to other African countries as well as to industrialized nations. President Clinton's recent visit to Africa and his agenda for that continent may result in more visible student and cultural exchanges between the USA and some African countries: these human movements and migrations, whether for education, business, or cultural exchanges, have their attendant psychological distress and need for psychiatric services.

The continent of Africa is large and its peoples varied, with different body types, religious backgrounds, lifestyles and dietary habits. The countries of the continent of Africa are at different levels of industrialization and have varying levels of relationship with the highly industrialized nations. The title of this chapter, therefore, will be meaningless unless we pay heed to the caveat by J.H. Orley, who stated:

> There does seem a tendency for some writers, especially psychiatrists, to talk of Africa and the 'African' when in fact they are referring only to their experiences and to their research among the patients with whom they have worked. Thus, they give an impression of making valuable generalizations about Africa, when they are doing nothing of the such.

Furthermore, although I am a Nigerian and therefore an African, my medical training and professional career have been entirely in the UK and USA, so my case

---

Cross Cultural Psychiatry. Edited by John M. Herrera, William B. Lawson and John J. Sramek.
© 1999 John Wiley & Sons Ltd.

histories are drawn from African patients whom I have consulted upon or treated in the USA.

The purpose of this chapter is fourfold:

1. To explore the interrelationship of factors likely to be influential in the pre-scription of psychotropics for Africans;
2. To review some ethnopharmacological findings which may have direct impli-cations for Africans;
3. To review some general ethnopharmacological findings of which anyone prescribing in a transcultural context should be aware;
4. To illustrate with case histories some guidelines for prescribing for Africans—whether they are foreign students, permanent residents, immigrants, or refugees.

FACTORS THAT INFLUENCE PRESCRIPTION OF MEDICATIONS AND THEIR ACCEPTANCE BY PATIENTS

The Pharmaceutical Industry

A major player in making any drug available to any country are the manufacturers, which are generally driven by profit motives. Many African countries do not have their own pharmaceutical houses and generally have to rely on importation of drugs. If these drugs are too expensive, they may represent a drain on the limited resources of such African countries. It is not surprising, therefore, that the avail-ability of some essential medicines is limited in some of these countries. Even when these medicines are available, they are very often in generic forms. Their bio-equivalence cannot be relied upon.

Drug Administration

Another influential factor in the availability and regulation of drugs is the drug administration agency of each country. The emphasis and influence of these agencies vary. Again, less industrialized countries do not generally have a budget, or they cannot generally set up a high-profile and well funded drug administration. Even in industrialized countries, the function of these agencies may differ, resulting in different drug policies, accessibility, and sometimes important outcomes. For example, the generally slow process of approval by the United States Food and Drug Administration was probably responsible for limiting the effects of thalidomide in the USA, while the experience in the UK was more severe.

Prescribing Habits

Another major factor in the interplay of prescription of drugs and the acceptance of these drugs is the habit of the prescriber. In Africa, because of the interdigitation of primary care and mental health, the average physician who is not a psychiatrist is in a position to prescribe a variety of psychotropics. Because of the limited number of physicians, pharmacists, and nurses, family members may play a significant role in the recommendation and prescription of medications.

Patient Beliefs and Attitudes

The belief systems and attitudes of the patients are also likely to be very important in the acceptance and compliance with medications. It is not unusual in Africa (and actually perhaps also elsewhere) that injections are regarded as more powerful than pills and tablets. Similarly, I have an impression that some patients often search for the all-powerful, omnipotent drug. In the Yoruba language this is referred to as 'gbogboloshi', which, translated literally, means 'It does it all'.

Drug Profile

The efficacy and side-effects profile of the drug are also important factors in compliance. An efficacious drug with severe adverse effects may not gain popularity. Drugs with adverse effects on sexual performance are generally at risk.

Therefore, the issues of cost, availability of the medication when the patient returns to his or her homeland, the efficacy of the medication, and beliefs regarding the cause of illness and the role of medications in its treatment all play a vital role in the prescription and acceptance of medications by Africans.

ETHNOPHARMACOLOGICAL FINDINGS WITH DIRECT IMPLICATIONS FOR AFRICAN PATIENTS

In 1969, Murphy, a pioneer in transcultural psychiatry, reported on ethnic differences in response to psychotropic medications [1]. That same year, Overall and his colleagues reported that Blacks experienced more improvement than Whites from a number of psychotropic medications [2]. In 1975, it was reported by Raskin and Crook that, when administered imipramine, a sample of Black patients showed relatively more improvement than a sample of White patients at the end of one week [3].

In 1980, we reported that red blood cells of Blacks concentrated lithium to a greater extent than the red blood cells of Whites [4]. Strickland and his colleagues have compared red blood cell/serum lithium in bipolar Black and White patients and, more recently, have related the ratio to the presence of adverse side effects [5].

Interest in the cytochrome P-450 enzymes has led to estimation of poor metabolizers (PMs) and extensive metabolizers (EMs) of CYP2D6 and CYP2C19—two enzymes that are important in psychotropic drug metabolism in different racial groups [6].

The metabolism of dexamethazone, tricyclics, antidepressants, selective serotonin reuptake inhibitors and thioridazine is dependent on the CYP2D6 system. Relling and colleagues have found that 7.7% of White children and 1.9% of Black children are deficient in this enzyme [7]. They are therefore PMs of diazepam, imipramine and hexobarbital, metabolism of which depends on CYP2C19. Significant differences have been observed in the deficiency of this enzyme in different groups. Individuals who have a deficiency in this enzyme system are PMs of the drugs that are metabolized by it. The distribution of PMs and EMs varies with ethnic group—for example, the frequency of PMs is higher in Orientals than in Blacks [6], which means that, for equivalent doses, Oriental people are likely to have higher plasma levels of these drugs than Blacks.

The above findings imply a need for caution in extrapolating clinical findings in non-African populations to Africans. In the above discussions, we have assumed that pharmacological findings in Afro-Americans may apply to Africans, but this in fact may not be so.

STUDIES WITH INDIRECT IMPLICATIONS FOR THE TREATMENT OF AFRICANS

Yamamoto and his colleagues reported that people of Asian origin generally required lower doses of neuroleptics than other groups [8]. Lin and Finder compared the maximum and stabilized doses given to an inpatient population in Los Angeles [9]. They found no difference in the incidence of extrapyramidal symptoms between the Asian and White subjects, and observed that the Asian patients were generally prescribed lower doses of neuroleptics. A similar study was conducted by Binder and his colleagues using a sample of patients in San Francisco [10]. They found that the dosages of neuroleptics in both Asian and White patients showed no differences; however, the incidence of extrapyramidal symptoms was higher among the Asian patients.

Sramek duplicated the study by Lin and Finder, but his results appeared to contradict theirs [9, 11], showing no difference between Asian and White subjects in terms of the maximum and stabilizing doses and the incidence of extrapyramidal symptoms. However, when their study sample was divided into two subgroups (those who had lived in the country for 5 years or more and those who had lived in the country for less than 5 years) a statistical significance was found. More recent surveys of dosages of psychotropic medications for Japanese, Korean, and Taiwanese patients living in their own country point to requirements of higher doses in these patients than in similar patients in the USA.

A number of lessons are to be learned from these studies, including:

• prescribing habits in any culture may change from time to time; and
• acculturation and length of stay in a foreign country may have some effect on a patient's neuroleptic requirements.

This latter point was underscored by a study by Potkin and colleagues [12], who demonstrated that recent immigrants had higher plasma levels of haloperidol and prolactin than American-born Asians. Such findings hint at the complex relationships between biochemical and environmental factors in drug metabolism.

Although the above studies compared Asian and White subjects, the lessons learned will have indirect applications for prescribing for Africans, both at home and abroad.

CLINICAL ASPECTS REQUIRING SPECIAL EMPHASIS IN TREATING AFRICANS

Case A

A was an African student in his twenties married to a West Indian woman. Both were in a professional school. The patient had presented with some thoughts of being controlled and influenced by external factors. His symptoms were so severe and disabling that he was hospitalized in a university hospital. He was referred to me because he is Nigerian.

During the first interview, I asked him which part of Nigeria he came from, and if he knew certain individuals. It transpired that he knew some members of the family of one of my classmates in medical school. For this reason (or for some other reason, including his suspiciousness), the patient was reticent in describing his symptoms. Subsequently, from interviews with his wife and in marital sessions, I was able to obtain more information. Firstly, his mother was unhappy about his decision to marry a foreigner, and he had attributed his illness to his mother's influence. Also, before his hospitalization, the couple had sought help from a West Indian 'bishop'. The experience was helpful, but the fees were exorbitant. With treatment, the symptoms cleared up and I discharged the patient; however, he did not keep his post-hospital appointment.

Discussion

It is often instructive for the therapist to explore with the patient the basis of his or her illness. This patient clearly related his illness to the magical activities of his affronted mother. He believed in magic, sorcery and witchcraft. Ness and Wintrop have stressed that this magical belief system also occurs in many religious societies in Western nations [13]. With acculturation and the adoption of non-traditional values, individual Africans may not, under ordinary circumstances, resort to a magical explanation for their human dilemmas. However, in times of emotional crises, and especially when confronted with chronic illness, they may search for a meaning by turning to witchcraft or sorcery. This couple probably participated in some ritualistic healing administered by the bishop to appease the patient's mother.

It is possible that this patient's initial discomfort with me could have been due to his fear of being stigmatized if he were treated by an individual who had an intimate knowledge of the patient's background.

It is imperative, in all cases, to also inquire as to the patient's history and previous attempts at treatment before immigration.

Case B

B was a Nigerian graduate student. Before he moved to the USA, his wife suffered a brief cardiovascular illness and died. Soon after his arrival, the patient began to feel isolated and depressed and developed concerns about his heart. He was referred to me informally and was willing to be hospitalized on the basis of the severity of his illness. He was seen in individual psychotherapy, he participated in group psychotherapy and was prescribed psychotropics. A nurse reported that he had difficulty adjusting in the group therapy sessions; however, the patient's own perception was that he was not given enough time during the group sessions.

With treatment, his condition improved. He gave up his studies in the USA and returned to Nigeria. I referred him to a colleague at the Lagos University Teaching Hospital and subsequently he made a full recovery.

Discussion

This case contrasts with Case A in many important areas.

1. He was relieved to have a fellow countryman as his physician.
2. Patient B was having problems adjusting to a new environment, but the man in case A had lived and studied here for some time.
3. This patient suspected that his illness was due to physiological (natural) causes; the patient in case A saw the root of his problem as external forces.

Case B's symptomatology was highly colored by somatization. The obvious connection between the cardiac cause of his wife's death and his own fear of death through cardiac symptoms did not appear to be obvious to him. This patient was grieving the loss of his wife, and he was deeply depressed. Many workers, including Kirmayer and Van Moffaert, have emphasized the complex relationship of somatoform, affective and anxiety disorders [14, 15]. Van Moffaert has emphasized the risk of misdiagnosis when immigrants present with highly dramatic symptoms. In her work with Mediterranean immigrants, she observed that such presentations did not necessarily mean a high frequency of somatoform or histrionic personalities in these populations.

Case C

C, a middle-aged Nigerian woman, was visiting her daughter and her daughter's family. Before coming to the USA, she had experienced some vague symptoms at the back of her head. She also had some 'creepy' feelings. Her symptoms became more severe during her stay. She had family and responsibilities in Nigeria and at the same time she was providing help to her daughter and her family in the USA. The patient did not appear to be fluent in day-to-day, or even pidgin, English and I had to use her daughter as an interpreter. I had some concerns with the quality of the interpretations. Nevertheless, I was able to treat her successfully with a combination of antidepressant and benzodiazepine.

Discussion

In this case there was some somatization: 'creepy' feelings in her head. Several workers have documented that sensations of 'hot' and 'peppery' feelings in the head, with or without sensations of crawling worms or a 'creepy' feeling are quite common throughout Africa and Asia and may occur in a wide range of psychiatric disorders [16–18]. A similar condition, 'brain fog', is a condition that has been described in students who are highly driven and separated from their parents. It is seen as an anxiety disorder [19]. Another aspect of this case is the patient's limited fluency in English, which made the task of treatment more difficult as the services of an interpreter were necessary: it will be difficult for the daughter (who probably has a vested interest to have her mother stay here) to be truly objective and neutral. Lastly, this patient, like the man described Case B, was having early adjustment difficulties in a foreign country. There were few opportunities for her to meet other Nigerians of her age and background.

Case D

A Sudanese man was staying in the USA to escape the civil war in the Sudan. He is a Christian, and the war there had a religious tone: a conflict between Moslems and Christians. This individual was a fairly young man and was sent to a local hospital by his primary care physician, who informed him that he had hepatitis. He believed he was about to die and complained of something in his blood, his brain, and his heart. Although he had a good educational background, he was working in housekeeping. The patient's wife was attending a professional graduate school in a neighboring African country. This patient was very depressed. He was successfully treated with a combination of antidepressant, neuroleptic and benzodiazepine.

Discussion

This patient, although very well educated, was not fluent in English—language was a barrier to his treatment. He was also underemployed, which is often a risk for immigrants and refugees. Several friends would often visit him in hospital simultaneously, sitting on his bed. A nurse communicated her (erroneous) suspicion that this patient could be homosexual.

The patient was seen by me on an outpatient basis and discovered that he was not complying fully with his medication regimen because he was experiencing financial difficulties. I gave him medications from my stock of samples—and before he paid a trip to his homeland I gave him 3 months supply of medications. A related point is that his compliance fell as the acute symptoms resolved. Such patients must be fully instructed as to their condition so that they realize they must continue to take medication even when symptoms lessen.

Another important aspect in this case is the fact that this patient was a refugee. African refugees living in industrialized nations seem to have received less attention than their Asian counterparts.

Case E

An adolescent girl from a French-speaking African country, whose parents were very well educated, alleged that she had been sexually molested. However, her father found some inconsistency in her story and did not believe her. The patient became very depressed and began to threaten suicide. I was consulted to help clarify the diagnosis. During the initial meeting with the patient and her parents, the girl's father, who was a senior civil servant in his home, dominated the conversation. One of the patient's brothers served as interpreter. The patient's father expressed dismay that the girl was being treated by a physician whom he did not know and was highly dissatisfied that the physician should have asked him about medications to be used because he was not a physician. He clearly misconstrued the physician's request for permission and informed consent before the use of psychotropics for advice on prescribing. He also indicated that the girl's problem could have been taken care of in her home country by one of her aunts.

Discussion

Once again, language was an obstacle as I had to use an interpreter. There are problems in using a family member as an interpreter as the translation may not always be unbiased. Additionally, there were some intergenerational and cultural difficulties between the adolescent patient and her father. The patient was threatening suicide. Suicide in Africa, especially in adolescent groups, is rare. Lastly, there were cultural clashes between the rights of the family and the rights of the psychiatrist.

Conclusion

The cases described here help to illustrate some general guidelines in prescribing and treating Africans in the transcultural context. Each case must be fully assessed in its own right with complete history, appropriate consultation (when possible) and appropriate diagnosis. The risk of misdiagnosis because of language barriers and the presence of dramatic symptoms and somatization should always be considered.

The presence of significant somatization is not synonymous with histrionic behavior or conversion symptoms. Rather, it may be caused by anxiety, depression, psychosis, and severe mental and family conflict. Africans tend to have strong family interest and responsibility not only to the immediate family members but also to members of the extended family. Inability to meet their obligations may result in considerable guilt. Thus, treatment approaches should be comprehensive and, whenever possible, should include family sessions.

Anyone prescribing for African patients should be aware of interindividual as well as ethnic differences in drug metabolism. Attention should be paid to compliance issues as well as problems with adverse effects, especially as they relate to sexual side-effects. Whether an individual is a refugee should also be ascertained, as refugees may suffer acute or chronic post-traumatic stress disorders.

Finally, with increased globalization and possible shifts of international policy, the presence of Africans abroad may continue to rise. The provision of appropriate mental health services to such populations is becoming a necessity.

REFERENCES

1. Murphy HEM. 1989. Ethnic variations in drug responses. *Transcult Psychiatr Res Rev* **6**: 6–23.
2. Overall JE, Hollister LE, Kimbell I, Shelton J. 1969. Extrinsic factors influencing responses to psychotherapeutic drugs. *Arch Gen Psychiatry* **21**: 89–94.
3. Raskin A, Crook TH. 1975. Antidepressants in black and white inpatients. *Arch Gen Psychiatry* **32**: 643–9.
4. Okpaku S, Frazer A, Mendels J. 1980. A pilot study of racial differences in erythrocyte lithium transport. *Am J Psychiatry* **137**: 120–1.
5. Strickland TL, Lin K-M, Fu P, Anderson D, Zheng Y. 1995. Comparison of lithium ratios between African-American and Caucasian bipolar patients. *Biol Psychiatry* **37**: 325–30.
6. Kinzie JD, Edeki T. 1998. Ethnicity and psychopharmacology. In: Okpaku SO, ed. *The Experience of Southeast Asians in Clinical Methods in Transcultural Psychiatry*. Washington DC: American Psychiatric Press.

7. Relling MV, Chessie J, Schell MJ, Petrus WP, Meyer WH, Evans WE. 1991. Lower prevalence of the debrisoquin oxidative poor metabolizer phenotype in American black versus white subjects. *Clinical Pharmacol Ther* **50**: 308–33.
8. Yamamoto J, Fung D, Lo S *et al.* 1979. Psychopharmacology for Asian Americans and Pacific Islanders. *Bycus Pharmacol Bull* **15**: 29–31.
9. Lin K-M, Finder E. 1983. Neuroleptic dosages for Asians. *Am J Psychiatry* **140**: 490–1.
10. Binder RJ, Levy R. 1981. Extrapyramidal reactions in Asians. *Am J Psychiatry* **138**: 1243–4.
11. Sramek JJ, Sayles MS, Simpson GM. 1986. Neuroleptic dosage for Asians: A failure to replicate. *Am J Psychiatry* **143**: 535–6.
12. Potkin SG, Shen Y, Pardes H, Phelps BH, Zhou D, Shu L *et al.* 1984. Haloperidol concentrations elevated in Chinese patients. *Psychiatry Res* **12**: 167–72.
13. Ness RC, Wintrob RM. 1981. Folk healing: A description and synthesis. *Am J Psychiatry* **138**: 1477–81.
14. Kirmayer LJ. 1998. Somatization and psychologization. In: Okpaku SO, ed. *Understanding Cultural Idioms of Distress in Clinical Methods in Transcultural Psychiatry*: Washington DC: American Psychiatric Press.
15. Van Moffaert M, Vereecken A. 1989. Somatization of psychiatric illness in Mediterranean migrants in Belgium. *Cult Med Psychiatry* **13**: 297–313.
16. Ebigo PO. 1986. A cross-sectional study of somatic complaints of Nigerian females using the emegu somatization scale. *Cult Med Psychiatry* **10**: 167–86.
17. Gureje O, Obikoya B. 1992. Somatization in primary care: pattern and correlates in a clinic in Nigeria. *Acta Psychiatr Scand* **86**: 223–7.
18. Srinivasan TN, Suresh TR. 1991. The non specific symptom screening method: detection of nonpsychotic morbidity based on nonspecific symptoms. *Gen Hosp Psychiatry* **13**: 106–14.
19. Jegede RO. 1983. Psychiatric illness in African students, 'brain fog' syndrome revisited. *Can J Psychiatry* **28**: 188–92.

6

Ethnicity and Psychopharmacology in Latin America

Luis F. Ramirez

Case Western Reserve University, Cleveland, OH, USA

INTRODUCTION

It has been reported anecdotally that patients from Latin American countries require less medication than Caucasian patients for the treatment of disorders such as major depression, panic, or schizophrenia. While these clinical observations have been questioned, clinicians in Latin American countries do use smaller doses of psychotropic medications than the amounts used by their colleagues in North America. Suffice it to say, ethnic differences in pharmacokinetics and pharmacodynamics are known to cause clinically observed differences in the effects of certain drugs, such as alcohol or beta-blockers, in different populations. These effects are most pronounced in Asian populations, but few studies have been carried out in Latin America. Fortunately several efforts are under way to study the importance of ethnicity in psychopharmacology.

PHARMACOKINETICS AND PHARMACODYNAMICS

Significant advances have been made in the study of pharmacokinetics and pharmacodynamics in different populations. For example, two of the most frequently encountered cytochrome P-450 isoenzymes, CYP2D6 (responsible for the metabolism of tricyclic antidepressants, selective serotonin reuptake inhibitors, and antipsychotic agents such as clozapine and risperidone) and YCYP2C19 (responsible for the metabolism of some benzodiazepines) are polymorphic in nature and have cross ethnic variations. In practical terms, when this polymorphism is manifested in some patients (who possess normally functioning enzymes), they are referred to as poor metabolizers (PMs)—as opposed to extensive metabolizers (EMs). The PM rate for CYP2D6 varies with ethnic group, from 0.8% for Asians, 1.9% for African Americans, 4.5% for Hispanics to 7% for Caucasians. The rates for CYP2C19 are

Cross Cultural Psychiatry. Edited by John M. Herrera, William B. Lawson and John J. Sramek.
© 1999 John Wiley & Sons Ltd.

20% for Asians, 18.5% for African Americans, 4.8% for Hispanics, and 3.3% for Caucasians [1]. Another ethnic factor of importance is body size and percentage of fat, since these influence the volume of distribution of lipophilic psychotropic agents. Differences in body size and fat distribution may explain some of the differences in doses between Latino and Anglo patients because of the high lipophilic profile of many psychotropic agents.

TYPICAL AND ATYPICAL ANTIPSYCHOTICS

Several studies have investigated plasma concentrations of medications in Asian populations. Healthy Asian volunteers and Asian patients with schizophrenia had been found to have significantly higher plasma haloperidol concentrations than their Caucasian counterparts. These differences cannot be explained at present [2]. A recent review of the literature showed no published studies on the blood levels of antipsychotic medications in Latin Americans who are healthy and/or who have schizophrenia.

Novartis Pharmaceuticals in Argentina is actively studying oral doses, blood levels, clinical response, and quality of life in patients treated with clozapine. Their hypothesis is that Argentinean patients will require less oral medication to achieve the therapeutic blood levels of clozapine described in the literature by Potkin et al. [3]. On the other hand, Gaviria et al. [4] have reported that the pharmacokinetics of nortriptyline in Hispanics is similar to the kinetics in Anglos, which casts some doubt on the hypothesis described above.

A study presented by Susana Viale-Hansen from Argentina, during the Pan American Congress of Psychiatry in Mexico City in 1994, showed that in 60 patients treated successfully with clozapine, the dose range was 25–600 mg per day during the acute phases, with a maintenance average dose of 300 mg per day. Similar results from a larger sample were presented by Veronica Larach from Chile. These dosages are smaller than the amounts used in North America, as reported by Meltzer and his group [5]. In a consensus meeting organized by Janssen Pharmaceuticals during the first reunion of the Latin American College of Neuropsychopharmacology in Brazil, psychiatrists from Colombia, Argentina, and Mexico reported that the dose of risperidone used to treat their patients with schizophrenia was similar to the amounts recommended by Janssen in the USA (6 mg daily), but there was a tendency toward the use of smaller dosages in a large number of patients.

Currently, the author is conducting a related study under the auspices of Novartis Argentina and with the collaboration of Doctors Susana Viale-Hansen and Pedro Gargoloff. This is a reasonably large multicenter study in which several hundreds of patients have been screened and only the treatment-resistant ones, according to the Kane criteria, selected for the study. The patients were treated in a naturalistic way and the dosage of medication adjusted according to each patient's clinical response. The clinical response was evaluated with standard diagnostic instruments (BPRS, PANSS and the Quality of Life Scale). Patients were treated for 1 year and blood levels of clozapine measured every 3 months.

At present the results are still being processed, but preliminary findings are available for about 150 patients. The symptoms and quality of life significantly improved in more than 60% of the patients and no cases of agranulocytosis were detected. The average daily oral dosage of clozapine was 300 mg and more than 60% of the patients had blood levels of 400 ng/ml or higher. The range of blood levels of clozapine was very wide, reaching up to 15-fold in some patients; however there was a trend towards reduction in blood levels of clozapine at the end of the study.

Some preliminary conclusions include the possibility that Argentineans need lower doses of clozapine than other ethnic groups to respond clinically and to develop therapeutic blood levels of the medication. Further, the reduction in the blood levels of the drug at the end of the study may be due to non-compliance or reduction by autoinduction of the metabolism—this needs to be studied further. At present, we are processing all the data for future publication.

COMMENTS

It is quite reasonable to state that there is a general belief, from Mexico to Argentina, that Latin American patients need less medication than their North American counterparts, although this generalization is not confirmed by published reports. It is important for us to realize that Latin Americans are not a homogeneous population but a melting pot of many different cultures, and many 'non-biological' factors influence treatment outcome. Factors such as availability of care, biases on the part of healthcare workers, special beliefs of patients, expectations, placebo effects, economics, and compliance are as important as the efficacy of the medication. For example, Escobar and Tuason [6] reported that non-Caucasians may respond better to placebo than Caucasians. The World Health Organization has also reported that the outcome of patients with schizophrenia is better in underdeveloped than in developed countries [7]. These, and other, examples make the information available about dosage and clinical response in Latin American patients difficult to interpret. Consequently, more epidemiological and cross cultural studies must be conducted to determine the accuracy of the clinical observation that less medication is needed to achieve remission in patients with Latin American ancestry.

REFERENCES

1. Lin K-M, Anderson D, Poland RE. 1995. Ethnicity and psychopharmacology. *Psychiatry Clin North Am* **18**: 3.
2. Potkin SG, Shen Y, Pardes H *et al.* 1984. Haloperidol concentrations elevated in Chinese patients. *Psychiatry Res* **12**: 167–72.

3. Potkin SG, Bera R, Culasekaram B *et al.* 1994. Plasma clozapine concentrations predict clinical response in treatment-resistant schizophrenia. *J Clin Psychiatry* **55**: 133–7.
4. Gaviria MA, Gill AA, Javaid JI. 1986. Nortriptyline kinetics in Hispanic and Anglo subjects. *J Clin Psychopharmacol* **6**: 227–31.
5. Meltzer HY, Alphs L, Bastani B *et al.* 1989. One year outcome of study of clozapine in treatment resistant schizophrenia. Presented at 8th World Congress of Psychiatry, Athens, October 13–19: 19–27.
6. Escobar J, Tuason V. 1980. Antidepression agents: A cross cultural study. *Psychopharmacol Bull* **16**: 49–52.
7. Jablensky A, Sartorious N, Emberg C *et al.* 1992. Schizophrenia: manifestations, incidence and course in different cultures. A World Health Organization ten-country study. *Psychol Med Monogr Suppl* **20**.

7

The Art and Science of Ethnopharmacotherapy

William B. Lawson

Indiana University School of Medicine, Indianapolis, IN, USA

INTRODUCTION

Extensive studies have shown that African Americans and other racial and ethnic minorities have higher rates of morbidity and mortality across the life span [1]. These differences have been related to ethnic differences in access to health care. However, few outcome studies have investigated the mental health of many ethnic minorities. Psychiatric disorders are of interest because of the stigma, cost, and modest treatment successes, which may be especially daunting for African Americans and Hispanics.

In the mental health system African Americans tend to receive the least desirable treatment [2]. African Americans and Hispanics are more likely to be hospitalized, to be involuntarily committed, and to be placed in seclusion or restraints [2–8] than other ethnic groups. Moreover, African Americans are more likely than Caucasians to receive PRN medication and higher doses of antipsychotic medication [9–12]. The reason for the differential dosing is not clear. However as noted in other papers, ethnic minorities may present with different or more symptoms that can lead to misdiagnosis [11], and African Americans are more likely to be perceived as being violent. We reported that the staff on an inpatient unit perceived African American patients to be more dangerous even though independent assessment of violent behavior showed that they were in fact significantly less likely to be violent to self or others [5]. African Americans in distress or with mental disorders often do not seek treatment [13–15] because of fear of hospitalization and involuntary committal [15]. Treatment delay may worsen symptoms at admission, and increase the likelihood of involuntary committal. However, racial differences in symptom presentation or degree are not reliably found, even in studies that have reported differences in the treatment that African Americans receive [2, 5–7, 16].

African Americans may perceive the mental health system differently than providers [10]: providers are often not African Americans, and differing perceptions of treatment may impair the therapeutic alliance. Consequently, when such people do

Cross Cultural Psychiatry. Edited by John M. Herrera, William B. Lawson and John J. Sramek.
© 1999 John Wiley & Sons Ltd.

seek treatment, it is usually not from mental health professionals [14]. A contributing factor to the unwillingness of African Americans to participate in the standard mental health treatment system is widespread awareness of the Tuskegee study [17], a federally sponsored study begun in the 1930s in which treatment was withheld from African American men diagnosed with syphilis without their knowledge. Only a newspaper exposé in the 1970s ended the study. As a consequence, psychotropic medication and mental health treatment may be viewed with suspicion. Suspiciousness or lack of knowledge about treatment may be additional contributors to treatment delay. Access to appropriate treatment issues are especially relevant with psychotropic medication.

Racial misdiagnosis often leads to the use of the wrong medications, which in turn could lead to poorer outcomes. As noted previously, African Americans and Hispanics are overdiagnosed with schizophrenia and consequently are more likely to receive antipsychotics when they are not needed [18–19]. Bell and Mehta [20–21], using case reports, showed that African American patients with clear-cut bipolar affective disorder and excellent lithium response were often initially diagnosed with schizophrenia and not given lithium therapy until much later. Mukherjee *et al.* [22], in a larger sample of admissions to an outpatient clinic, reported that African Americans and Hispanics with confirmed manic-depressive illness were far more likely to receive an initial diagnosis of schizophrenia; consequently, they would be less likely to receive lithium and other antimanic agents [23]. The author studied a group of Hispanic patients with English as their second language and with a presumptive diagnosis of schizophrenia. Using a Spanish translator, we found that half of the patients met DSM-IIIR criteria for delusional depression but had been treated exclusively with antipsychotics. When an antidepressant was added they improved and were able to be discharged. African Americans with affective disorders are more likely to show psychotic symptoms [24]. Affective disorders in general are more likely to present with psychotic symptoms, mania may present with more irritable symptoms, and depression may present with suspiciousness [25, 26]. Thus, antipsychotics may be used more frequently to treat perceived psychotic symptoms.

An adverse consequence of the excessive use of antipsychotics is the increased risk for development of adverse effects such as abnormal involuntary movements. The worst consequence is the development of tardive dyskinesia, characterized by choreoathetoid movements that may persist for a lifetime and for which there is no reliable cure. Glazer reported that African Americans patients were more likely to develop tardive dyskinesia than Caucasian patients [27, 28]. One possibility is that African Americans may have some, as yet unrecognized, genetic or enzymatic defect that may predispose to tardive dyskinesia. However, these patients are also more likely to be medicated differently: African Americans are more likely than Caucasians to receive neuroleptic medication, and to receive higher doses [2, 9, 13, 29]. Dosing is more likely to be intermittent—from PRN medication, more frequent medication interruptions due to poor compliance, or lack of access to regular treatment. Exposure to neuroleptic medication, excessive dosing and intermittent treatment are all risk factors for tardive dyskinesia [30]. The diagnosis of an affective disorder is another risk factor for tardive dyskinesia in individuals exposed to neuroleptics.

Different ethnic groups may require different dosages. Asian providers often prescribe lower doses of many different psychotropic agents, including antipsychotic medication, and tricyclic antidepressants, to Asian patients [31, 32]. Part of the reason for this is that Asians report more adverse effects and show higher plasma levels than Caucasians given the same dose, due to ethnic differences in drug metabolism [33, 34]. Early multicenter studies have showed that African Americans tend to respond more quickly to antipsychotic medication and tricyclic antidepressants than Caucasian patients [3, 23, 35]. We have reported that African Americans may show slightly higher serum levels of thiothixene [5]; others have reported an increased risk of toxic side-effects and higher plasma levels of tricyclic antidepressants in African Americans than in Caucasians [36]. Rudorfer and Robins [37] showed that African Americans who had taken a lethal dose of tricyclics had higher plasma levels than Caucasians who had overdosed. These findings suggest that African Americans may be at a greater risk of toxic side-effects when treated with tricyclic antidepressants [35].

These differences in clinical response and pharmacokinetics have been attributed to ethnic differences in metabolism, mediated through the cytochrome P-450 microsomal enzyme system, of most psychotropic medication [34, 35, 38]. Although African Americans are sometimes given excessive medication the pharmacokinetic data does not justify this practice. Ethnic differences have also been reported in lithium metabolism. African Americans tend to show a higher red blood cell to plasma ratio of lithium than either Asians or Caucasians [23, 39, 40], which suggests increased cellular egress, but similar plasma levels. The clinical significance of this was unknown until Strickland et al. [40] found that African Americans on lithium therapy reported more adverse effects during a standardized interview than Caucasians. Moreover, ratings of adverse effects were directly related to the patient's red blood cell to plasma ratio. Other reports suggest that a plasma to high red blood cell ratio increases the risk of other adverse effects such as lithium neuroleptic toxicity [23]. It is not clear if African Americans require a lower clinical dose but more caution may be warranted when lithium treatment is initiated.

The lithium ratio in African Americans has been attributed to the mechanism that accounts for the increased risk for hypertension in African Americans. Many of the ancestors of today's African Americans died while crossing the Atlantic in slave ships probably due to hyponatremia. The survivors tend to handle sodium differently and are more likely to conserve sodium, which would lead to an increased risk of hypertension [41]. This differential response to a sodium load presumably also accounts for the difference in lithium ratio [23].

Newer agents such as the serotonin reuptake inhibitors (SSRIs) do not have the side-effect profile, particularly the cardiovascular toxicity, of older agents: while someone could successfully suicide using SSRIs, they are generally far safer. This is especially important given the risk of toxicity that the tricyclics possess for ethnic minorities. Many of the newer SSRIs have less effect on the hepatic cytochrome P-450 system, which might further reduce their likelihood of overdose and toxicity for ethnic minorities. Drugs such as divalproex and carbamazepine, and other agents used to treat partial complex seizures, are alternatives to lithium in the treatment of bipolar affective disorder [33]. As noted above, lithium may not be as well tolerated among African Americans as other agents but unfortunately there is as yet no information about the relative tolerability of the alternative agent in African Americans, and whether it should be prescribed instead of lithium to treat mania.

New pharmacotherapeutic approaches may address some of the consequences of overprescribing for psychotic disorders. The new antipsychotic clozapine has become a model for atypical agents [42]. It is effective in many patients unresponsive to treatment by 'typical' antipsychotics. It also seems to have few extrapyramidal effects and a lower risk for tardive dyskinesia. Clozapine, however, has other features that limit its availability to African Americans. First it is expensive [43]. Clozapine is not alone in this because many of the newer agents do not yet have generic equivalents because their patents have not yet expired. In addition, part of the cost of clozapine is due to the significantly greater risk of agranulocytosis it causes [44] and the weekly leukocyte counts which are required before clozapine can be started despite the lack of evidence that pre-existing counts predict agranulocytosis. However, African Americans are known to have a leukocyte count whose normal range can extend well below listed normal values—a 'benign leukopenia' [45]. As a result the overly cautious clinician may choose not to start otherwise healthy African American patients on clozapine. A recent study did in fact show that clozapine is more likely to be discontinued in African Americans than in other groups [46]. A contributing factor may have been the lower baseline leukocyte counts of the African Americans.

Other new atypical antipsychotics do not increase the risk of agranulocytosis but they are less likely to cause acute extrapyramidal symptoms and probably are at a lesser risk of causing tardive dyskinesia. We reported that one agent, olanzapine, was not associated with more abnormal involuntary movements among ethnic minorities [47]. Unfortunately, all of these agents are more costly than the standard agents and often are excluded from formularies. African Americans and Hispanics, particularly, are more likely to be on Medicaid—and Medicaid tends to have restrictive formularies, which further limit the availability of new agents. More needs to be done to educate policy makers about assessing total cost of care in determining the cost of including newer agents on formularies. Newer agents can cut the overall cost of care and may be especially beneficial for ethnic minorities.

CONCLUSION

More research is needed with African American and other ethnic minorities: African Americans are often not well represented in pharmaceutical trials [48], and most psychiatric journals that do publish biological research do not include racial data [49]. The argument is often made that racial groupings are not scientifically valid or promote prejudice. Clearly this argument has merit when race is used as an explanatory concept; however, race can serve as a proxy for other variables not previously identified as significant, such as a gross approximation or 'first cut' of phenotypic variables, or of access to service. Also, the argument that race is irrelevant leads to the equally fallacious assumption that information derived from exclusively Caucasian samples can be generalized to all ethnic groups. New treatment approaches may be the answer to ethnic disparities in mental health services and outcome. The decision to use new treatments should be determined by their costs in the total healthcare system.

REFERENCES

1. Malone T. 1985. Chairman, Report of the secretary's task force on black and minority health. Washington, DC: US Department of Health and Human Services.
2. Flaherty JA, Meagher R. 1980. Measuring racial bias in inpatient treatment. *Am J Psychiatry* **137**: 679–82.
3. Lawson WB. 1986. Racial and ethnic factors in psychiatric research. *Hosp Community Psychiatry* **37**: 50–4.
4. Lawson WB, Hepler N, Holladay J, Cuffel B. 1994. Race as a factor in inpatient and outpatient admissions and diagnosis. *Hosp Community Psychiatry* **45**: 72–4.
5. Lawson WB, Yesavage JA, Werner RD. 1984. Race, violence, and psychopathology. *J Clin Psychiatry* **45**: 294–7.
6. Lindsey KP, Paul GL, Mariotto MJ. 1989. Urban psychiatric commitments: Disability and dangerous behavior of black and white recent admissions. *Hosp Community Psychiatry* **40**: 286–94.
7. Paul GI, Menditto AA. 1992. Effectiveness of inpatient treatment programs for mentally ill adults in public psychiatric facilities. *Appl Prevent Psychol* **1**: 41–63.
8. Strakowski SM, Lonczak HS, Sax K, West SA, Crist A, Mehta R, Thienhaus OJ. 1995. The effects of race on diagnosis and disposition from a psychiatric emergency service. *J Clin Psychiatry* **56**: 101–7.
9. Chung H, Mahler JC, Kakuna T. 1995. Racial differences in the treatment of psychiatric inpatients. *Psychiatr Serv* **46**: 586–91.
10. Flaherty JA, Naidu J, Lawton R, Pathak D. 1981. Racial differences in perception of ward atmosphere. *Am J Psychiatry* **138**: 815–17.
11. Lawson WB. 1986. Clinical issues in the pharmacotherapy of African-Americans. *Psychopharmacol Bull* **32**: 275–81.
12. Strakowski SM, Shelton RC, Kolbrener ML. 1993. The effects of race and comorbidity on clinical diagnosis in patients with psychosis. *J Clin Psychiatry* **54**: 96–102.
13. Brown DR, Feroz A, Gary LE, Milburn NG. 1995. Major depression in a community of African Americans. *Am J Psychiatry* **152**: 373–8.
14. Neighbors HW. 1984. The distribution of psychiatric morbidity in black Americans: a review and suggestion for research. *Community Ment Health J* **20**: 169–81.
15. Sussman LK, Robins LN, Earls F. 1987. Treatment-seeking for depression by black and white Americans. *Soc Sci Med* **24**: 187–96.
16. Strakowski SM, Flaum M, Amador X, Bracha HS, Pandurangi AK, Robinson D, Tohen M. 1996. Racial differences in the diagnosis of psychosis. *Schizophrenia Res* **21**: 117–24.

17. Roy B. 1995. The Tuskegee syphilis experiment: biotechnology and the administrative state. *J Natl Med Assoc* **87**: 56–67.
18. Lawson WB. 1986. The black family and chronic mental illness. *Am J Soc Psychiatry* **6**: 57–61.
19. Strickland TK, Ranganath V, Lin K-M, Poland RE, Mendoza R, Smith MW. 1991. Psychopharmacologic considerations in the treatment of black American populations. *Psychopharmacol. Bull* **27**: 441–8.
20. Bell CC, Mehta H. 1980. The misdiagnosis of black patients with manic-depressive illness. *J Natl Med Assoc* **72**: 141–5.
21. Bell CC, Mehta H. 1981. Misdiagnosis of black patient with manic-depressive illness: Second in a series. *J Natl Med Assoc* **73**: 101–7.
22. Mukherjee S, Shukla S, Woodline J. 1983. Misdiagnosis of schizophrenia in bipolar patients: A multi-ethnic comparison. *Am J Psychiatry* **140**: 1571–4.
23. Strickland TL, Lawson WB, Lin K-M. 1993. Interethnic variation in response to lithium therapy among African-American and Asian-American populations. In: Lin K-M, Poland RE, Nakasaki G, eds. *Psychopharmacology and Psychobiology of Ethnicity*. Washington DC: American Psychiatric Association, pp. 107–23.
24. Strakowski SM, McElroy SL, Keck PE Jr, West SA. 1996. Racial influences on diagnosis in psychotic mania. *J Affect Disord* **39**: 157–62.
25. Adebimpe VR. 1981. Overview: White norms and psychiatric diagnosis of black patients. *Am J Psychiatry* **138**: 279–85.
26. Adebimpe VR, Hedlund JL, Cho DW *et al.* 1982. Symptomatology of depression in Black and White patients. *J Natl Med Assoc* **74**: 185–90.
27. Glazer WM, Morgenstern H, Doucette J. 1994. Race and tardive dyskinesia among outpatients at a CMHC. *Hosp Community Psychiatry* **45**: 38–42.
28. Morgenstern H, Glazer WM. 1993. Identifying risk factors for tardive dyskinesia among chronic outpatients maintained on neuroleptic medications: results of the Yale tardive dyskinesia study. *Arch Gen Psychiatry* **50**: 723–33.
29. Price N, Glazer W, Morgenstern H. 1985. Demographic predictors of the use of injectable versus oral antipsychotic medications in outpatients. *Am J Psychiatry* **142**: 1491–2.
30. Jeste DV, Wyatt RJ. 1982. *Understanding and Treating Tardive Dyskinesia*. New York: Guilford Press.
31. Lin K-M, Finder E. 1983. Neuroleptic dosage for Asians. *Am J Psychiatry* **140**: 490–1.
32. Yamashita I, Asano Y. 1979. Tricyclic antidepressants: therapeutic plasma level. *Psychopharmacol Bull* **15**: 40–1.
33. Bond WS. 1990. Therapy update: ethnicity and psychotropic drugs. *Clin Pharmacology* **10**: 467–70.
34. Lin K-M, Poland RE. 1995. Ethnicity, culture, and psychopharmacology. In: Bloom FE, Kupler DJ, eds. *Psychopharmacology: The Fourth Generation of Progress*. New York: Raven Press.
35. Silver B, Poland RE, Lin K-M. 1993. Ethnicity and the pharmacology of tricyclic antidepressants. In: Lin K-M, Poland RE, Wallasaki G, eds. *Psychopharmacology and Psychobiology of Ethnicity*. Washington, DC: American Psychiatric Association, pp. 61–89.
36. Ziegler VE, Biggs JT. 1977. Tricyclic plasma levels—effect of age, race, sex and smoking. *JAMA* **238**: 2167–9.
37. Rudorfer MV, Robins E. 1982. Amitriptyline overdose: clinical effects on tricyclic antidepressant plasma levels. *J Clin Psychiatry* **43**: 457–60.
38. Lin K-M, Poland RE, Silver B. 1993. Overview: The interface between psychobiology and psychiatry. 151: 825–35, 1994. In: Lin K-M, Poland RE, Nakasi G, eds. *Psychopharmacology and Psychobiology of Ethnicity*. Washington, DC: American Psychiatric Association, pp. 11–35.

39. Okpaku S, Frazer A, Mendels J. 1980. A pilot study of racial differences in erythrocyte lithium transport. *Am J Psychiatry* **137**: 120–1.
40. Strickland TL, Lin K-M, Fu P, Anderson D, Zheng Y. 1995. Comparison of lithium ratio between African-American and caucasian bipolar patients. *Biol Psychiatry* **37**: 325–30.
41. Wilson TW, Grim CE. 1991. Biohistory of slavery and blood pressure differences in blacks today. *Hypertension* **17** (Suppl 1): 122–8.
42. Kane J, Honifield G, Singer J, Meltzer H, The Clozaril Collaborative Study Group. 1988. Clozapine for the treatment resistant schizophrenic: a double-blind comparison versus chlorpromazine. *Arch Gen Psychiatry* **45**: 789–96.
43. Griffith EEH. 1990. Clozapine: Problems for the public sector. *Hosp Community Psychiatry* **41**: 837.
44. Alvir JMJ, Lieberman JA, Safferman AZ, Schwimmer JL, Schaaf JA. 1993. Clozapine-induced agranulocytosis: incidence and risk factors in the United States. *N Engl J Med* **329**: 162–7.
45. Caramikat E, Karayalcin G, Aballi A, Lunzkowsky P. 1973. Leukocyte count differences in healthy white and black children 1 to 5 years of age. *J Pediatric* **86**: 252–75.
46. Moeller FG, Chen YW, Steinberg JL, Petty F, Ripper GW, Shah N, Garver DL. 1995. Risk factors for clozapine discontinuation among 805 patients in the VA hospital system. *Ann Clin Psychiatry* **7**: 167–73.
47. Lawson WB, Shavers E, Bergstrom R, Anderson S. 1999. Antipsychotic Treatment Of African Americans. *Psychopharmacol Bull* In Press.
48. Svenson CK. 1989. Representation of American blacks in clinical trials of new drugs. *JAMA* **261**: 263–5.
49. Lawson WB. 1990. Biological markers in neuropsychiatric disorders: Racial and ethnic factors. In: Sorel E, ed. *Family, Culture, and Psychobiology.* New York: Levas.

C
Diagnosis

8

American Indians and Mental Health: Issues in Psychiatric Assessment and Diagnosis

Ilena M. Norton

University of Colorado, Denver Health Medical Center, Denver, CO, USA

The description of psychiatric disorders in DSM-IV and earlier versions reflects the nature of the mind, behavior, and the self as experienced in Western European cultures [1]. This is acknowledged in DSM-IV by the statement in the introduction that the symptoms and course of psychiatric disorders are influenced by cultural and ethnic factors [2]. Clinicians need to be knowledgeable about the cultural factors that determine the patient's presentation of illness in order to effectively assess and treat mental disorder.

The aim of this chapter is to describe issues that arise in the psychiatric diagnostic assessment of American Indian patients. The chapter begins with a description of the American Indian and Alaska Native populations. This is followed by specific clinical examples to illustrate how American Indian cultural values and orientations influence the patients' presentation of illness, using the framework of the cultural formulation in DSM-IV. Particular attention is given to those sections of the cultural formulation that relate to diagnosis. These include the predominant idioms of distress, perceived causes of illness or the explanatory models, and the meaning and perceived severity of the individual's symptoms in relation to norms of the cultural reference group.

American Indians and Alaska Natives constitute a vibrant and growing population within the USA. At the time of the 1990 census, the population of American Indians and Alaska Natives had reached 1 937 391—a figure that had nearly doubled since the mid-1970s. There are signs, too, that this growth will continue, given the overall youth of the population; in 1990, the median age was only 27 years.

American Indians and Alaska Natives are geographically disbursed throughout the USA. Forty-eight percent of American Indians and Alaska Natives live in the West; the states with the largest concentration are Oklahoma, California, Arizona, New Mexico, and Alaska [3]. According to the census, 22% of American Indians

Cross Cultural Psychiatry. Edited by John M. Herrera, William B. Lawson and John J. Sramek.
© 1999 John Wiley & Sons Ltd.

and Alaska Natives live on reservation and trust lands, but many live in towns and cities bordering their reservations to take advantage of better employment opportunities.

After World War II, many American Indians living on reservations were forced to resettle in urban centers by the Bureau of Indian Affairs' relocation program. Significant migration between reservations and urban areas continues. The largest number of urban-dwelling American Indians and Alaska Natives are found in New York City, Oklahoma City, Phoenix, Los Angeles, Tulsa, Anchorage, Minneapolis, and Albuquerque. In view of the population growth and the wide geographic distribution, mental health clinicians throughout the USA should be skilled in the assessment of psychiatric disorders among American Indians and Alaska Natives.

American Indians and Alaska Natives are a diverse group of over 550 federally recognized tribes and Alaska Native villages. The largest of these tribes are the Navajo and Cherokee, numbering more than 200 000 members; however the vast majority of tribes have fewer than 1000 members. These tribes have important differences in language, customs, family structure, illness experiences, and healing traditions. At the same time, they have a shared history of extermination through disease and warfare, loss of traditional lands and means of obtaining food, shelter, and clothing, forced residence on reservations, mandated education in White boarding schools, and cultural extermination through the repression of traditional languages, ceremonies, and religions.

One of the ways that this knowledge of demographics and history is incorporated into the assessment is that tribal affiliation is often a key aspect of identity. Asking about tribal affiliation will communicate that the clinician understands that this is an important aspect of American Indian and Alaska Native identity. Secondly, the relationship between the non-Indian clinician and the patient will be influenced by the history of Indian–White relations. The history of White oppression and betrayal, in addition to today's racism, may cause patients to be wary of trusting a mental health clinician who is unknown within their community. There are many other considerations in counseling American Indians and Alaska Natives, and these are not reviewed here in detail. Interested readers are referred to works by Carolyn Attneave [4] and Joseph Trimble and his colleagues [5] for comprehensive reviews of this topic.

In 1965, Johnson described a syndrome of 'totally discouraged' among the Standing Rock Sioux, which included symptoms of the traveling of one's thoughts to the dwelling place of one's dead relatives; facilitating sending one's spirit on to the ghost camp by willing death, committing suicide, or drinking to excess; and being preoccupied with ideas of ghosts or spirits [6]. This disorder was associated with suicide attempts or excessive drinking. In contrast to the symptoms described above, normative cultural beliefs encompassed the nearness of the ghost world, the desire to be in contact with the spirits of departed relatives, and the positive valuing of dreams and visions. In this description, Johnson characterized the spiritual beliefs of this tribe, and differentiated these beliefs from pathological symptoms characteristic of mental disorder.

The differentiation of normative versus non-normative spiritual experiences in the syndrome 'totally discouraged' is an example of how culture shapes the diagnostic process. The following sections further illuminate issues in the diagnostic assessment of American Indians using excerpts from transcriptions of a semi-structured diagnostic interview, the Structured Clinical Interview for DSM-III-R (SCID) [7]. The SCID was administered by the author as part of a community survey of Vietnam veterans on Northern Plains and Southwest reservations.

The clinician's diagnostic assessment begins with observing the patient's appearance and non-verbal behavior. This includes the patient's hygiene and dress, posture, physical activity, eye contact, affect, quality of expression, and the manner of greeting. The assessment of these characteristic social behaviors is based on the clinician's knowledge of the norms in his or her culture of reference. When the clinician and patient are from different cultures, these norms may vary significantly. Among American Indians physical activity may be more restrained and eye contact avoided in normal social contact. Greetings may be friendly but reserved, and with a gentle instead of a firm handshake [4, 8]. These differences in normative social behavior may be misinterpreted in the clinical setting as depression, low intelligence, or lack of interest in treatment.

An essential element of psychiatric diagnosis is the use of psychiatric language to describe symptoms. The influence of the language of psychiatry on mainstream American culture is seen in movies, television, and literature, and persons exposed to the mainstream culture are familiar with terms such as anxiety, depression, and mania. Some American Indians have less familiarity with this terminology either because they speak English as a second language or because they have little exposure to mainstream culture. In this case, the patient may not comprehend phrases such as 'feeling depressed' or 'feeling anxious' as the language used to assess psychiatric disorder. The following dialogue is an example of this sort of miscommunication.

Dr Norton: In the last six months have you been particularly nervous or anxious?
Mr Jones: The last six months—nervous? Well, the only thing that I was anxious was for me to, when I took that class, I wanted to be enrolled right away. What I was most anxious about was winter being half way over with, you know, instead of the beginning, you know, because I know I'll have to be getting up all hours of the morning and maybe all hours of the day.

In this example, nervous or anxious are interpreted as looking forward to or anticipating an event. This is typical of the usage of these phrases in this Northern Plains tribe. The psychiatrist in this case would need to explain to the patient the intended meaning of the terms nervous or anxious.

Another aspect of psychiatric diagnosis is the assessment of pathological emotional states. Characteristic emotional experience and the norms for expression of emotion vary in different cultures. In Western cultures, the emotions elation and its opposite, depression, are considered central to emotional experience, and the expression of these emotions in the appropriate contexts is encouraged. However, many American Indian children are guided from an early age to refrain from expressing strong emotion such as crying. Children are not taught labels for emotions, nor are they encouraged to talk about their emotions [9]. As a result, American Indian patients may be less likely to express depressed or euphoric emotions, and therefore clinicians may miss psychiatric disorders. This was demonstrated by the experience of the mental health program at the Tohono O'odham Indian reservation. Patients who were identified as seriously disturbed and requiring hospitalization by the program staff would behave in a shy and quiet manner when assessed at the public hospital off the reservation. As a result, the patient would not be admitted to the hospital [10].

American Indians tend to express psychological distress in terms of impairment in social relations instead of reporting an internal emotional state such as feeling depressed, anxious, or manic. Several authors have described the relative centrality of social and community relationships to American Indian identity [4, 11, 12]. This is manifest as the preferences of the group taking precedence over individual preferences, and as a sense of obligation to share individual wealth and material goods. As a result, American Indians may communicate their distress in the context of a disturbance in social relations, instead of focusing on their internal emotional state or problems in individual functioning. Among the Flathead, distress is often communicated in stories about being neglected or abused by family members, and loneliness is an idiom of distress. Normal loneliness involves feelings of pity, compassion, and loneliness for others, but pathological loneliness consists of statements about the lack of compassionate feelings of others for oneself, associated with feelings of worthlessness or one's own lack of compassionate feelings for others [12]. O'Nell indicates that 'not caring' about others is a more serious indicator of pathology than dysphoric mood.

The following example from a Southwest veteran illustrates the importance of disordered social relationships as an idiom of distress among American Indians.

Dr Norton: In the last four weeks, has there been a period of time when you were feeling depressed, down, lonely or lonesome most of the day, nearly every day?
Mr Smith: Nearly every day.
Dr Norton: What was that like?
Mr Smith: People not visiting, I guess. I know they had their own jobs, business to take care of, never had the intention. I don't know. They said I have cancer. People don't want to see you. They think cancer or someway they're afraid of it or something.

Although many persons with cancer in mainstream American society may be concerned about no one caring for them, the primary complaint is more likely to be fear of the cancer progressing, fear of dying, concerns about disability or pain, and concerns about loss of independence and being a burden to others. This Southwest man's primary concern is being neglected by others, which is characteristic of how disordered social relationships is a common idiom of distress among American Indians.

Another important diagnostic issue is what are the perceived causes or explanatory models of illnesses that are common within a particular culture. For example, in mainstream American society the biological explanatory model is predominant, as when alcohol dependence is characterized as a disease instead of a social problem. In the Navajo religion, people are surrounded by potential dangers, and there are many taboos related to antagonizing ghosts. When a Navajo person becomes ill, a traditional diagnostician called a hand trembler may diagnose the problem as caused by breaking a taboo. The prescribed treatment is a ceremony by a medicine man [13]. When a Navajo man reported panic attacks and chronic anxiety, he traced his problems to having touched the coffin of a friend who died. He sought treatment from both a medicine man and a psychiatrist, obtaining some relief from both sources but continuing to be symptomatic. The psychiatrist in this case needed to be cognizant of the patient's explanation of his illness. Prescribing medication without recognizing the need to address the broken taboo would probably result in a limited response to treatment, and closer collaboration with the medicine man may potentiate the effect of psychiatric treatment.

Equally as important is recognizing whether the patient's symptoms are normative or abnormal within the cultural context. Clinicians are at risk of making errors in judging whether a symptom is abnormal when they are unfamiliar with the norms of behavior within a particular culture. It is also likely that the clinician will have difficulty in eliciting symptoms that are culturally specific for the same reason. For example, among traditional Navajo men drinking often occurs in groups and a bottle is shared among all the members of the group until the supply is depleted. These drinking episodes are spontaneous and can be interrupted if there is work or religious ceremonies to attend to [14]. However, the DSM criteria for alcohol dependence are oriented towards persons who plan or think ahead about drinking, who drink individual glasses of wine/liquor or cans of beer, and who are able to quantitate the amount that they drink. The following exchange with a Northern Plains man illustrates this point.

Dr Norton: Did you spend a lot of time drinking, being high, or hung over?
Mr Clark: Maybe, but off and on, yes. But not always. I didn't like that beer.
Dr Norton: So sometimes when you were on a binge it was a lot of time, but then there were times when you didn't drink at all?
Mr. Clark: If someone had the money and would buy the booze, I would drink it. As long as someone didn't start a fight and get all hostile.

The patient's description of his drinking style may be representative of drinking patterns among men in his tribe, and is an example of how symptom expression is determined by the cultural context. Kunitz *et al.* [15] suggest that many of the Navajo men who maintain this drinking style as young adults will later become abstainers and will not have long-term consequences of their drinking. Instead, a solitary drinking style is more frequently associated with long-term consequences.

Differentiating normal from abnormal behavior within a given culture is not just an issue for symptom assessment, but is also important when assessing the presence or absence of psychiatric diagnoses. As a case in point, clinicians may overdiagnose social phobia among American Indians because the avoidance of direct eye contact may be misinterpreted as phobic behavior. In the following dialogue a Northern Plains man endorses the symptoms of social phobia, but with further exploration the psychiatrist discovers that he is referring to normative social behavior of avoiding direct eye contact.

> Dr Norton: Is there anything that you were ever afraid to do or felt uncomfortable doing in front of other people—like speaking, eating, or writing?
>
> Mr Thomas: Talking in front of people. I can't do it all. I mean I just don't like people staring at me, especially when I'm talking. I turn and look at something.
>
> Dr Norton: What were you afraid would happen when you talked in front of people? Were you afraid something bad would happen or embarrassing would happen?
>
> Mr Thomas: Probably embarrassing cause you, I would probably forget what I, probably wouldn't even bring up the words. I just probably can't say at all. Maybe I'm not talking straight, not talking sense, something like that.
>
> Dr Norton: Do you think you are more uncomfortable than most people are in public, speaking in public?
>
> Mr Thomas: Talking in public? Like I said, I don't like talking in front of people. I don't know some people can do that.
>
> Dr Norton: How much does this interfere with your life, being afraid of talking in public?
>
> Mr Thomas: How much does it interfere?
>
> Dr Norton: Does it cause any problems for you?
>
> Mr Thomas: Just if I have to talk in front of people. I try not to talk in front of people. I try to get out of it, you know.
>
> Dr Norton: So you basically avoid these situations. Does it cause any problems at work or with your friends?
>
> Mr Thomas: No, I just talk with them. I don't look at them directly.
>
> Dr Norton: So that doesn't prevent you from having friends.
>
> Mr Thomas: No, it's just like if I'm talking to one of my co-workers, I don't stand there and look at them directly in the eye or right to his face, or stand there exactly in front of him. I turn the other way, or don't even look. I just look far enough so he can hear me, you know, or hear what I'm saying or something like that.

This case illustrates the importance of understanding the influence of culture on social behavior, expression of symptoms, and the experience of illness. A mere difference in non-verbal social behavior such as the amount of eye contact has a significant impact on the diagnostic assessment. The clinician evaluating an American Indian patient should be aware of the potential for misdiagnosis and the inappropriate treatment of patients. This requires an awareness that the DSM is biased towards the elicitation of pathology from patients in Western cultures.

The previous discussion illustrates some key issues in the diagnostic assessment of American Indian patients. As part of the assessment, the clinician should also consider the degree to which an American Indian patient has assimilated the values and traits of the mainstream culture. Much of the population of American Indians is widely dispersed in urban areas throughout the USA. Interracial marriages have also contributed to increased assimilation into mainstream American society. Some

American Indian patients will describe symptoms such as feeling depressed or anxious, and will not have any traditional beliefs or other characteristics of traditional cultures—although, even among patients who have been assimilated into the mainstream culture, there are likely to be some issues in the assessment that are linked to aspects of traditional American Indian cultures.

American Indians do not share one culture and one identity, but are members of many different tribes with differing cultures. A clinician working on a reservation may become familiar with the norms of an individual tribe, but the clinician working in an urban setting has fewer opportunities to gain experience with individual tribal cultures. The clinician needs to be aware that there are differences between tribal cultures, and that these differences may be important in the diagnostic assessment. He or she may need to consult with a cultural expert to understand the meaning of a specific symptom or behavior within the tribal cultural context. Cultural experts may be found in urban and reservation agencies that focus on providing services to American Indians, such as urban Indian health centers and reservation mental health programs within the Indian Health Service.

Why is it necessary to take into account these issues in the diagnostic assessment? There is evidence that American Indians are more likely to terminate treatment after the initial contact than Whites [16, 17]. Previously, this phenomenon has been explained as due to differing values, beliefs, and expectations regarding interventions [18]. Also, counselor traits such as flexibility and trust are thought to be important [5, 19, 20]. The environment where the treatment takes place is also a factor [21, 22]. An understanding of the nature of the problem, and an ability to meaningfully assess symptoms and the degree of functional impairment are also important in establishing an alliance with American Indian patients. When the questions that form the diagnostic assessment appear irrelevant to the patient or cause the patient to feel misunderstood, she or he will have no investment in continuing treatment.

During the psychiatric diagnostic assessment the patient presents with a complaint of illness, and the clinician then interprets the patient's presentation of illness within the diagnostic framework of DSM. Patients from non-Western cultures may present idioms of distress, explanatory models, and abnormal behavior that differ from what is characteristic in Western cultures. This chapter has provided insight into cultural factors that influence the presentation of illness among traditional American Indian patients. However, this discussion is not comprehensive in that there are probably many diagnostic issues that have not been included in this chapter, and which require further elucidation.

It occurs to me in writing the conclusion to this chapter, that I have chosen to use 'clinician' as the descriptive term for the provider of care. The use of this term is an example of how the medical model pervades the field of psychiatric diagnosis. However, the concepts underlying DSM and the medical model do not allow for the cultural construction of pathological emotions and disorder, although the cultural formulation in DSM-IV begins to incorporate this perspective. This chapter illustrates that there is variability across cultures in how mental disorder is experienced and expressed, and specifically characterizes these differences among the vibrant cultures of American Indians.

REFERENCES

1. Fabrega H. 1996. Cultural and historical foundations of psychiatric diagnosis. In: Mezzich JE, Kleinman A, Fabrega H, Parron DL, eds. *Culture & Psychiatric Diagnosis: A DSM-IV Perspective*. Washington, DC: American Psychiatric Press.
2. American Psychiatric Association. 1994. *Diagnostic and Statistical Manual, Fourth Edition*. Washington, DC: American Psychiatric Association.
3. US Bureau of the Census: Race and Hispanic Origin. 1991. *1990 Census Profile, Profile 2*. Washington, DC: US Government Printing Office.
4. Attneave C. 1982. American Indians and Alaska Native families: Emigrants in their own homeland. In: McGoldrick M, Pearce JK, Giordano J, eds. *Ethnicity and Family Therapy*. New York: Guilford Press.
5. Trimble JE, Fleming CM, Beauvais F, Jumper-Thurman P. 1996. Essential cultural and social strategies for counseling Native American Indians. In: Pederson PB, Draguns JG, Lonner WJ, Trimble JE, eds. *Counseling Across Cultures*. Thousand Oaks, California: Sage Publications.
6. Johnson DL, Johnson CA. 1965. Totally discouraged: A depressive syndrome of the Dakota Sioux. *Transcult Psychiatr Res* 2: 141–3.
7. Spitzer RL, Williams J, Gibbon M. 1987. *Structured Clinical Interview for DSM-III-R, version NP-V*. New York: Psychiatric Institute, Biometrics Research Department.
8. McShane D. 1987. Mental health and North American Indian/Native communities: Cultural transactions, education, and regulation. *Am J Community Psychol* 15: 95–116.
9. Minde R, Minde K. 1995. Socio-cultural determinants of psychiatric symptomatology in James Bay Cree children and adolescents. *Can J Psychiatry* 40: 304–12.
10. Kahn MW, Lejero L, Antone M, Francisco D, Manuel J. 1988. An indigenous community mental health service on the Tohono O'odham (Papago) Indian reservation: Seventeen years later. *Am J Community Psychol* 16: 369–79.
11. Dana RH. 1993. *Multicultural Assessment Perspectives for Professional Psychology*. Boston: Allyn and Bacon.
12. O'Nell TD. 1996. *Disciplined Hearts: History, Identity, and Depression in an American Indian Community*. Berkeley: University of California Press.
13. Adair J. 1963. In: Galdston I, ed. *Physicians, medicine men and their Navaho patients, in Man's Image in Medicine and Anthropology, Monograph IV*. New York: International Universities Press.
14. Levy JE, Kunitz SJ. 1974. *Indian Drinking: Navajo Practices and Anglo-American Theories*. New York: John Wiley & Sons.
15. Kunitz SJ, Levy JE, Andrews T, DuPuy C, Gabriel KR, Russell S. 1994. *Drinking Careers: A Twenty-five year study of Three Navajo Populations*. New Haven: Yale University Press.
16. Sue S, Allen DB, Conaway L. 1978. The responsiveness and equality of mental health care to Chicanos and Native Americans. *Am J Community Psychol* 6: 137–46.
17. Walker RD, Howard MO, Anderson B, Lambert MD. 1994. Substance dependent American Indian veterans: A national evaluation. *Publ Health Rep* 109: 235–42.
18. McCormick R. 1996. Culturally appropriate means and ends of counseling as described by the First Nations people of British Columbia. *Int J Adv Counsel* 18: 163–72.
19. Everett F, Proctor N, Cartmell B. 1983. Providing psychological services to American Indian children and families. *Prof Psychol Res Pract* 14: 588–603.

20. LaFromboise TD, Dixon DN. 1981. American Indian perception of trustworthiness in a counseling interview. *J Counsel Psychol* **28**: 135–9.
21. Katz P. 1981. Psychotherapy with native adolescents. *Can J Psychiatry* **26**: 455–9.
22. Norton IM, Manson SM. 1997. Domestic violence intervention in an urban Indian health center. *Community Ment Health J* **33**: 331–7.

9

Structured Diagnostic Instruments in Cross Cultural Psychiatric Epidemiology: The Experience in Hispanic Communities and Other Groups

Maritza Rubio-Stipec and Milagros Bravo
University of Puerto Rico, San Juan, Puerto Rico

CULTURAL AND CONTEXTUAL ISSUES

The biological model of psychiatric disorders is not as well known as that of other physical diseases. Two nosologies available to the field, DSM-IV and ICD10, provide a detailed description of the essential and associated features for each defined disorder and the necessary criteria to be classified as a case [1, 2]. However, operationalization of these criteria by diagnostic instruments constitutes a major challenge.

Cross cultural studies in the field of psychiatry strengthen our capacity to generalize findings to multiple ethnic groups and multiple settings. What is contextual and what is intrinsic to the condition is still a matter of discussion in the field of psychiatry. Restricting analyses to one culture, or one setting, can result in restricting the analyses by the interaction with environment. Generalizability and validity of the findings are not as easily disentangled in psychiatry as in other fields of medicine. Findings that are replicated across cultures and settings lend validity to the outcomes of the research. Culture and setting represent such an important role in the description of the condition that they can either lend or take away validity of the findings.

Ascertainment of a psychiatric condition has been enhanced by the development of structured diagnostic instruments. These instruments are designed with the purpose of either classifying a subject within a specific nosology, such as DSM or ICD, or tapping the presence of a set of symptoms related to a psychiatric

Cross Cultural Psychiatry. Edited by John M. Herrera, William B. Lawson and John J. Sramek.
© 1999 John Wiley & Sons Ltd.

condition. They can be used as screening instruments in clinical practice and in the evaluation of different intervention programs, but they have been more widely used in the field of psychiatric epidemiology to assess the prevalence of disorders in the community. Assessment instruments can provide uniform classification for all subjects in the study: a uniform classification of all subjects is necessary to achieve a homogenous definition of the psychiatric condition [3].

When it is necessary to replicate a study in different cultures, an instrument that can measure the presence or absence of the condition independent of the culture is crucial. The selected diagnostic instrument should identify, not necessarily the same set of behavioral expressions, but the same latent construct independent of the culture—otherwise the study cannot disentangle measurement error from cultural differences. The Composite International Diagnostic Instrument (CIDI) was designed by the World Health Organization [2] to account for cultural variability [4, 5].

Operationalizations of the nosology that are not culturally consonant can result in different definitions of the same disorders in different cultures and contexts. For example, when the diagnosis of interest is alcoholism, the criterion is the social consequences of drinking. The structured diagnostic instrument elicits a set of questions to measure the criterion; endorsement of one or more is required. The instrument should provide a 'fixed menu' of possible consequences. However, this set of potential consequences might vary from one country to another, or even within different groups in the same country.

To illustrate the issue, let us consider different items listed in the instrument as potential social consequences. For example, in a country where few people drive 'the probability of being arrested for drunken driving' is low and therefore the probability of meeting criteria and being identified as a case is also low. When contrasting prevalence between two such countries it is possible that the results are measuring differences in the judicial system rather than differences in number of disorders. Furthermore, an increase in incidence could simply mean that more people drive with time. Similarly, when comparing gender differences in a country 'losing one's job due to drinking' can reflect different participation rates by gender, not different prevalence of alcoholism, and an increase in incidence rates of alcoholism could reflect more women joining the labor force. On the other hand, alcohol dependence is a criteria more 'medically defined' and less prone to this type of error [3].

Another example is the validity of findings in genetic psychiatric epidemiology with a classification not based on the presence of a gene. When we aim at the identification of a phenotype in psychiatric genetics differential misclassification by level of acculturation can diminish the accuracy in our estimations of the heterogeneity of the disorder. Phenotypic heterogeneity, for example, has been associated with age in different studies dealing with migrant populations. Migrant subjects in a research project can have various levels of acculturation to the host culture. Hence, people from different generations in the same family can be classified differently, not because they have different diagnostic status but because the manifestation of the illness varies with the generation. This can bring a new source of misclassi-fication, incorrectly classifying people with and without a putative genetic illness [3].

Case assessment in psychiatric epidemiology usually requires an interview and is prone to measurement error from various sources. Measurement error in case assessment refers to the difference between the true mental health status of the subject and the operational classification given in the study. Information necessary to determine case status is provided by the interviewed subject, either to the clinician or to a lay person. At times more than one informant is needed; when children are the population of interest multiple informants, such as parents, teachers or the children themselves are considered necessary. Once the information is gathered case status is determined either by the clinician or a computerized diagnostic algorithm using a standard nosology. Measurement errors can result in information biases; due to inaccurate response on the part of the informant(s), poor coverage of manifestations of illness in the structured diagnostic instrument, or inaccurate operationalization of the nosology. This misclassification can be sys-tematic or not, differential or non-differential.

ECONOMIC CONSIDERATIONS

The use of structured diagnostic instruments responds to several needs, not only to increase comparability between different cultures and different settings but also for economic considerations. Structured diagnostic instruments can be administered by trained lay interviewers, who are more readily available in a variety of settings at a lower cost than psychiatrists. Thus, such instruments may be the classification scheme of choice when conducting large survey research and when screening in a clinical setting.

Types of Diagnostic Instrument

Traditionally, in order to provide adequate treatment a clinician interviews a patient and, based on the results of the interview, gives a diagnosis (or diagnoses). This way of classifying persons is called a clinical diagnosis because the classification is based on clinical judgment. The classification is as good as the judgment of the clinician. This seems to be an appropriate classification scheme when the clinician has the opportunity of interviewing the patient several times during treatment. However, in epidemiologic studies, where there is usually only one encounter between clinician and interviewee, this approach is not reliable. Furthermore, the sources of dis-crepancies are not transparent. The argument in favor of this approach is that when the clinician is familiar with the nosology and with the culture, adequate validity is obtained. However, this argument can be challenged when one considers that multiple studies have reported poor reliability between different clinicians inter-viewing the same subject. When one considers reliability as a prerequisite to validity the first argument loses credibility. Structured and semistructured instruments aim at addressing the needs of epidemiological studies.

There is a variety of diagnostic instruments in the field. We will focus in this chapter on those that can produce a diagnostic classification based on a specific nosology. Not addressed are those that generate data on symptoms that are not tapped to a specific nosology. Instruments that tap a specific nosology can be classified into two distinct categories: informant or interviewer based. These categories respond to different approaches to the classification of subjects.

Interviewer-based Instruments

Interviewer-based instruments are those where the classification is based on the judgment of the interviewer, usually a clinician, using a semistructured instrument.

The SCAN is a good example of an interviewer-based instrument developed for use in multiple cultures. It provides a structure to conduct the interview, but requires training and must be administered by a clinician. Because the structure requires a judgment on the part of the interviewer this instrument is considered as semistructured. The final diagnosis is a combination of both the clinician's judgment on whether the criteria have been met and the computer's algorithm based on the nosologies. Adequate to good reliability and validity has been reported by various studies.

Respondent-based Instruments

Respondent-based instruments are usually fully structured. The interviewer's role is to gather the symptom information without departing from the guidelines of the instrument. A computerized algorithm based on the existing nosology then generates the final diagnosis. Correspondence with the nosology is attained by using a set of questions that tap different symptoms related to a specific nosological criterion. The 'menu of symptoms' is determined by those that develop the instrument and can be culture specific. Prevalence estimates are therefore affected by the types of symptoms included. These can be contrasted to the results of a clinical interview, where the questions are determined by the psychiatrist and the cultural relevance depends on his or her ability to ask culturally relevant questions. These clinical interviews, when they are not structured, can be adequate to treat a patient, but tend to generate information that is not useful for epidemiologic purposes.

Structured Diagnostic Instruments

The first large epidemiologic study in the USA using a fully structured diagnostic instrument was the Epidemiologic Catchment Area Study, commonly referred to as the ECA. In this study, the diagnostic instrument of choice was the Diagnostic Interview Schedule (DIS). The DIS is a highly structured diagnostic instrument that was developed for use in the ECA [6]. It mimics a psychiatric interview by using a Probe Flow Chart (PBF) to sort reported symptoms into five categories:

1. absent;
2. not clinically significant;
3. explained by use of drugs or alcohol;
4. explained by a physical illness;
5. a psychiatric symptom. Psychiatric symptoms can then be joined into diagnostic criteria and diagnoses.

Multiple modifications to the original version have been made mainly to respond to changes in the nosology. The latest version can generate DSM-IV diagnoses.

The Composite Diagnostic Interview (CIDI) is a fully standardized, structured interview for the assessment of psychiatric disorders according to two nosologies, DSM and ICD. It follows the same structure as its parent instrument, the DIS [6]. It was developed for cross cultural comparisons and has enhanced coverage of the manifestation of the illness [7]. The development of this interview has been the collaborative effort of researchers from 18 sites around the world. In both the DIS and in the WHO-CIDI a symptom is not clinically significant if does not interfere with everyday life, if the person did not consult a doctor or any other professional and did not take medications for it. The CIDI also makes use of the probe flow chart to separate probable psychiatric symptoms from positive responses that are not clinically significant, from symptoms that can be fully explained by use of drugs, medicines or alcohol, or from symptoms that can be fully explained by the presence of a medical condition [8].

The UM-CIDI was developed from the CIDI by a group of investigators from the University of Michigan to be used in the National Co-morbidity Survey [9]. The UM-CIDI modified the order of the interview, and redesigned the stem question administration procedures to minimize the 'no' responses. It does not use the probe flow chart but incorporates a similar approach in the body of the interview for some of the targeted diagnoses. The main modification was placing the stem questions for mood and anxiety disorders at the beginning of the inter-view, where in the WHO-CIDI each diagnostic module is self-contained with stem questions at the start of each module. In addition, in the UM-CIDI three stem questions for mood disorders are placed at the start of the interview and there are also some wording differences in several questions.

Prevalence Estimates With Structured Instruments

Most of the data available in the USA has been based either on the DIS or on the CIDI. These instruments have generated a wealth of information that has been analyzed and published in many journals. We will classify these findings into the following categories:

- consistency through time;
- consistency through cultures and contexts;
- acculturation issues;
- the effects of time (cohort, period effect, and aging effects);
- the effects of gender

Consistency Through Time

The data discussed in this chapter refer to the two large epidemiological studies with structured instruments, the ECA in 1980 and the NCS in 1990 [9, 10]. The ECA interviewed persons 18 years of age or older in five catchment areas and the rates were standardized to the 1980 US census population. The study consisted of two waves; however, in this chapter we discuss only the findings of the first wave to avoid the use of the assumptions necessary for 'adding' the results of the two waves. Moreover, the NCS survey 10 years later consisted of only one wave [11]. Each wave is subject to random measurement error that a simple addition of cases would ignore. Previous studies using the DIS alcoholism module showed measurement error to be larger than 3 years incidence [12]. In this way, prevalence estimates differences can be explained either by effect of time or by differences in the two instruments and not by the assumptions made in joining the two waves (we do not know what the prevalence estimates would have been had the NCS consisted of two waves; probably much larger). In the first wave, a total of 20 206 people were interviewed. The standardized rates reported for the ECA were:

- a total of 15.7% of the population had at least one mental and addictive disorder in the last month;
- 21.8% had at least one in the last 12 months; and
- 32.7% had one in their lifetime [10].

The NCS interviewed 7599 people of 15–54 years of age in a probability sample of English speaking persons in the USA. They reported 28.5% as having had at least one mental and addictive disorder in the last 12 months and 48% in their lifetime [9].

When comparing the two surveys differences in prevalence estimates could be explained by differences in the age group included. The NCS is a younger cohort and younger people were found to have lower rates in the ECA. To compare the two sets of rates the prevalence for the 18–54 group in each sample was estimated [11]. Outstanding differences remained, with the NCS estimates consistently higher. In the first wave of the ECA the 12-month prevalence of any mental and addictive disorders for those aged 18–54 was 24.1% and the lifetime prevalence was 36.1%, while in the NCS the prevalence estimates for the same age group were 28.5% and 48% respectively. The rates in the NCS are 18% higher for any disorder in the last 12 months and 33% higher for any lifetime disorder than those in the first wave of the ECA [11].

The differences vary with type of disorder. When we compare prevalence estimates in the NCS with those of the first wave of the ECA by diagnostic categories we see that the larger differences are:

- for social phobia (12 months: 7.4% vs. 1.6%; lifetime 13.3% vs. 2.5%) about a fivefold increase;
- for major depression episode (12 months: 10.1% vs. 4.2%; lifetime 17.3% vs. 7.2%) more than a twofold increase;
- substance abuse and/or dependence (12 months: 11.5% vs. 9.5%; lifetime 28.1% vs. 19.9%) an increase of around 20% in the 12-month estimates and 40% in the lifetime estimates;
- for any anxiety disorder (12 months: 11.8% vs. 9.9%; lifetime 22.8% vs. 14.2%).

Can we attribute these differences to an increase in 10-year incidence of disorders? As changes in lifetime prevalence estimates are even larger than in the 12-month estimates, can we also conclude that the duration of the disorder is also longer? At the time this book goes to press, we cannot confidently disentangle whether these differences are explained by the effect of time or by changes in the structure of the instrument.

CROSS CULTURAL FINDINGS

Once methodological artifacts have been minimized using culturally equivalent methods and measures, the comparison of prevalence rates across cultures yields differences and similarities which are important for a full understanding of psychiatric disorders. These comparisons are more fruitful when they include many and varied cultures.

Prevalence Rates

Various studies have produced prevalence rates estimates using the DIS. Comparisons between these estimates have generated assorted results. Contrasts between such diverse areas as Asia, Europe and North America for the diagnoses of alcoholism [12], major depression and bipolar disorder [13], panic disorder [14], social phobia [15], and obsessive-compulsive disorder [16] have been reported. Lifetime prevalence rates have been found to vary widely for some disorders— alcoholism (0.45–23%) and major depression (1.5–19%)—but more consistent results have been observed for others—specifically, bipolar disorder (0.3–1.5%), social phobia (0.5–2.6%), panic disorder (0.4–2.9%) and obsessive-compulsive disorder (1.9–2.5%). It has been suggested that these disorders may be rather invariant to contextual risk factors.

Illness Course and Expression of Symptoms

Although prevalence estimate rates may differ widely, similarities may be found in the course and symptomatic expression of the disorders. This has been the case for alcoholism [17]: similarities were observed in 13 sites in mean age of onset (early to mid twenties), mean number of symptoms (four to six), duration of the illness (8–10 years), and pattern of symptoms. Regarding this last, similar symptom frequency rankings were found in countries in the same region (e.g. rank-order correlation >0.80 in North American and Asian sites), and even across sites in very different cultural regions (for example, Puerto Rican and Asian sites rank-order correlations >0.70). The authors concluded that these results suggest that alcoholism is a disorder with considerable consistency in manifestation, even in culturally and technologically diverse countries (highly industrialized vs. rural agrarian economies).

Age of onset is a component of the course of the disorder that has been analyzed in many cross cultural studies. Findings for many other disorders have been similar to those reported for alcoholism. Regardless of differences in prevalence rates, reasonably consistent age of onset has been observed across sites for all disorders: social phobia (mid teens to early twenties) [15], bipolar disorder (late teens to mid twenties) [13], panic disorder (early twenties to mid thirties) [14]; obsessive-compulsive (early twenties to mid thirties) [16], and major depression (mid twenties to early thirties) [13].

On the other hand, the symptomatic expression of obsessive-compulsive disorder has been shown to vary across cultures, a difference that cannot be explained by differences in lifetime and 1-year prevalence rates. While the majority of those interviewed at the four sites (Munich, Taiwan, Korea and the USA) reported only obsessions, obsessions were as frequent as compulsions in Munich and Taiwan, and more compulsions than obsessions were reported in Korea [15]. The authors concluded that cultural factors may explain this variability in symptomatic expression.

Risk Factors and Correlates

Although, several common risk factors have been reported for diverse cultures and settings, many differences have also been observed.

Gender

When prevalence rates are compared by gender, similar patterns are observed. However, the magnitude of female to male ratios vary considerably. Showing a remarkable consistency throughout the studied sites, major depression [13], panic disorder [14], and social phobia [18] have been found to be female prevalent, alcoholism to be male prevalent [17], and bipolar disorder to be gender balanced [19]. In these cross cultural studies the only disorders for which gender patterns are not similar across sites are obsessive-compulsive [16] and somatization [8]. Panic disorders appears to be as common in males as in females in all sites—with the exception of Munich, where it appears to be a male disorder; authors attributed this difference to the sample size and age composition (Munich's sample is the smallest and oldest). For somatization, the ECA found that women had higher prevalence rates than men, except in Puerto Rico where the rates were similar. Differences in educational level appears to be the best explanation: in Puerto Rico women had more years of education than men and education has been recognized as a protective factor for psychiatric disorders [20].

Male:female prevalence ratio of disorders vary across sites and cultures. The prevalence ratio ranges for major depression are 1.6:1–3.5:1 and for panic disorder 1.3:1–5.8:1. The gender differences in alcoholism are more pronounced across cultures, varying from 4:1 to 25:1. Nevertheless, similar ratios are observed for some disorders; specifically, bipolar disorder (range 0.3:1–1.2:1) and social phobia (range 1.4:1–1.6:1 in three of four sites).

Although an explainable consistent pattern was not observed for major depression [18], the variations in gender ratios in alcoholism may be explained by sociocultural factors [17]. The male:female ratio was particularly high in the Asian and Hispanic cultures compared with Western and Anglo-Saxon cultures (12–25 times greater in males compared with 4–6). The fact that this rate was considerably higher in Mexican American immigrants to the USA (25:1) than Mexican Americans native to the USA (4:1) could suggest an important cultural effect, such as a social stigma attached to drinking among women. Nevertheless, other complementary explanations such as genetic risk and lower tolerance for alcohol among women cannot be ruled out without further study. Furthermore, as discussed above, the differences could be artifactual due to differential misclassification by gender. The set of symptoms under each criterion for each disorder could be culture and context specific: fewer women working, fewer lose their jobs due to drinking; fewer women driving, fewer arrested for drunken driving. On the other hand, the symptomatic expressions described for depression in the diagnostic instrument could be geared more towards women in some contexts and not in others.

Age

Age is an important factor because it reflects not only the effect of 'aging' (getting older) but also the effect of time (older people have been at risk for a disorder for a longer period of time). The lifetime prevalence of alcoholism and depression by age shows interesting differences across countries. For alcoholism, most of the 13 sites studied show a fall in lifetime prevalence with age. This finding is counterintuitive because lifetime prevalence is cumulative over the entire time period at risk [17]. However, the expected increase with age was observed in four sites (Puerto Rico, Seoul, rural Korea and Munich). Lifetime prevalence rate estimates of major depression by age are reported by Klerman and Weissman for seven sites [21]; they also show a tendency to decrease with age. Various explanations have been contemplated by the authors, including differences in mortality rates and recall bias by age, such as diminished recall of earlier problems or decreased willingness to admit such difficulties by older respondents. However, these explanations have been deemed as inadequate [17]. The most widely accepted explanation is the presence of a cohort effect. At the same age the new cohorts are at greater risk than the older cohorts when they were that age. In the case of alcoholism, this interpretation is consistent with rising per capita consumption of alcohol. A liberalization of attitudes toward alcohol consumption could differentially affect youths since their habits are not well established and they may be profoundly affected by social attitudes. The lack of a cohort effect in some sites is attributed by the authors to a more longstanding attitude toward drinking, such that older members of society could have been exposed to heavy drinking from an early age. Thus, sociocultural factors are again used to explain a risk factor for two widely studied disorders.

Migration

The study of migration has been used to try to understand the influence of sociocultural factors in psychopathology. A study, also based on the DIS, compared various Hispanic groups from Puerto Rico and Los Angeles and Anglos from Los Angeles that have been differently exposed to migration [22]. Results suggest that factors associated with immigration are more important than country of origin in explaining risk for disorders. Immigrant Mexican Americans had the fewest mental health problems of all groups. Puerto Ricans were generally intermediate between them and Mexican Americans native to the USA (after controlling for age, education and household size). Explanations for these findings include the thought that immigrant Mexican Americans are more resilient because they have to overcome substantial obstacles to move successfully from Mexico to the USA; persons with psychopathology would not be likely to succeed in overcoming the obstacles (selective migration). Mexican American natives may feel more deprived in Los Angeles than the immigrants because they lack the immigrants' frame of reference of a hard life in Mexico, and feel more deprived than Island Puerto Ricans because socioeconomic differences are not as large in Puerto Rico as in Los Angeles (relative socioeconomic deprivation). They are also more likely to be discriminated against in Los Angeles than Puerto Ricans in their own country (social discrimination).

SUMMARY

In summary, the use of common instruments in psychiatric epidemiology research has enabled comparison of rates and risk factors across different countries and between different cultures within the same country. This research increases our understanding of the etiology of disorders and the role of culture. However, the role of measurement error needs to be further addressed. Differences in the adequacy of the coverage of the manifestation of the illnesses in dissimilar cultures cannot be ruled out as an explanation. Further cross cultural research, both in the psychometric properties of the available instruments and in the etiology of disorders, is needed.

REFERENCES

1. American Psychiatry Association. 1994. *Diagnostic and Statistical Manual for Mental Disorders*, 4th edition. Washington, DC: American Psychiatric Association.
2. World Health Organization. 1992. *International Classifications of Diseases*, 10th Revision (ICD-10). Geneva: World Health Organization.
3. Rubio-Stipec M, Hicks M, Tsuang M. 1998. Cultural factors influencing the selection, use and interpretation of psychiatric measures and outcomes. In: *Handbook of Psychiatric Measures and Outcomes* (in press).
4. Robins LN, Wing J, Wittchen HU, Babor TF, Farmer A, Jablensky A *et al.* 1988. The Composite International Diagnostic Interview: an epidemiologic instrument suitable for use in conjunction with different diagnostic systems and in different cultures. *Arch Gen Psychiatry* **45**: 1069–77.
5. Wittchen HU, Robins LN, Cottler L, Sartorius N, Burke J, Regier D *et al.* 1991. Cross-cultural feasibility, reliability and sources of variance of the Composite International Diagnostic Interview (CIDI)—Results of the multicentre WHO/ADAMHA field trials (Wave I). *Br J Psychiatry* **159**: 645–53.
6. Robins LN, Helzer J, Croughan J, Ratcliff KS. 1981. The NIMH Diagnostic Interview Schedule: Its history, characteristics and validity. *Arch Gen Psychiatry* **38**: 3819.
7. Robins LN, Wing J, Wittchen HU, Helzer JE, Babor TF, Burke J *et al.* 1988. The Composite International Diagnostic Interview. An epidemiologic instrument suitable for use in conjunction with different diagnostic systems and in different cultures. *Arch Gen Psychiatry* **45**: 1069–77.
8. Rubio-Stipec M, Canino G, Robins LN, Wittchen HU, Sartorius N, Torres de Miranda C *et al.* 1993. The somatization schedule of the composite diagnostic interview: The use of the Probe Chart in 17 different countries. *Int J Meth Psychiatr Res* **3**: 129–36.
9. Kessler RC, McGonangle KA, Zhao S, Nelson CB *et al.* 1994. Lifetime and 12 Month Prevalence of DSM-III-R Psychiatric Disorders in the US: results from the National co-morbidity survey. *Arch Gen Psychiatry* **51**: 8–19.
10. Robins LN, Locke BZ, Regier DA, eds. 1991. *Psychiatric Disorders in America*. New York: Free Press.
11. Regier D, Kaebler C, Rae D, Farmer M, Knauper B, Kessler R, Norquist G. 1998. Limitations of diagnostic criteria and assessment instruments for mental disorder: Implications for research and policy. *Arch Gen Psychiatry* **55**: 109–15.
12. Rubio-Stipec M, Freeman D, Robins L, Shrout PE, Canino G, Bravo M. 1992.

Response error and the estimation of lifetime prevalence and incidence of alcoholism: Experience in a community survey. *Int J Meth Psychiatr Res* **2**: 217–24.

13. Weissman MM, Bland RC, Canino GJ, Faravelli C, Greenwald S, Hwu HG *et al.* 1996. Cross-national epidemiology of major depression and bipolar disorder. *JAMA* **276**: 293–9.

14. Weissman MM, Bland RC, Canino GJ, Faravelli C, Greenwald S, Hwu HG *et al.* 1997. The cross-national epidemiology of panic disorder. *Arch Gen Psychiatry* **54**: 305–9.

15. Weissman MM, Bland R, Canino G, Greenwald S, Lee CK, Newman SC *et al.* 1998. The cross national epidemiology of social phobia: a preliminary report. *Int J Clin Psychopharmacol* (in press).

16. Weissman MM, Bland MB, Canino GJ, Greenwald S, Hwu HG, Lee CK *et al.* 1994. The cross national epidemiology of obsessive compulsive disorder. *J Clin Psychiatry* **55** (Suppl 3): 5–10.

17. Helzer JE, Canino G. 1992. Comparative analysis of alcoholism in ten cultural regions. In: Helzer J, Canino G, eds. *Alcoholism—North America, Europe and Asia: A Coordinated Analysis of Population from Ten Regions*. Oxford: Oxford University Press, pp. 289–308.

18. Weissman MM, Bland RC, Canino GJ, Greenwald S, Lee CK, Newman SC *et al.* 1996. The cross-national epidemiology of social phobia: a preliminary report. *Int Clin Psychopharmacol* **11** (Suppl 3): 9–14.

19. Weissman MM, Bland R, Canino G, Faravelli C, Greenwald S, Hwu HG *et al.* 1998. International aspects of the epidemiology of bipolar disorder and major depression. *J Depression* (in press).

20. Canino I, Escobar J, Canino G, Rubio-Stipec M. 1992. Functional somatic symptoms: a cross-ethnic comparison. *Am J Orthopsychiatry* **62**(4): 605–12.

21. Klerman GL, Weissman MM. 1989. Increasing rates of depression. *JAMA* **261**: 2229–35.

22. Shrout PE, Canino GJ, Bird HR, Rubio-Stipec M, Bravo M, Burnam MA. 1992. Mental health status among Puerto Ricans, Mexican Americans, and Non-Hispanic Whites. *Am J Community Psychol* **20**: (6) 729–52.

10

Psychiatric Diagnosis of African Americans

William B. Lawson

Indiana University School of Medicine, Indianapolis, IN, USA

Racial differences for diagnostic categories were consistently reported in the psychiatric literature until quite recently. In a review over a decade ago, Adebimpe [1] reported that African Americans were more likely than Caucasians to receive the diagnosis of schizophrenia and less likely to be diagnosed with affective disorders. Schizophrenia is a disorder characterized by hallucinations, delusions, and/or thought disorganization and generally has the worst prognosis of any psychiatric disorder. On the other hand, African Americans were less likely to receive diagnoses of mood disorders such as mania or depression, the prognosis for which is usually more favorable. As a result African Americans have been disproportionately treated with antipsychotic medication and considered poor candidates for psychotherapy [2].

This overdiagnosis of schizophrenia and underdiagnosis of mood disorders in African Americans may be a consequence of 'true' differences in prevalence, of differences in phenomenology rather than prevalence (i.e. African Americans with the same disorder as Caucasians may have different presenting symptoms), or may be a consequence of misdiagnosis (African Americans with mania may be misdiagnosed as having schizophrenia) [3]. Empirical studies have shown that racial differences tend to disappear when structured interviews rather than clinical diagnoses are used, probably because such interviews require strict adherence to diagnostic criteria [4, 5].

The Epidemiological Catchment Area (ECA) Study, a five-city door-to-door survey using a structured interview to determine diagnosis, was the first large-scale effort to make an objective determination of the prevalence of mental disorders in the USA [6]. No significant differences in the prevalence of affective disorders were found between African Americans and Caucasians. Racial differences in the prevalence of schizophrenia disappeared when socioeconomic class was controlled. Moreover, any ethnic differences were far smaller than previous clinical reports had indicated.

Cross Cultural Psychiatry. Edited by John M. Herrera, William B. Lawson and John J. Sramek.
© 1999 John Wiley & Sons Ltd.

The National Comorbidity Study (NCS), a more recent national randomized survey, utilized more reliable (and presumably more valid) assessment instruments that led to diagnosis based on the most up-to-date criteria [7]. The NCS found no diagnostic categories containing more African Americans than other racial or ethnic groups. Although differences were small, African Americans showed lower prevalence of most disorders including schizophrenia. No socioeconomic effect was seen. Some of the discrepancy between the ECA and NCS may be due to the fact that the NCS included only non-institutionalized respondents. African Americans are more likely to be institutionalized [8], so any study that does not include institutionalized patients may under-report African Americans with severe mental illness. Nevertheless, both the ECA and the NCS are consistent in showing that African Americans are over-diagnosed with schizophrenia, while affective disorders are, if anything, under-diagnosed [4]. Recent studies, even with the use of modern diagnostic criteria such as the DSM IIIR and DSM IV, which are presumed to be more empirically based, unfortunately show that African Americans continue to be overdiagnosed with schizophrenia [2, 8–11]. The reason for the misdiagnosis remains unclear but a recent study suggests that information variance (the quality or type of history and symptoms used) rather than criterion variance (disagreement about the diagnostic criteria used) accounted for most of the diagnostic disagreement around race [12]. Culture, class, and ethnicity may contribute to information variance. Often patients with affective disorders are misdiagnosed as having schizophrenia or simply not diagnosed at all, perhaps because of differences in the presentation of ancillary symptoms that are not included in the core symptoms necessary for diagnosis. Moreover, core symptoms could be misinterpreted or simply not recognized [2]. Differences in presenting symptoms may account for some of the misdiagnosis, even though key symptoms used for diagnosis may not differ. African Americans tend to score differently on the MMPI, endorsing more items consistent with paranoid symptoms than do Whites [13]. Part of the problem is that the MMPI was standardized on an almost exclusively White Midwestern sample. African Americans tend to show a culturally based wariness, called by some a 'healthy paranoia', that skews MMPI results and clinically has been misinterpreted as frank psychosis [2].

Affective disorders are more likely to present with psychotic symptoms, mania may present with more irritable symptoms or hostility, and depression may present with suspiciousness or hostility [1, 9, 14–16]. In fact, therapists unfamiliar with African Americans misrepresent cultural differences as psychopathology [4], and as a consequence the risk for the misdiagnosing of schizophrenia is increased [4, 17, 18]. African Americans may feel fewer social constraints to discuss unusual intra-psychic experiences and may be labeled psychotic. The author once was part of a treatment team who kept a patient longer because he continued to see the 'haunts'. When his family from Louisiana visited, we quickly discovered that the patient's entire community of origin believed in the ongoing presence of dead ancestors appearing as 'haunts' who may cause the curtains to unexpectedly flutter.

African Americans who are depressed may report primarily somatic or neuro-vegetative symptoms [5, 15, 19, 20]. Depressed or stressed African Americans may describe such somatic symptoms as 'falling out'. Depressive symptoms are often minimized or underreported, especially in elderly African Americans [21, 22]. This focus on somatic complaints and tendency to minimize depressive symptoms may help to explain the tendency of African Americans to go to providers of primary medicine rather than mental health providers when despondent or in distress [4, 23]. Socioeconomic factors may contribute as much as cultural factors to some of these differences in symptom presentation [14, 24, 25]. However, the cultural differences could be underestimated. For example, African Americans may be less likely to present with symptoms of guilt [5, 19, 15, 26]; guilt is more a Western European concept because it assumes a more individualistic view of the world and focuses on individual responsibility but people from tribal cultures assume more communal responsibility. Shame is more likely than guilt to be experienced by depressed inhabitants of sub-Saharan Africa [27], and depressed African Americans may not report guilt feelings often because of their cultural heritage.

Recent reviews also suggest that a number of anxiety disorders, including obsessive-compulsive disorder, panic disorder, phobic disorders, and post-traumatic stress disorder (PTSD) are often underrecognized or underdiagnosed in African Americans. These clinical observations are important because empirical studies suggest that these disorders have a prevalence that is the same as, or higher than, that in Caucasians [28–31]. Misdiagnosis and underrecognition probably leads to inappropriate treatment because panic disorder and phobic disorders are often mistaken for general medical disorders [30, 31]. The ego dsytonic obsessions in obsessive-compulsive disorder may easily be misinterpreted as delusions or a thought disturbance, while the compulsions may be mistaken for psychotic behavior. The flashbacks in PTSD may be mistaken for hallucinatory experiences and the emotional blunting for a flattened affect or the hyperreactivity for psychotic excitement. Patients with these disorders are consequently at risk of misdiagnosis with a psychotic disorder such as schizophrenia [28, 32]. Unfortunately no studies have examined the problem of misdiagnosis of these disorders in African Americans [30].

The incidence of PTSD in African American populations has generated increased recent interest. Differences in symptom manifestation between African Americans and Caucasians have been reported [33–35]; in particular, more psychotic symptoms have been reported in African Americans. Substance abusers in people of African descent who had experienced heavy combat exposure were reported to be more disturbed than a similar group of White subjects, scoring higher on the MMPI scales for paranoid and psychotic symptoms [36, 37]. A later study using the MMPI-2, which has been normed on diverse ethnic groups, found higher levels of psychotic symptoms and paranoid ideation in Black than in White subjects with PTSD [38]. Together these findings suggest that the different presentation of African Americans with PTSD, perhaps with more psychotic symptoms, might contribute to overdiagnosis of schizophrenia.

African Americans often present with isolated sleep paralysis: an altered state of consciousness experienced while falling asleep or on awakening, usually lasting a few seconds or minutes [30, 39–41]. Individuals report waking up and not being able to move. Isolated sleep paralysis is reported far more often in African Americans than Caucasians, often in association with panic disorder, and is frequently accompanied by auditory or visual illusions and panic-like symptoms. It may be seen in association with hypertension [42]. The etiology is unknown and the phenomenon has been related to nocturnal panic attacks, narcolepsy, and stress. Generally it is considered an anxiety disorder or anxiety syndrome; however, African Americans refer to it as 'the witch is riding you', which, along with the perceptual experiences and panic, can lead the culturally unsophisticated investigator to diagnose schizophrenia.

Finally, issues related to treatment utilization are also important. Mental health treatment is often greeted with suspicion or fear by African Americans [23]. As a result, treatment may be delayed and symptoms may become more dramatic: disorders such as mania may be difficult to distinguish from schizophrenia, and somatic symptoms probably become more prominent when treatment is delayed.

In today's managed care environment the time taken to do a thorough assessment when the diagnosis is questionable increases short-term costs. Consequently, the clinician may have difficulty in performing the semistructured assessment of the DSM-IV and misdiagnosis can result [43]. The long-term costs of patient care may thus be high because the patient may be given the wrong treatment. For patients with bipolar disorder misdiagnosed with schizophrenia, the result may be delayed treatment with antimanic agents [44, 45]. The patient may face more relapses and more hospitalizations. The problem of underdiagnosis of depression is a well known national problem that has led to 'depression screens' and various public awareness concerns. The problem of misdiagnosis of depression or anxiety as psychosis is not as well appreciated and could have the same adverse consequences.

In conclusion, despite the development of the DSM-III and its predecessors, misdiagnosis of African Americans remains a mental health concern. More needs to be done to educate clinicians and mental health administrators about the role of ethnicity in the diagnosis of psychiatric disorders. Research is needed to assess the cost of misdiagnosis. Finally, efforts should continue to improve access of African Americans to mental health services that the African American community will perceive as being user friendly.

REFERENCES

1. Adebimpe VR. 1981. Overview: White norms and psychiatric diagnosis of black patients. *Am J Psychiatry* **138**: 279–85.
2. Jones BE, Gray BA. 1986. Problems in diagnosing schizophrenia and affective disorders among blacks. *Hosp Community Psychiatry* **37**: 61–5.
3. Neighbors HW. 1984. The distribution of psychiatric morbidity in black Americans: A review and suggestion for research. *Community Mental Health J* **20**: 169–81.
4. Adebimpe VR. 1994. Race, racism, and epidemiological surveys. *Hosp Community Psychiatry* **45**: 27–31.

5. Simon R, Fleiss J. 1973. Depression and schizophrenia in hospitalized patients. *Arch Gen Psychiatry* **28**: 509–12.
6. Robins LN, Locke B, Regier DA. 1991. An overview of psychiatric disorders in America. In: Robins LN, Regier DA, eds. *Psychiatric Disorders in America: The Epidemiologic Catchment Area Study*. New York: The Free Press, pp. 328–66.
7. Kessler RC, McGonogle KA, Zhao S, Nelson CB, Hughes M, Eshleman S *et al*. 1994. Lifetime and 12 month prevalence of DSM III-R psychiatric disorders in the United States. *Arch Gen Psychiatry* **51**: 8–19.
8. Lawson WB, Hepler N, Holladay J, Cuffel B. 1994. Race as a factor in inpatient and outpatient admissions and diagnosis. *Hosp Community Psychiatry* **45**: 72–4.
9. Adebimpe VR, Klein HE, Fried J. 1981. Hallucinations and delusions in Black psychiatric patients. *J Natl Med Assoc* **73**: 517–20.
10. Strakowski SM, Shelton RC, Kolbrener ML. 1993. The effects of race and comorbidity on clinical diagnosis in patients and psychosis. *J Clin Psychiatry* **54**: 96–102.
11. Strakowski SM, Lonczak HS, Sax K, West SA, Crist A, Mehta R, Thienhaus OJ. 1995. The effects of race on diagnosis and disposition from a psychiatric emergency service. *J Clin Psychiatry* **56**: 101–7.
12. Strakowski SM, Hawkins JM, Keck PE, McElroy SL, West SA, Bourne ML *et al*. 1997. The effects of race and information variance on disagreement between psychiatric emergency service and research diagnoses in first-episode psychosis. *J Clin Psychiatry* **58**: 457–63.
13. Adebimpe VR, Gigardet J, Harris E. 1979. MMPI diagnosis of Black psychiatric patients. *Am J Psychiatry* **135**: 85–7.
14. Adebimpe VR, Hedlund JL, Cho DW *et al*. 1982. Symptomatology of depression in Black and White patients. *J Natl Med Assoc* **74**: 185–90.
15. Fabrega H, Mezzich J, Ulrich RF. 1988. Black-white differences in psychopathology in an urban psychiatric population. *Comprehensive Psychiatry* **29**: 285–97.
16. Raskin A, Crook TH, Herman KD. 1975. Psychiatric history and symptom differences in black and white depressed inpatients. *J Consult Clin Psychol* **43**: 73–80.
17. Lawson WB. 1990. Biological markers in Neuropsychiatric disorders: Racial and ethnic factors. In: Sorel E, ed. *Family, Culture, and Psychobiology*. New York: Levas.
18. Strickland TK, Ranganath V, Lin K-M, Poland RE, Mendoza R, Smith MW. 1991. Psychopharmacologic considerations in the treatment of black American populations. *Psychopharmacol Bull* **27**: 441–8.
19. Carter JH. 1974. Recognizing psychiatric symptoms in black Americans. *Geriatrics* **29**: 95–9.
20. Hanson B, Klerman G. 1974. Interracial problems in the assessment of clinical depression: Concordance differences between white psychiatrists and black and white patients. *Psychopharmacol Bull* **10**: 65–6.
21. Callahan CM, Wolinsky ED. 1994. The effect of gender and race on the measurement properties of the CES-D in older adults. *Med Care* **32**: 341–56.
22. Koenig H, Meador K, Goli V, Shelp F, Cohen H, Blazer D. 1992. Self-rated depressive symptoms in medical inpatients: Age and racial differences. *Int J Psychiatry Med* **22**: 11–31.
23. Sussman LK, Robins LN, Earls F. 1987. Treatment-seeking for depression by black and white Americans. *Soc Sci Med* **24**: 187–96.
24. Jones-Webb RJ, Snowden LR. 1993. Symptoms of depression among blacks and whites. *Am J Public Health* **83**: 240–4.
25. Neff JA, Hoppe SK. 1993. Race/ethnicity, acculturation, and psychological distress: Fatalism and religiosity as cultural resources. *J Community Psychol* **21**: 3–20.
26. Lawson WB. 1986. Racial and ethnic factors in psychiatric research. *Hosp Community Psychiatry* **37**: 50–4

27. German GA. 1972. Aspects of clinical psychiatry in sub-Saharan Africa. *Br J Psychiatry* **121**: 461–79.
28. Allen IM. 1986. Posttraumatic stress disorder among black Vietnam veterans. *Hosp Community Psychiatry* **37**: 55–61.
29. Brown DR, Eaton WW, Sussman L. 1990. Racial differences in prevalence of phobic disorders. *J Nerv Ment Dis* **178**: 434–41.
30. Neal AM, Turner SM. 1991. Anxiety disorders research with African Americans: Current status. *Psychol Bull* **109**: 400–10.
31. Paradis CM, Hatch M, Friedman S. 1994. Anxiety disorders in African Americans: An update. *J Natl Med Assoc* **86**: 609–12.
32. Hwang MY, Hollander E. 1993. Schizo-obsessive disorders. *Psychiatry Ann* **23**: 396–401.
33. Allen IM. 1996. PTSD among African Americans. In: Marsella AJ, Friedman MJ, Gerrity ET, Scurfield RM, eds. *Ethnocultural Aspects of Posttraumatic Stress Disorder: Issues, Research, and Clinical Applications.* Washington, DC: American Psychological Association, pp. 209–38.
34. Parson ER. 1985. Ethnicity and traumatic stress: the intersecting point in psychotherapy. In: Figley CR, ed. *Trauma and its Wake: The Study and Treatment of Posttraumatic Stress Disorder.* New York: Brunner/Mazel.
35. Penk WE, Allen IM. 1991. Clinical assessment of post-traumatic stress disorder (PTSD) among American minorities who served in Vietnam. *J Traumatic Stress* **4**: 41–66.
36. Penk W, Robinowitz R, Black J, Dolan M, Bell W, Doresett D *et al.* 1989. Ethnicity: Post-traumatic stress disorder (PTSD) differences among Black, White, and Hispanic veterans who differ in degrees of exposure to combat in Vietnam. *J Clin Psychol* **45**: 729–35.
37. Penk W, Robinowitz R, Dorsett D, Bell W, Black J. 1988. Postraumatic stress disorder: Psychometric assessment and race. In: Miller T, ed. *A Primer on Diagnosing and Treating Vietnam Combat-related Post Traumatic Stress Disorders.* New York: International Universities Press.
38. Frueh BC, Smith DW, Libet JM. 1996. Racial differences on psychological measures in combat veterans seeking treatment for PTSD. *J Personality Assessment* **66**: 41–53.
39. Bell CC, Dixie-Bell DD, Thompson B. 1986. Further studies on the prevalence of isolated sleep paralysis in Black subjects. *J Natl Med Assoc* **78**: 649–59.
40. Bell CC, Hildreth CJ, Jenkins EJ, Carter C. 1988. The relationship of isolated sleep paralysis and panic disorder to hypertension. *J Natl Med Assoc* **80**: 389–94.
41. Bell CC, Shakoor B, Thompson B, Dew D, Hughley E, Mays R, Shorter-Gooden K. 1984. Prevalence of isolated sleep paralysis in Black Subjects. *J Natl Med Assoc* **76**: 501–8.
42. Paradis CM, Friedman S, Hatch M. 1997. Isolated sleep paralysis in African Americans with panic disorder. *Cult Diversity Mental Health* **3**: 69–76.
43. Mukherjee S, Shukla S, Woodline J. 1983. Misdiagnosis of schizophrenia in bipolar patients: A multi-ethnic comparison. *Am J Psychiatry* **140**: 1571–4.
44. Bell CC, Mehta H. 1980. The misdiagnosis of black patients with manic-depressive illness. *J Natl Med Assoc* **72**: 141–5.
45. Bell CC, Mehta H. 1981. Misdiagnosis of black patients with manic-depressive illness: Second in a series. *J Natl Med Assoc* **73**: 101–7.

Schizophrenia

11

Review of Neuroleptic Dosage in Different Ethnic Groups

Edyta J. Frackiewicz[a], John J. Sramek[a], John M. Herrera[b], and Neal R. Cutler[a]

[a]California Clinical Trials, Beverly Hills, CA, USA;
[b]Eli Lilly and Company, Indianapolis, IN, USA

INTRODUCTION

Changes in demographics in the USA will require that clinicians become increasingly involved in the pharmacological management of schizophrenic patients with diverse ethnic and racial backgrounds and become aware of possible interethnic/racial differences in antipsychotic response [1]. Most comparative studies of ethnicity/race in relation to differences in drug response or side-effect profile have been conducted in Caucasian and Asian populations, with fewer studies conducted in Hispanic and African-American populations (Tables 11.1 and 11.2). Despite methodological flaws, reports of differences in response to antipsychotic medications emerge from the literature, with certain ethnic groups requiring lower dosages of antipsychotics [2, 5–7]. Proposed mechanisms for these differences encompass pharmacokinetic and pharmacodynamic variations and non-pharmacological explanations such as cultural and societal variations in the way psychiatry is practiced.

PROPOSED EXPLANATIONS FOR ETHNIC DIFFERENCES IN DRUG RESPONSE

A number of explanations have been proposed to elucidate why alterations in drug response exist between different ethnic and racial groups. Rosenblat [19], in a drug history review and international opinion survey, asked psychiatrists to offer their opinions explaining the existence of these variations: they felt that these differences were due to drug metabolism, frequency and severity of side-effects, and body weight. Other reasons included diet, social support systems, attitude towards

Cross Cultural Psychiatry. Edited by John M. Herrera, William B. Lawson and John J. Sramek.
© 1999 John Wiley & Sons Ltd.

TABLE 11.1 Demographic data for studies assessing antipsychotic response in ethnic groups

Reference	No. in study	Race	Ethnicity*	Gender	Diagnosis
[2]	106	Asian	Chinese	51 men, 55 women	Schizophrenia
[3]	71	Caucasian (34) Chinese (10) Hispanic (27)		18 men, 16 women 10 women 4 men, 23 women	Schizophrenia
[4]	18	Non-Hispanics (8)	Indian (3), Jamaican (1), Pakistani (1), Filipino (1), Romanian (1), American (1)	4 men, 4 women	Schizophrenia
		Hispanics (10)	Colombian (2), Dominican Republican (1) Ecuadorian (2), Mexican (3), Puerto Rican (1), San Salvadorian (1)	5 men, 5 women	
[5]	26	Caucasian (13) Asian (13)	Japanese (4), Vietnamese (4), Chinese (3), Filipino (2)	6 men, 7 women 6 men, 7 women	Schizophrenia (18); psychosis (8)
[6]	34	Caucasian (12) American-born Asian (11) Foreign-born Asian (11)	Filipino (5), Chinese (3), Japanese (2), Korean (1) Filipino (5), Chinese (3), Korean (2), Japanese (1)	Male	Healthy

[7]	29	Caucasian (13), Asian (16)	Chinese (5), Japanese (4), Filipino (2), Vietnamese (4), Korean (1)	3 men, 10 women; 6 men, 10 women	Schizophrenia/
[8]	24	Caucasian (7), Asian (17)	Korean American	6 men, 1 woman; 11 men, 6 women	Schizophrenia/ schizophreniform schizoaffective
[9]	21	Caucasian (9)		male	Schizophrenia/ schizophreniform
[10]	36	Asian (18), Non-Asian (18)	Han Chinese (18), Caucasian (15), African American (3)	12 men, 6 women; 12 men, 6 women	Schizophrenia
[11]	140	Non-Hispanic, non-Asian (64), Asian (48), Hispanic (27)		26 men, 38 women; 21 men, 27 women; 11 men, 16 women	Schizophrenia
[12]	60	Caucasian (30), Asian (30)	Korean (11), Chinese (10), Japanese (9)	17 men, 13 women; 17 men, 13 women	Schizophrenia (42), psychosis (18)

* If specified

TABLE 11.2 Demographic data for studies assessing antipsychotic-induced side-effects in ethnic groups

Reference	No. in study	Race	Ethnicity*	Gender	Diagnosis
[5]	26	Caucasian (13 Asian (13)	Japanese (4), Vietnamese (4), Chinese (3), Filipino (2)	6 men, 7 women 6 men, 7 women	Schizophrenia (18), psychosis (8)
[7]	29	Caucasian (13) Asian (16)	Chinese (5), Japanese (4), Filipino (2), Vietnamese (4), Korean (1)	3 men, 10 women 6 men, 10 women	Schizophrenia/ schizophreniform
[12]	60	Caucasian (30) Asian (30)	Korean (11), Chinese (10), Japanese (9)	17 men, 13 women 17 men, 13 women	Schizophrenia (42), psychosis (18)
[13]	126	Asian	Japanese		Schizophrenia (119), psychiatric disorder; not specified (7)
[14]	398	Asian	Chinese		Schizophrenia (167), schizoaffective (67), affective disorder (60), other (64), mixed diagnosis (40)

[15]	80	Caucasian (40) African American (20) Asian (20)	Chinese (17), Korean (1), Japanese (2)	19 men, 21 women 12 men, 8 women 11 men, 9 women	Schizophrenia, schizoaffective, bipolar
[2]	917	Asian	Chinese	503 men, 414 women	Schizophrenia (602), manic depressive (44), demented (97), mentally retarded (97), other (77)
[16]	31	Jewish (22) Non-Jewish Caucasian (8) Non-Caucasian (1)		21 men, 8 women	Schizophrenia/ schizoaffective
[17]	491	Caucasian (280) African American (112) Hispanic (99)		185 men, 95 women 74 men, 38 women 74 men, 25 women	
[18]	11	Jewish (7) Non-Jewish (4)	Ashkenazi		Schizophrenia

* If specified

mental illness, prescribing habits and social practices. Some psychiatrists also felt that there may be differences in the central nervous system and physical and chemical structures that may contribute to these differences. Several proposed explanations for ethnic differences in drug response will be presented in more detail below.

The Cytochrome P-450 Enzyme System

Genetic polymorphism of cytochrome P-450 (CYP) enzymes plays a role in variability of drug response because these enzymes are involved in the oxidative metabolism of a wide variety of medications [20]. The CYP enzymes responsible for the metabolism of psychiatric drugs include CYP1A2, CYP2C, CYP2D6, and CYP3A4 [20]. CYP2D6 is responsible for the metabolism of haloperidol, risperidone, olanzapine, perphenazine, and thioridazine [21]. It is also responsible for the metabolism of a number of other psychotropics such as the tricyclic antidepressants and selective serotonin reuptake inhibitors. Individuals possessing a mutation at the CYP2D6 locus lack a functional form of the enzyme and are referred to as poor metabolizers because these mutations result in a slower metabolic rate; individuals possessing normal functioning enzymes are referred to as extensive metabolizers. Poor metabolizers may accumulate potentially toxic blood concentrations after taking recommended doses of medications that are metabolized by the CYP2D6 enzyme [22] and the incidence of adverse effects is considerably higher in poor metabolizers [23]. As many antipsychotic drugs (such as haloperidol) have a very high first-pass effect, a poor or slow metabolizer phenotype could account for variations in steady-state blood levels; to avoid increased adverse effects poor metabolizers will require a lower than usual dose.

Studies estimate that approximately 6–10% of European and North American Caucasians possess mutations at the CYP2D6 enzyme causing them to be unable to effectively metabolize drugs that are substrates for this enzyme [24–27]. The estimated frequency rate for poor metabolizers in Chinese, Japanese, and other Asian populations is less than 1% [28, 29]. The frequency of poor metabolizers in African populations varies considerably, 0.7–5% for Ghanaians [30, 31], 3–8% for Nigerians [32, 33], and 19% for Sans Bushmen [34]. A more recent study found that 7.7% of Caucasians are poor metabolizers, compared with 1.9% of African Americans [35]; another study reported that the prevalence of poor metabolizers in African Americans is 6.1% [36]. Limited studies have been conducted with Hispanic populations; however, the estimated prevalence rate for poor metabolizers in Spaniards is estimated at 5–10%, which is similar to the rate in Caucasians [37], and the prevalence of poor metabolizers in Hispanics has been estimated at 4.5% [38]. More studies need to be conducted to examine the prevalence rate for poor metabolizers in different Hispanic populations.

Genetic polymorphism is complex and alterations at the DNA level may result in CYP2D6 enzyme activity that is absent (poor metabolizers), increased (ultrarapid metabolizers) or decreased (slow metabolizers) compared with the homozygous form of the enzyme. Approximately 37% of Asian extensive metabolizers possess a mutation at the CYP2D6 gene causing them to exhibit a significantly lower metabolic capacity than that of Caucasian extensive metabolizers [39]. Individuals with this mutation are referred to as slow metabolizers, and they have an intermediate metabolic rate that makes them less efficient metabolizers than extensive metabolizers—and therefore also makes them more sensitive to the effects of drugs metabolized by CYP2D6 [20].

PROPOSED PHARMACODYNAMIC AND RECEPTOR-MEDIATED FACTORS

Pharmacodynamic variables have become the focus of investigation for determining if there are ethnic variations in psychotropic drug response. The possibility exists that there may be an ethnic influence in receptor-mediated responses, with different ethnic groups having alterations in the number of receptors for the active drug [40]. Therefore, these individuals would require different blood or end-organ drug concentrations for a therapeutic effect. A recent study found a dopamine D4 receptor variant present in Africans that was not present in Caucasians. Even though the study could not find any association between this variant and schizophrenia, findings of this type may eventually link altered drug response with receptor-mediated differences in different ethnic groups. Other evidence to support the concept of pharmacodynamically based differences in drug response include the more prominent prolactin responses that were found in Asians following haloperidol administration [6]. Blockade of dopamine receptors in the hypothalamus with typical antipsychotics results in elevated prolactin concentrations; therefore prolactin levels are used to gauge the effectiveness of typical antipsychotics. Further research is necessary to determine whether ethnic differences in receptor-mediated responses exist.

PLASMA PROTEIN BINDING

In order to exert an antipsychotic effect, a drug must cross the blood–brain barrier and interact with receptors in the central nervous system. Because only the unbound fraction is able to cross the blood–brain barrier, slight variations in the concentration of drug-binding proteins in the plasma could result in differences in responsiveness and side-effects [1]. α_1-Acid glycoprotein is a protein that binds many basic compounds, including haloperidol, chlorpromazine, fluphenazine, loxapine, and thioridazine [41]. Acutely psychotic schizophrenic patients treated with haloperidol had significantly lower α_1-acid glycoprotein levels than patients treated with placebo. Haloperidol binds to α_1-acid glycoprotein, and thus a decrease in α_1-acid glycoprotein over time would lead to an increase in unbound drug. Therefore, in individuals with reduced serum concentrations of α_1-acid glycoprotein the unbound fraction of the drug will be greater, possibly contributing to variations in therapeutic and adverse effects [41]. Zhou *et al.* [42] found that plasma binding of certain drugs to α_1-acid glycoprotein is significantly lower ($p < 0.05$) in Chinese subjects than in Caucasians. Therefore the possibility exists that Chinese patients could be expected to have an altered pharmacological response when taking antipsychotics with a high affinity for α_1-acid glycoprotein. Further research is needed to determine whether a decrease in α_1-acid glycoprotein concentrations is associated with any change in the quantity of drug bound at the site of action, or whether it causes any changes in antipsychotic response.

DIETARY, ENVIRONMENTAL AND OTHER FACTORS

Smoking

Smoking, alcohol intake, concurrent drug use, and exposure to environmental or occupational toxins are associated with an increased drug elimination rate [43]. Jann *et al.* [44] found that smokers who consumed more than one pack of cigarettes per day had significantly lower concentrations of haloperidol and reduced haloperidol than non-smokers, and that clearance of haloperidol was significantly greater in smokers than in non-smokers. Smoking has also been determined to decrease serum levels of chlorpromazine [45–47] and fluphenazine [48]. These effects may be due to induction of liver enzymes, which leads to increased clearance and decreased concentration of a number of medications [49].

Interethnic/racial differences in the frequency and prevalence of smoking also exist. Hymowitz *et al.* [50], in a comparison of Caucasians, African Americans, Mexicans, and Puerto Ricans found that Caucasian men and women were more likely to be heavy smokers than members of the other three groups. Rogers *et al.* [51] reported similar findings when comparing Caucasians with African Americans and Mexican Americans. The lower incidence of smoking in these ethnic groups could result in increased sensitivity due to higher plasma drug concentration of antipsychotic medication.

Alcohol Consumption

Alcohol affects the clearance rate and metabolism of a number of drugs [52, 53]. Short-term consumption of alcohol inhibits the CYP oxidase system and decreases the clearance rate of drugs with a high first-pass effect that undergo oxidative metabolism [54]. Chronic alcohol use, on the other hand, induces the CYP oxidative system so that the clearance rate of many drugs increases [55]. Long-term, heavy alcohol use causes cirrhosis of the liver for many patients. This later results in a diminished capacity for oxidative metabolism [56].

Studies have reported that Asians consume significantly lower amounts of alcohol than Caucasians [57, 58]. This has been attributed to cultural and physiological factors because Chinese cultural values stress moderation and self-restraint, leading to a lower incidence of alcohol drinking [59, 60]. Asians also experience a high incidence of facial and neck flushing after alcohol consumption that is very unpleasant and accompanied by increased heart rate [60]. The incidence of alcohol-induced flushing in Asians is in the range of 70–83%, whereas that for Caucasians is 3–13% [61–64]. The increased sensitivity to alcohol resulting in flushing is thought to be linked to a deficiency in aldehyde dehydrogenase activity. This causes a higher level of acetaldehyde to be produced following alcohol metabolism [65].

Diet and Nutritional Status

Diet and nutritional status affect the pharmacokinetics of medications. Poor nutritional status causes deficiencies in coenzymes and vitamins, which may play important roles in biochemical reactions, including the absorption, metabolism and excretion of medications [66]. Certain groups of foods—such as the cruciferous vegetables (cabbage, broccoli, and brussels sprouts)—induce chemical oxidation and increase the activity of CYP1A2 [67, 68]. Therefore individuals who consume such vegetables may have lower plasma concentrations of antipsychotics, such as haloperidol and clozapine, which are metabolized by CYP1A2 [20]. Polycyclic aromatic hydrocarbons formed during charcoal broiling also increase drug oxidation rates [69]; grapefruit juice inhibits CYP1A2 and causes increases in the serum concentration of certain medications [20].

The amount of protein consumed in the diet can also affect drug plasma levels. A high-protein, low-carbohydrate diet has been shown to decrease the half-life and increase the elimination rate of medications such as antipyrine and theophylline [52, 69]. Dollery et al. [52] examined the metabolism of phenazone and acetaminophen following single doses in 96 London factory workers of varying ethnicities. They found that the metabolic clearance of both drugs was significantly greater in those subjects who ate meat more than once a week than in those who ate meat less frequently. Interestingly, 90% of the meat eaters were of European descent, whereas most of the vegetarians were Asians. Studies have also reported that as immigrant peoples adopt the lifestyle and diet of their new homeland their rates of metabolism come to more closely resemble that of the native peoples [70]. Further studies are warranted to determine how diet can affect the pharmacokinetics of antipsychotics because there is considerable variability in the food choices [71] and dietary practices [72] of different ethnic groups.

Certain medicinal herbs used in traditional Chinese medicine—such as muscone, panax ginseng, and glycyrrhiza—are able to induce or inhibit CYP enzymes [73]. They therefore have the potential for interacting with prescribed drugs, possibly having additive pharmacodynamic effects. Clinicians should be aware that traditional herbal and natural medicines are often used in combination with prescription and over-the-counter drugs [1].

Other Factors

Body weight and size are important in influencing plasma drug concentrations because, for a given dose of drug, the greater the volume of distribution the lower the concentration of drug reached in the fluid compartments of the body. Therefore, small individuals may require lower doses than large individuals in order to produce comparable plasma levels. Dosage adjustments in very lean or very obese individuals should be made on the basis of body surface area [74]. Body fat distribution and obesity are also known to affect the pharmacokinetics of many drugs. In obese individuals apparent volumes of distribution for highly lipophilic drugs such as haloperidol are increased, necessitating higher doses [75, 76].

Age also plays an important factor, because the rates of absorption, metabolism and excretion can be altered in elderly people [74, 77], in part due to age-related changes in body composition, protein binding and renal clearance [76].

Prescribing Practices

The recommended daily dose of antipsychotic drugs can vary from country to country because dose–response relationships for antipsychotics such as haloperidol have been difficult to demonstrate [78, 79] and even the minimum effective dose of antipsychotics remains unresolved [79]. Therapeutic plasma concentrations for antipsychotics such as haloperidol, chlorpromazine, and thioridazine have not been defined, and there is very little evidence correlating therapeutic response with plasma levels [80–83]. Lower doses have been shown to be just as just as effective in treating psychotic symptoms as higher doses [84]. A study by Kapur et al. [85] revealed that low doses of haloperidol (2 mg/day) resulted in high levels of D_2 receptor occupancy, in the range of 53–74% (as measured by positron emission tomography). At this dose most patients showed substantial clinical improvement with minimal side-effects. These researchers believe that clinicians should be encouraged to start treatment with antipsychotics at low doses. In Japan, polypharmacy is common and Japanese psychiatrists often utilize a combination of antipsychotics to combat target symptoms; the recommended daily dose of antipsychotic drugs is lower in Japan than in Western countries [86].

Ethnic differences in dosing may arise from attitudes or habits affecting assessment and prescribing practices rather than from actual differences in response due to physiological differences. If clinicians believe that one ethnic or racial group should receive less medication, that group is likely to receive less [12]. Studies have reported that African Americans are more likely than Caucasians to be misdiagnosed [87, 88], to be treated with antipsychotic agents irrespective of diagnosis [14], to be diagnosed with a more severe diagnosis such as schizophrenia [14, 89], and to be treated with significantly higher doses of antipsychotic agents [90]. Therefore they may be at a greater risk for inappropriate psychiatric treatment [91]. Few studies assessing prescription patterns have been conducted in Hispanics;

however, greater diagnosis rates of schizophrenia have been reported in Hispanic Americans than in non-Hispanics even though Hispanics have the same (or even slightly lower) prevalence rates [92]. This has been attributed to cultural miscommunication, which causes providers to diagnose schizophrenia in a patient who may be suffering from hypomania or depression [93]. Several studies have reported that Hispanics tend to underuse mental health services [94, 95], possibly due to cultural insensitivity on the part of the healthcare professional [96, 97]. Finally, there are other 'non-biological' factors—such as patient expectations, special beliefs of patients, placebo response, quality of care, and economic and compliance issues—which are subject to ethnic and racial variation and which are nevertheless important in determining the effectiveness of antipsychotics [38].

ANTIPSYCHOTIC DOSING STUDIES

Response of Asians to Antipsychotic Medication

A search of the literature revealed that most of the studies examining differences in antipsychotic dosing have compared Asians with Caucasians (see Table 11.1 for demographic data). Rosenblat and co-workers [19] assessed differences in the dosages of several different psychotropics (chlorpromazine, haloperidol, trifluoperazine, amitriptyline, phenelzine, diazepam, chlordiazepoxide) for Asians and Caucasians. They examined 33 patient pairs and collected data from 14 psychiatrists practicing in Asia and North America and found that the initial starting doses for the four agents did not differ between the two groups. However, they did find that during the course of treatment there was a tendency for Asians to receive lower maintenance dosages of chlorpromazine, haloperidol, and amitriptyline.

In a retrospective study of Chinese schizophrenic patients in Hong Kong, Chiu et al. [2] found that the mean daily dose of antipsychotics was 2–3 times lower than the dosage reported in an American study of Caucasian patients. The dose for Asians remained lower even after the differences in body weight were taken into consideration, with the mean daily dose in chlorpromazine equivalents in Asians being 568.5 (±371.5) mg, compared with 1428 (±1260) mg chlorpromazine equivalents in Caucasians.

Lin and Finder [5], in a controlled, comparative, prospective study of Asian patients and Caucasian patients with diagnoses of schizophrenia and psychosis who were matched for age, sex, diagnosis, and date of discharge, found that Asian psychotic patients required significantly lower doses of antipsychotic medication than Caucasians to control their symptoms (mean maximum dose $p < 0.05$; mean stabilized dose $p < 0.02$). Subsequently, Potkin et al. [10], in a prospective, 6-week fixed-dose oral haloperidol treatment compared Han Chinese schizophrenic patients with American schizophrenics who were matched for sex and body weight. The Han Chinese schizophrenic patients had 52% higher plasma haloperidol concentrations than the American schizophrenic patients ($p < 0.024$).

A prospective study conducted by Lin *et al.* [6] measured haloperidol and prolactin concentrations in normal male volunteers who were administered 0.5 mg intramuscularly and 1 mg oral dosages of haloperidol. All of the subjects were physically healthy, and none had a history of psychiatric illness or substance abuse. All subjects were non-smokers, did not drink alcoholic beverages on a regular basis, and there were no significant differences in the age or percentage of body fat among the three groups. After controlling for body surface area, they found that Caucasians had significantly lower serum haloperidol concentrations ($p < 0.01$) and less prominent prolactin responses than did Asians ($p < 0.025$). There were no significant differences between the two Asian groups, and the authors concluded that genetic rather than environmental factors appear to be responsible for variations in antipsychotic response.

Lin *et al.* also investigated haloperidol serum concentrations in Asian and Caucasian schizophrenic patients who were treated with weight-adjusted fixed doses of haloperidol (0.15 mg/kg per day) for a period of 2 weeks, followed by a clinically determined dose for the remainder of the 3-month study period [7]. The researchers found that during the fixed-dose phase the Asians' serum haloperidol concentrations were slightly higher than those of the Caucasians ($p < 0.02$). During the variable dose phase, because doses were clinically determined, Asian patients required a lower dose of haloperidol, resulting in lower steady-state serum haloperidol concentrations ($p < 0.05$). They also found differences after controlling for any differences in body surface area. The authors concluded that there were ethnic differences in therapeutic response; however, the differences in steady-state serum concentrations between the two groups were not significant. These results differ significantly from the results of Potkin *et al.* [10], and the differences may be attributable to the fact that Lin *et al.* [7] used weight-adjusted and clinically determined doses.

Not all retrospective studies support the hypothesis that Asians may require lower doses of antipsychotics. Sramek *et al.* [12], in a retrospective chart review of Asian patients and matched Caucasian patients with diagnoses of schizophrenia or acute psychosis, did not find any statistically significant differences in the antipsychotic dosage requirements of either group. They also found that the frequency of adverse events did not differ between the two groups. They believe that the chronic nature of illness in the patients may have created a dosage requirement different from that needed in less chronically ill patients.

Response of Hispanics and African Americans to Antipsychotic Medication

Our literature search found fewer studies conducted with Hispanic and African American patients. Ruiz *et al.* [11] examined the prescribing pattern of antipsychotic medication to Asian and Hispanic schizophrenic outpatients. A matched sample of Caucasian schizophrenics was drawn for comparison and for all three samples antipsychotic doses were converted to chlorpromazine equivalents and corrected for body weight. The results revealed that significantly larger doses of antipsychotics were prescribed to Caucasian patients than either of the two ethnic minority samples ($p < 0.002$ for Asians; $p < 0.029$ for Hispanics), although the two ethnic samples did not significantly differ from each other ($p > 0.05$). In a second study, these authors identified samples of Hispanic and Chinese inpatients and a matched sample of Caucasian patients [3]. These results also revealed that Caucasian schizophrenic patients were prescribed significantly larger doses of antipsychotic medication than either of the two ethnic minority samples ($p < 0.002$ for Chinese; $p < 0.009$ for Hispanics).

Even fewer studies have been conducted in the African American population. Studies determining the pharmacokinetics of fluphenazine [9] and haloperidol [98] between healthy African American and Caucasian subjects found no statistically significant differences between the two groups. However, in a clinical setting steady-state dosing occurs, and it is not always possible to extrapolate the results of a single dose study.

Ethnic Response to Atypical Antipsychotics

Newer, atypical antipsychotic agents have become available in recent years and are used frequently in the treatment of psychotic illness; however research examining ethnic differences in response to these newer agents is limited. Recent anecdotal reports from Latin America state that dosages of antipsychotics such as risperidone used to treat patients with schizophrenia are lower than the doses used in the USA [38]. Most recently, Frackiewicz *et al.* [4] examined the efficacy of risperidone (6 mg four times or 3 mg twice daily) in matched sample(s) of Hispanic and non-Hispanic schizophrenic patients. They reported a significantly faster rate of symptom improvement ($p < 0.02$) concurrent with more frequently occurring extrapyramidal symptoms (EPS) on the part of the Hispanics, under recommended dosing conditions.

One study conducted in Caucasian and Korean American schizophrenics/schizoaffectives evaluated the efficacy and safety of clozapine [8]. Asians showed greater improvement on the Brief Psychiatric Rating Scale at lower dosages ($p < 0.025$), had significantly lower mean clozapine concentrations than Caucasians, and had a significantly greater incidence of anticholinergic and other adverse effects. The findings of these studies suggest that these novel chemical compounds at lower doses may be preferable in the treatment of ethnic minorities by offering the benefits of reduced EPS and/or other adverse effects and rapid onset of action in addition to alleviation of positive and negative symptoms. However, further studies need to be conducted in order to fully ascertain the role of these atypical antipsychotic agents in the treatment of ethnic patients.

Many of the studies discussed above are confounded by methodological issues. Most controlled for obvious factors such as age and body weight; however, many of the researchers conducting the studies did not consider equally important factors, such as prior antipsychotic use and exposure to enzyme-inducing and enzyme-inhibiting agents, environmental factors, length of illness, observer bias, and gender differences. Well designed, double-blind, controlled clinical trials are needed in order to confirm that ethnic differences in response to antipsychotics exist. Recommendations for designing these types of trials will be discussed below.

Ethnic Differences in the Prevalence of Antipsychotic Side-effects

Differences in the incidence and intensity of adverse effects in ethnic populations have also been described, and most of these studies have been conducted in Asians (see Table 11.2 for demographic data). Binder et al. [13] evaluated the frequency of extrapyramidal reactions in Asians and compared them to those in African Americans and Caucasians; all patients received haloperidol for 22 months during the course of the study. They discovered that, after 2 weeks of haloperidol treatment, 95% of the Asian subjects developed extrapyramidal symptoms (acute dystonic reactions, parkinsonian rigidity and akathisia), whereas the incidence of extrapyramidal side-effects in the African American and Caucasian patients was 60% and 75%, respectively. The differences in the incidence of reactions between the Asians and the other groups were statistically significant ($p < 0.05$), even though there were no statistically significant differences between the groups in regards to demographic variables such as age or sex.

Lin and Finder [5], in a study of Asian and Caucasian patients matched for age, sex, diagnosis, and date of discharge, found that the percentages of patients developing extrapyramidal symptoms were almost identical (69% in Asians; 77% in Caucasians); however, the Asian patients developed extrapyramidal symptoms at a lower dose than the Caucasian patients (574 mg/day for Asians vs. 1079 mg/day of chlorpromazine equivalents for Caucasians). In another study, Lin et al. [7] found during the fixed-dose phase that there was a significantly higher incidence of extrapyramidal symptoms in Asians than in Caucasians ($p < 0.03$). During the phase of the study when the serum haloperidol concentrations were lower, they found that the side-effect profiles of the two groups were strikingly similar. One probable explanation for the increased incidence of side-effects could be that a greater proportion of the Asian patients were poor or slow metabolizer phenotypes. This metabolic impairment could result in higher plasma concentrations of anti-psychotics and a greater chance of developing adverse effects.

Ethnic differences in the incidence of tardive dyskinesia have also been assessed; however, the results are inconsistent (see Table 11.2 for demographic data). Sramek et al. [12] have evaluated the prevalence of tardive dyskinesia in African Americans, Caucasians, and Hispanics and found that the overall prevalence of tardive dyskinesia in chronic psychiatric patients was 17.7%, although there were no significant differences in the prevalence of tardive dyskinesia between the three groups ($p > 0.06$). The prevalence of tardive dyskinesia did, however, increase with increasing age. Binder *et al.* [13] studied the antipsychotic drug response in inpatient schizophrenics in Japan. They found the prevalence of tardive dyskinesia in this population to be 14–21%. This finding was similar to studies in Europe and North America, which stated a prevalence of 0.5–56%, with a mean prevalence of 20% [99, 100]. They also found no significant association between tardive dyskinesia and the dose of antipsychotics or the sex of the patient. Chiu *et al.* [2] found that the prevalence rate of tardive dyskinesia in Chinese patients was 9.3%, which they felt was significantly lower than the rates found in Western studies. Glazer *et al.* [14], in a prospective analysis found that non-Caucasian patients were 1.83 times as likely to develop tardive dyskinesia as Caucasian patients ($p = 0.025$); however, they also found that non-Caucasian patients were given higher doses of antipsychotics than Caucasian patients. Non-Caucasian patients were also more likely to receive high-potency antipsychotic medication, which causes a higher incidence of tardive dyskinesia. Sramek *et al.* [17] also suggest that higher doses of antipsychotics mask the appearance of tardive dyskinesia because they increase dopaminergic blockade; therefore optimally one would have to systematically withdraw patients from antipsychotic drugs in prospective studies in order to assess for tardive dyskinesia. In the studies we reviewed none of the patients were withdrawn from their antipsychotic or EPS medications before assessment for tardive dyskinesia.

Ethnic variations are also seen with side-effects other than extrapyramidal symptoms. Lieberman *et al.* [16] found that there is a major histocompatibility complex haplotype that is known to occur significantly more frequently ($p = 0.0007$) in patients who develop agranulocytosis with clozapine treatment. This particular haplotype (HLA-B38, DR4, DQw3) occurs more frequently in the Ashkenazi Jewish population, and therefore Jewish schizophrenic patients may be at greater risk for developing agranulocytosis when being treated with clozapine. Individuals of non-Jewish descent have also been found to posses this haplotype but at a lower prevalence rate. Yunis *et al.* [18] also studied a group of patients who developed agranulocytosis with clozapine treatment; of the Jewish patients, 100% were positive for the associated haplotype (compared with 19% of the non-agranulocytotic patients).

RECOMMENDATION FOR FURTHER RESEARCH

An emerging body of evidence suggests that ethnic pharmacogenetic, pharmaco-dynamic, and pharmacokinetic differences exist which influence individuals' responses to antipsychotic drugs. Studies conducted to date offer valuable insight, but none are unequivocal. Future studies must accommodate such factors as consistency in diagnosis, disease chronicity, differences in body fat and weight, hepatic and renal function, prior exposure to enzyme inducing and inhibiting agents and other variables that can effect drug metabolism, distribution, and elimination.

Ensuring the Ethnic/Racial Homogeneity of Subjects

One major confounding factor concerns the homogeneity of the ethnic and racial groups (see Tables 11.1 and 11.2). In several of the studies reported [5–7, 11, 12] homogeneous groups of Asians were not studied; instead a number of different ethnic groups—such as Chinese, Japanese, and Korean—were included under the racial classification of 'Asian'. Anecdotal claims of lower antipsychotic dosages in Latin America are difficult to interpret because Latin American countries are melting pots of many different ethnic groups [38]. 'Caucasian' is also a broad racial classification that may encompass genetically and culturally dissimilar individuals of European, Middle Eastern, Near Eastern and Jewish descent.

'Race' is a term that groups individuals who share distinct genetic characteristics; ethnic groups are subpopulations who differ in religion, language, ancestry, language, culture or nationality [101]. Grouping individuals into a broadly defined racial group can confound the results of studies because of intraracial and inter-ethnic variability; even within a relatively well defined group differences exist, such as in the incidence of agranulocytosis among Ashkenazi Jewish patients receiving clozapine or the variations in the prevalence of CYP2D6 polymorphism among different Africans [16, 18].

Culture is also of paramount importance because different cultures have different diet and food preparation habits, exposure to pesticides and toxins and use of nicotine, medication, and alcohol in different ways [101]. Studies of Mexican Americans, Cuban Americans, and mainland Puerto Ricans found that the groups differed significantly in regards to diet even though racially they are all Hispanics [102]. Additionally, the level of acculturation within an individual ethnic group plays an important role in the dietary practices, alcohol consumption and smoking behavior [72]. For example, the diet and nutritional intake of second-generation Mexican-American women differs significantly from that of first-generation Mexican-American women, approximating that of White non-Hispanic women [103]. Future studies are needed to evaluate homogeneous ethnic groups and should avoid categorizing different ethnic groups under a racial classification [40]. The precise identification of ethnic groups associated with differences in response could greatly assist in the ultimate goal of identifying the genetic and/or cultural factors responsible for these differences.

Need for More Antipsychotic Dosing Studies in Minority Groups

Most of these studies were conducted in Asian populations; fewer studies have been conducted with Hispanics and African Americans. Few compelling reasons have been proposed for excluding minorities from clinical research in general. Studies have shown that racial and ethnic minorities are less likely to be included in pharmaceutical trials [104]. The NIH Revitalization Act of 1993 mandates the inclusion of minorities and women in clinical research studies [105]; therefore pharmaceutical companies and their researchers need to focus on conducting studies in many diverse ethnic groups, particularly Hispanics and African Americans, in order to gain a better understanding of the actions of the new antipsychotic agents in these populations. This will ensure that individuals of different ethnic and racial groups will be able to obtain medication and feel secure in the knowledge that the latest scientific information regarding treatment of their disease includes information that is directly applicable to them [105].

Gender as a Factor in Antipsychotic Dosing Studies

Another variable of increasingly recognized importance is gender, because gender differences exist in efficacy, dosage, and side-effects of antipsychotic medication [106]. Women seem to require lower doses of antipsychotic symptoms [107], have higher plasma concentrations of certain antipsychotics when administered similar dosages [108, 109], and exhibit a greater incidence of tardive dyskinesia [110, 111] than men. Several of the studies reviewed accounted for gender and matched patients on this basis; however, their final analysis treated male and female patients as one group [5, 7, 12]. In these studies, the ratio of males to females was similar, but the researchers did not determine if there were any statistically significant differences between the male and female groups in regards to antipsychotic response. One study found significant gender differences among their ethnic samples, which they believe may have confounded their results [3]. Future studies should control for gender by conducting and analyzing data from males and females separately.

Advantages of Pharmacogenetic Testing

Recent advances in the area of pharmacogenetic testing have made it possible to ascertain whether individuals are metabolically similar. The activity of CYP2D6 can be assessed by metabolic phenotyping, which requires the intake of a probe drug such as debrisoquine or dextromethorphan [23]. Pharmacokinetic parameters (e.g. half life, clearance, or drug metabolites) can be measured and based on the findings; individuals may be deemed poor or extensive metabolizers or placed in an intermediate heterozygous group. Poor metabolizers will tend to have increased plasma levels of medication that are substrates for CYP2D6 and, as a consequence, may experience a greater drug response and/or increased number or severity of side-effects [112]. Because CYP2D6 activity has important therapeutic significance in determining the metabolism of medications that are substrates for this enzyme, and because significant variations exist in the incidence of CYP2D6 activity, it is recommended that future studies employ phenotype testing. Preliminary determination of a patient's phenotype ensures that a group of subjects is phenotypically homogeneous. Genotyping can also be undertaken to distinguish genetic polymorphism from environmentally induced polymorphism. None of the studies reviewed determined the metabolic phenotypes or genotypes of the subjects.

Impact of Past and Current Concomitant Medication Use

Current and previous exposure to enzyme-inducing and inhibiting agents is an important variable, which must be controlled. Studies have revealed that the clearance of antipsychotic drugs can be significantly decreased by inhibiting agents or increased by inducing agents [113, 114]. The popular antidepressant fluoxetine and some of the other selective serotonin reuptake inhibitors have demonstrated high affinity for the CYP2D6 enzyme and consequently inhibit the metabolism of other drugs [115]. Even certain antipsychotics have been found to competitively inhibit the CYP2D6 enzyme. One study has shown that the proportion of poor metabolizers among patients treated with antipsychotics is 46% [115]. Because psychiatric patients are often prescribed combinations of psychotropic medications that might interact with one another, in future studies concurrent drug administration should be avoided [74].

SUMMARY

Ethnic and racial differences in response to antipsychotic medications may be due to genetics, kinetic variations, dietary or environmental factors or variations in prescribing practices. The literature suggests that interracial variability exists in antipsychotic dosing particularly between Asian and Caucasian patients. Too few pharmacokinetic and pharmacodynamic studies to examine biological mechanisms of antipsychotic response have targeted Hispanic and African American populations to make any conclusions in these groups. Differences in antipsychotic dosing and/or response in Hispanics and African Americans may be due to variations in psychiatric assessment and prescription practices rather than differences in biological mechanisms. Advances in pharmacogenetics, along with renewed interest in ethnic variability, may provide the impetus necessary to validate these findings in carefully designed and well controlled studies. Future studies designed to validate these hypotheses should focus on homogenous ethnic groups, utilize recent advances in genetic testing, and try to control for such variables as gender, disease chronicity, dietary and environmental factors, and concomitant medication use. Until such studies have been carried out, clinicians need to be aware of the possible existence of interracial and interethnic differences in drug response when formulating antipsychotic medication regimens for the treatment of psychotic illness.

REFERENCES

1. Smith MW, Mendoza R. 1996. Ethnicity and pharmacogenetics. *Mt Sinai J Med* 63(5&6): 285–90.
2. Chiu H, Lee S, Leung CM, Wing YK. 1992. Antipsychotic prescription for Chinese schizophrenics in Hong Kong. *Aust NZ J Psychiatry* 26(2): 262–4.
3. Collazo J, Tam R, Sramek JJ, Herrera J. 1996. Neuroleptic dosing in Hispanic and Asian inpatients with schizophrenia. *Mt Sinai J Med* 63(5&6): 310–13.
4. Frackiewicz EJ, Sramek JJ, Collazo Y, Rotaru E, Herrera JM. Risperidone in the treatment of Hispanic schizophrenic patients. *Cult Med Psychiatry* (submitted).
5. Lin KM, Finder E. 1983. Antipsychotic dosage for Asians. *Am J Psychiatry* 140(4): 490–1.
6. Lin KM, Poland RE, Lau JK, Rubin RT. 1988. Haloperidol and prolactin concentrations in Asians and Caucasians. *J Clin Psychopharmacol* 8(3): 195–201.
7. Lin KM, Poland RE, Nuccio I, Matsuda K, Hathuc N, Su TP et al. 1989. A longitudinal assessment of haloperidol doses and serum concentrations in Asian and Caucasian schizophrenic patients. *Am J Psychiatry* 146(10): 1307–11.
8. Matsuda KT, Cho MC, Lin KM, Smith MW, Young AS, Adams JA. 1996. Clozapine dosage, serum levels, efficacy, and side-effect profiles: a comparison of Korean-Americans and Caucasian patients. *Psychopharmacol Bull* 32(2): 253–7.
9. Midha KK, Hawes E, Hubbard J, Korchinski ED, McKay G. 1988. Variation in the single dose pharmacokinetics of fluphenazine in psychiatric patients. *Psychopharmacology* 96(2): 206–11.
10. Potkin SG, Shen Y, Pardes H, Phelps BH, Zhou D, Shu L et al. 1984. Haloperidol concentrations elevated in Chinese patients. *Psychiatry Res* 12: 167–72.
11. Ruiz S, Chu P, Sramek JJ, Herrera J. 1996. Neuroleptic dosing in Asian and Hispanic outpatients with schizophrenia. *Mt Sinai J Med* 63(5&6): 306–9.
12. Sramek JJ, Sayles MA, Simpson GM. 1986. Antipsychotic dosage for Asians: a failure to replicate. *Am J Psychiatry* 143: 535–6.
13. Binder RL, Kazamatsuri H, Nishimura T, McNeil DE. 1987. Tardive dyskinesia and antipsychotic-induced parkinsonism in Japan. *Am J Psychiatry* 144(11): 1494–6.
14. Glazer WM, Morgenstern H, Doucette J. 1994. Race and tardive dyskinesia among outpatients at a CMHC. *Hosp Community Psychiatry* 45(1): 38–42.
15. Binder RL, Levy R. 1981. Extrapyramidal reactions in Asians. *Am J Psychiatry* 138(9): 1243–4.
16. Lieberman JA, Yunis J, Egea E, Canoso RT, Kane JM, Yunis EJ. 1990. HLA-B38, DR4, Dqw3 and clozapine-induced agranulocytosis in Jewish patients with Schizophrenia. *Arch Gen Psychiatry* 47(1): 945–8.
17. Sramek JJ, Roy S, Ahrens T, Pinanong P, Cutler NR, Pi E. 1991. Prevalence of tardive dyskinesia among three ethnic groups of chronic psychiatric patients. *Hosp Community Psychiatry* 42(6): 590–2.
18. Yunis JJ, Lieberman J, Yunis EJ. 1992. Major histocompatibility complex associations with clozapine-induced agranulocytosis. *Drug Saf* 7(1): 7–9.
19. Rosenblat R, Tang SW. 1987. Do Oriental psychiatric patients receive different dosages of psychotropic medication when compared with Occidentals. *Can J Psychiatry* 32: 270–4.
20. Jefferson JW, Greist JH. 1996. Brussels sprouts and psychopharmacology (understanding the cytochrome P450 enzyme system). In: Jefferson JW, Greist JH, eds. *Annual of Drug Therapy*, Vol. 3. Philadelphia: WB Saunders, pp. 2–22.
21. Nemeroff CB, Devane CL, Pollock BG. 1996. Newer antidepressants and the cytochrome P-450 system. *Am J Psychiatry* 153(3): 311–20.
22. Lin KM, Anderson D, Poland RE. 1995. Ethnicity and psychopharmacology: Bridging the gap. *Psychiatr Clin North Am* 18(3): 635–47.

23. Siddoway LA, Thompson KA, McCallister CB, Wang T, Wilkinson GR, Roen DM *et al.* 1987. Polymorphism of propafenone metabolism and disposition in man: clinical and pharmacokinetic consequences. *Circulation* **75**(4): 785–91.

24. Kroemer HK, Eichelbaum M. 1995. 'It's the genes, stupid'. Molecular basis and clinical consequences of genetic cytochrome P450 2D6 polymorphism. *Life Sci* **56**(26): 2285–99.

25. Lou YC, Ying L, Bertilsson L, Sjoqvist F. 1987. Low frequency of slow debrisoquine hydroxylation in a native Chinese population. *Lancet* **2**: 852–3.

26. Horai Y, Nakano M, Ishizaki T, Ishikawa K, Zhou HH, Zhou BJ *et al.* 1989. Metoprolol and mephenytoin oxidation polymorphisms in Far Eastern Oriental subjects Japanese versus mainland Chinese. *Clin Pharmacol Ther* **46**: 198–207.

27. Woolhouse NM, Andoh B, Mahgoub A, Sloan TP, Idle JR, Smith RL. 1979. Debrisoquin hydroxylation polymorphism among Ghanaians and Caucasians. *Clin Pharmacol Ther* **26**: 584–91.

28. Woolhouse N, Eichelbaum M, Oates NS, Idle JR, Smith RL. 1985. Dissociation of coregulatory control of debrisoquin/phenformin and sparteine oxidation in Ghanaians. *Clin Pharmacol Ther* **37**: 512–21.

29. Mbanefo D, Babbunkmi EA, Mahgoub A, Sloan TP, Idle Jr, Smith RL *et al.* 1980. A study of the debrisoquine hydroxylation polymorphism in a Nigerian population. *Xenobiotica* **10**: 811–18.

30. Iyun AO, Lennard MS, Tucker GT, Wood HJF. 1986. Metoprolol and debrisoquin metabolism in Nigerians: lack of evidence for polymorphic oxidation. *Clin Pharmacol Ther* **40**: 387–94.

31. Sommers K, Moncrieff J, Avenant J. 1988. Polymorphism of the 4-hydroxylation of debrisoquin in Bushmen of Southern Africa. *Hum Toxicol* **7**: 273–6.

32. Reling MV, Cherrie J, Schell MJ, Petros WP, Meyer WH, Evans WE. 1991. Lower prevalence of the debrisoquine oxidative poor metabolizer phenotype in African American versus Caucasian subjects. *Clin Pharmacol Ther* **50**: 308–13.

33. Marinac JS, Foxworth JW, Willsie SK. 1995. Dextromethorphan polymorphic hepatic oxidation (CYP2D6) in healthy Black American adult subjects. *Ther Drug Monit* **17**: 120–4.

34. Benitez J, Llerena A, Cogaled, J. 1988. Debrisoquine oxidation polymorphism in a Spanish population. *Clin Pharmacol Ther* **44**: 74–7.

35. Ramirez F. 1996. Ethnicity and psychopharmacology in Latin America. *Mt Sinai J Med* **63**(5&6): 330–1.

36. Johansson I, Yue QY, Dahl ML, Heim M, Säwe J, Bertilsson L *et al.* 1991. Genetic analysis of the interethnic differences between Chinese and Caucasians in the polymorphism of debrisoquine and codeine. *Eur J Clin Pharmacol* **40**(6): 553–6.

37. Lin KM, Poland RE, Lesser IM. 1986. Ethnicity and psychopharmacology. *Cult Med Psychiatry* **10**(2): 151–65.

38. Seeman P, Ulpian C, Chouinard G, Van Tol HHM, Dwosh H, Lieberman JA. 1994. Dopamine D4 receptor variant, D4GLYCINE194, in Africans, but not in Caucasians: no association with schizophrenia. *Am J Med Genet* **54**(4): 384–90.

39. Sramek JJ, Simpson GM. 1994. Antipsychotic drugs in schizophrenia. In: Cutler NR, Sramek JJ, Narang PK, eds. *Pharmacodynamics and Drug Development.* Chichester: Wiley, pp. 181–200.

40. Mendoza R, Smith MW, Poland RE, Lin KM, Strickland TL. 1991. Ethnic psychopharmacology: The Hispanic and Native American perspective. *Psychopharmacol Bull* **27**: 449–61.

41. Crabtree BL, Jann MW, Pitts WM. 1991. Alpha-1 acid glycoprotein levels in patients with schizophrenia: effect of treatment with haloperidol. *Biol Psychol* **29**: 70A.

42. Zhou HH, Adedoyin A, Wilkinson G. 1990. Differences in plasma binding of drugs between Caucasians and Chinese subjects. *Clin Pharmacol Ther* **48**(1): 10–7.

43. Conney AH, Pantuck EJ, Hsiao KC, Kuntzman R, Alvares AP, Kappas A. 1977. Regulation of drug metabolism in man by environmental chemicals and diet. *Fed Proc* **36**(5): 1647–52.

44. Jann MW, Saklad SR, Ereshefsky L, Richards AL, Harrington CA, Davis CM. 1986. Effects of smoking on haloperidol and reduced haloperidol plasma concentrations and haloperidol clearance. *Psychopharmacology* **90**(4): 468–70.

45. Pantuck EJ, Pantuck CB, Anderson K, Conney AH, Kappas A, Nutley N. 1982. Cigarette smoking and chlorpromazine disposition and action. *Clin Pharmacol Ther* **31**(4): 533–8.

46. Stimmel GL, Falloon IR. 1983. Chlorpromazine plasma levels, adverse effects, and tobacco smoking: case report. *J Clin Psychiatry* **44**: 420–2.

47. Sramek JJ, Herrera J, Swati R, Parent M, Hudgins R, Costa J et al. 1987. An analysis of steady state chlorpromazine plasma levels in the clinical setting. *J Clin Psychopharmacol* **7**(2): 117–18.

48. Ereshefsky L, Jann MW, Saklad SR, Davis CM, Richards AL, Burch NR. 1985. Effects of smoking on fluphenazine clearance in psychiatric inpatients. *Biol Psychiatry* **20**: 329–32.

49. Jusko WJ. 1978. Role of tobacco smoking in pharmacokinetics. *J Pharmacokinet Biopharm* **6**: 7–39.

50. Hymowitz N, Corle D, Royce J, Hartwell T, Corbett K, Orlandi M et al. 1995. Smokers' baseline characteristics in the COMMIT trial. *Prev Med* **24**(5): 503–8.

51. Rogers RG, Nam CB, Hummer RA. 1995. Demographic and socioeconomic links to cigarette smoking. *Soc Biol* **42**(1–2): 1–21.

52. Dollery CT, Fraser HS, Mucklow JC, Bulpitt CJ. 1979. Contribution of environmental factors to variability in human drug metabolism. *Drug Metab Rev* **9**(2): 207–20.

53. Naranjo CA, Bremner KE. 1993. Behavioral correlates of alcohol intoxication. *Addiction* **88**: 25–35.

54. Lane EA, Guthrie S, Linniola M. 1985. Effects of ethanol on drugs and metabolite pharmacokinetics. *Clin Pharmacokinet* **10**: 228–47.

55. Muhoberac BB, Roberts RK, Hoympa AM Jr, Schenker S. 1984. Mechanism(s) of ethanol–drug interaction. *Alcohol Clin Exp Res* **8**: 583–93.

56. Meir PJ. Alcohol, alcoholism and drugs. 1985. *Schweiz Med Wochenschr* **115**: 1792–803.

57. O'Hare T. 1995. Differences in Asian and White drinking: consumption level, drinking contexts, and expectancies. *Addict Behav* **20**(2): 261–6.

58. Higuchi S, Parrish KM, Dufour MC, Towle LH, Harford TC. 1994. Relationship between age and drinking patterns and drinking problems among Japanese, Japanese-Americans, and Caucasians. *Alcohol Clin Exp Res* **18**(2): 305–10.

59. Li HZ, Rosenblood L. 1994. Exploring factors influencing alcohol consumption patterns among Chinese and Caucasians. *J Stud Alcohol* **55**(4): 427–33.

60. Cheung YW. 1993. Beyond liver and culture: a review of theories and research in drinking among Chinese in North America. *Int J Addict* **28**(14): 1497–513.

61. Wolff PH. 1972. Ethnic differences in alcohol sensitivity. *Science* **175**: 449–50.

62. Ewing JA, Rouse BA, Perllizzari ED. 1974. Alcohol sensitivity and ethnic background. *Am J Psychiatry* **131**(2): 206–10.

63. Ewing JA, Rouse A, Aderhold RM. 1979. Studies of the mechanism of Oriental hypersensitivity to alcohol. *Curr Alcohol* **5**: 45–52.

64. Seto A, Tricomi S, Goodwin DW, Kolodney R, Sullivan T. 1978. Biochemical correlates of ethanol-induced flushing in Orientals. *J Stud Alcohol* **39**: 1–11.

65. Wall TL, Ehlers CL. 1995. Acute affects of alcohol on P300 in Asians with different ALDH2 genotypes. *Alcohol Clin Exp Res* **19**(3): 617–22.

66. Olatawara MO. 1978. The effects of psychotropic drugs in different populations. *Bull World Health Organ* **56**: 519–23.
67. Michnovicz JJ, Bradlow HL. 1991. Altered estrogen metabolism and excretion in humans following consumption of indole-3-carbinol. *Nutr Cancer* **16**(1): 59–66.
68. Pantuck EJ, Pantuck CB, Garland WA. 1979. Stimulatory effect of brussels sprouts and cabbage on human drug metabolism. *Clin Pharmacol Ther* **25**(1): 88–95.
69. Kappas A, Anderson KE, Conney AH, Alvares AP. 1976. Influence of dietary protein and carbohydrate on antipyrine and theophylline metabolism in man. *Clin Pharmacol Ther* **20**(6): 643–53.
70. Kalow W. 1982. Ethnic differences in drug metabolism. *Clin Pharmacokinet* **7**(5): 373–400.
71. Patterson BH, Harlan LC, Block G, Kahle L. 1995. Food choices of Whites, Blacks and Hispanics: data from the 1987 National Health Interview Survey. *Nutr Cancer* **23**(2): 105–19.
72. Otero-Sabogal R, Sabogal F, Perez-Stable EJ, Hiatt RA. 1995. Dietary practices, alcohol consumption, and smoking behavior: ethnic, sex, and acculturation differences. *J Natl Cancer Inst Monogr* **18**: 73–82.
73. Liu GT. 1991. Effects of some compounds isolated from Chinese medicinal herbs in hepatic microsomal cytochrome P-450 and their potential biological consequences. *Drug Metab Rev* **23**(3&4): 439–65.
74. Luscombe DK. 1977. Factors influencing plasma drug concentrations. *J Int Med Res* **5**(Suppl 1): S82–97.
75. Lawson GM. 1994. Monitoring of serum haloperidol. *Mayo Clin Proc* **69**(2): 189–90.
76. Anderson, KE. 1988. Influences of diet and nutrition on clinical pharmacokinetics. *Clin Pharmacokinet* **14**: 325–46.
77. O'Mahony MS, Woodhouse, KW. 1994. Age, environmental factors and drug metabolism. *Pharmacol Ther* **61**(1–2): 279–87.
78. Garver DL, Griffith J, Hirschowitz J. 1994. Minimum effective dose of haloperidol in treatment of psychoses [abstract]. *Biol Psychiatry* **35**: 667.
79. Janicak PG, Javaid JI, Sharma RP, Leach A, Dowd S, Blake L *et al*. 1994. Random assignment to three haloperidol plasma levels for acute psychosis [abstract]. *Biol Psychiatry* **35**: 366.
80. Bjorndal N, Bjerre M, Gerlach J, Kristjansen P, Magelund G, Oestrich IH *et al*. 1980. High dosage haloperidol therapy in chronic schizophrenic patients: a double-blind study of clinical response, side-effects, serum haloperidol, and serum prolactin. *Psychopharmacology* **67**(1): 17–23.
81. Potkin SG, Shen YC, Zhou DF, Pardes H, Shu L, Phelps BH *et al*. 1985. Does a therapeutic window for plasma haloperidol exist?: Preliminary Chinese data. *Psychopharmacol Bull* **21**: 59–61.
82. Smith RC, Baumgartner R, Ravichandran GK, Shvartsburd A, Schoolar JC, Allen P *et al*. 1984. Plasma and red cell levels of thioridazine and clinical response in schizophrenia. *Psychiatry Res* **12**(4): 287–96.
83. Van Putten T, May PR, Jenden DJ. 1981. Does a plasma level of chlorpromazine help? *Psychol Med* **11**(4): 729–34.
84. Neborsky R, Janowsky D, Munson E, Depry D. 1981. Rapid treatment of acute psychotic symptoms with high and low dose haloperidol. *Arch Gen Psychiatry* **38**: 195–9.
85. Kapur S, Remington G, Jones C, Wilson A, Da Silva J, Houle S *et al*. 1996. High levels of dopamine D_2 receptor occupancy with low-dose haloperidol treatment: a PET study. *Am J Psychiatry* **153**(7): 948–50.
86. Baldessarini RJ, Katz B, Cotton P. 1984. Dissimilar dosing with high potency and low potency antipsychotics. *Am J Psychiatry* **141**(6): 748–52.

87. Adebimpe VR. 1981. Overview: white norms and psychiatric diagnosis of Black patients. *Am J Psychiatry* **138**(3): 279–85.
88. Mukherjee S, Shukla S, Woodle J, Rosen AM, Olarte S. 1983. Misdiagnosis of schizophrenia in bipolar patients: a multiethnic comparison. *Am J Psychiatry* **140**(12): 1571–4.
89. Strakowski SM, Lonczak HS, Sax KW, West SA. 1995. The effects of race on diagnosis and disposition from a psychiatric emergency service. *J Clin Psychiatry* **56**(3): 101–7.
90. Segal SP, Bola JR, Watson MA. 1996. Race, quality of care, and antipsychotic prescribing practices in psychiatric emergency services. *Psychiatr Serv* **47**(3): 282–6.
91. Lawson WB, Yesavage JA, Werner PD. 1984. Race, violence, and psychopathology. *J Clin Psychiatry* **45**: 294–7.
92. Cheung FK, Snowden LR. 1990. Community mental health and ethnic minority populations. *Community Ment Health J* **26**: 277–91.
93. Woodward AM, Dwinell AD, Arons BS. 1992. Barriers to mental health care for Hispanic Americans: A literature review and discussion. *J Ment Health Admin* **19**(3): 224–36.
94. Hough RL, Landsverk JA, Karno M, Burman MA, Timbers DM, Escobar JI. 1987. Utilization of health and mental health services by Los Angeles Mexican-American and non-Hispanic sites. *Arch Gen Psychiatry* **44**: 702–9.
95. Sue S, Fujino DC, Hu LT, Tekeuchi DT, Zane NW. 1991. Community mental health services for ethnic minority groups: a test of the cultural responsiveness hypothesis. *J Consult Clin Psychol* **59**: 533–40.
96. Adams GL, Dworkin RJ, Rosenberg SD. 1984. Diagnosis and pharmacotherapy issues in the care of Hispanics in the public sector. *Am J Psychiatry* **141**: 970–4.
97. Miranda J, Azocar F, Organista KC, Munoz FR, Lieberman A. 1996. Recruiting and retaining low-income Latinos in psychotherapy research. *J Consult Clin Psychol* **64**: 868–74.
98. Midha KK, Chakraborty BS, Ganes DA, Hawes EM, Hubbard JW, Keegan DL *et al.* 1989. Intersubject variation in the pharmacokinetics of haloperidol and reduced haloperidol. *J Clin Psychopharmacol* **9**(2): 98–104.
99. Kane JM, Smith JM. 1982. Tardive dyskinesia: prevalence and risk factors, 1959– 1979. *Arch Gen Psychiatry* **39**: 473–81.
100. Tepper SJ, Haas JF. 1979. Prevalence of tardive dyskinesia. *J Clin Psychiatry* **40**: 508– 16.
101. Sramek JJ, Pi EH. 1996. Ethnicity and antidepressant response. *Mt Sinai J Med* **63**: 320–5.
102. Loria CM, Bush TL, Carroll MD, Looker AC, McDowell MA, Johnson CL, Sempos CT. 1995. Macronutrient intakes among adult Hispanics: a comparison of Mexican Americans, Cuban Americans, and mainland Puerto Ricans. *Am J Public Health* **85**(5): 684–9.
103. Abrams B, Gundelman S. 1995. Nutrient intake of Mexican-American and non-Hispanic White women by reproductive status: results of two national studies. *J Am Diet Assoc* **95**(8): 916–18.
104. Svensson CK. 1989. Representation of American Blacks in clinical trials of new drugs. *JAMA* **261**: 263–5.
105. LaRosa JH, Seto B, Caban CE, Haynga EG. 1995. Including women and minorities in clinical research. *Appl Clin Trials* **4**(5): 31–8.
106. Lewis-Hall F. 1996. Gender differences in psychotropic medications. *Mt Sinai J Med* **63**(5&6): 326–9.
107. Chouinard G, Annabele I. 1982. Pimozide in the treatment of newly schizophrenic patients. *Psychopharmacology* **76**: 13–19.

108. Simpson GM, Yakalam KG, Levinson DF, Stephanos J, Sing Lo EE, Cooper TB. 1990. Single dose pharmacokinetics of fluphenazine after fluphenazine decanoate administration. *J Clin Psychopharmacol* **10**: 417–21.

109. Ereshefsky L, Saklad SR, Watanabe MD, Davis CM, Jann MW. 1991. Thiothixene pharmacokinetic interactions: a study of hepatic enzyme inducers, clearance inhibitors, and demographic variables. *J Clin Psychopharmacol* **11**: 269–301.

110. Smith JM, Dunn DD. 1979. Sex differences in the prevalence of severe tardive dyskinesia. *Am J Psychiatry* **136**: 1080–2.

111. Chouinard G, Annable I, Ross-Chouinard A, Nestoros JN. 1979. Factors related to tardive dyskinesia. *Am J Psychiatry* **136**: 79–83.

112. Edeki T. 1996. Clinical importance of genetic polymorphism of drug oxidation. *Mt. Sinai J Med* **63**(5&6): 291–300.

113. Ereshefsky L, Saklad SR, Watanabe MD, Davis CM, Jann MW. 1991. Thiothixene pharmacokinetic interaction: A study of hepatic enzyme inducers, clearance inhibitors, and demographic variables. *J Clin Psychopharmacol* **11**: 269–301.

114. Jann MW, Ereshefsky L, Saklad SR, Seidel DL, Davis CM, Burch NR *et al.* 1985. Effects of carbamazepine on plasma haloperidol levels. *J Clin Psychopharmacol* **5**: 106–9.

115. Llerena A, Herraiz AG, Cobaleda J, Johansson I, Dahl ML. 1993. Debrisoquine and mephenytoin hydroxylation phenotypes and CYP2D6 genotype in patients treated with neuroleptic and antidepressant agents. *Clin Pharmacol Ther* **54**: 606–11.

12

Treatment of the African-American Patient with Novel Antipsychotic Agents

Pierre V. Tran[a], William B. Lawson[b], Scott Andersen[a] and Erina Shavers[a]

[a]Eli Lilly and Company, Indianapolis, IN, USA;
[b]Indiana University School of Medicine, Indianapolis, IN, USA

AFRICAN AMERICAN DEMOGRAPHICS

According to the US Census Bureau, the African-American population was estimated at 33 million (or 12.7% of the total American population) in 1994, and is predicted to reach 35.5 million (12.8%) in the year 2000. The African-American population has grown faster than either the total or the Caucasian population since the 1980 decennial census [1]. Assuming a lifetime prevalence rate of approximately 1%, the number of African Americans suffering from schizophrenia may be estimated to be around 330 000. This represents a large and important minority group among patients with schizophrenia.

DIAGNOSIS OF SCHIZOPHRENIA AND ANTIPSYCHOTIC TREATMENT AMONG AFRICAN AMERICANS

It is often difficult to recognize and diagnose psychiatric illnesses in African-American patients. Several studies suggest that African-American patients are more likely than Caucasians to receive a diagnosis of psychotic illness, such as schizophrenia, rather than a mood disorder [3–5]. The difficulty in diagnosis may lie in a number of factors including social stigma and failure of therapists to recognize that African Americans constitute a culturally distinct group of patients with unique needs [2]. However, the trend in diagnosing African-American patients with psychotic illness rather than mood disorder is evident even though more formal structured diagnostic instruments are used [5]. African-American schizophrenic patients were found to suffer from more severe first-rank symptoms than Caucasian patients during a DSM-IV Field Trial for schizophrenia and other psychotic disorders [5].

Cross Cultural Psychiatry. Edited by John M. Herrera, William B. Lawson and John J. Sramek.
© 1999 John Wiley & Sons Ltd.

In addition to the problem of overdiagnosis of schizophrenia, African Americans are more likely than other groups to be admitted into a psychiatric institution involuntarily, confined in seclusion and restraints, and medicated more often and with higher doses of antipsychotics [6]. Patients of African descent have a higher non-compliance rate with antipsychotic medications and receive more injectable neuroleptic medications than patients of other ethnic groups [7]. A study of the prescription practices over a 5-year period at four urban general hospitals in California shows that clinicians, composed primarily of Caucasians, prescribe more psychotropics to African-American patients. They also write more prescriptions for oral and injectable antipsychotic medications. In this study, African-American patients received a mean 24-hour dosage of antipsychotics of 1321 mg in chlor-promazine equivalents (compared with 825 mg for other patients; the difference is statistically significant) [8]. This tendency to overmedicate could result in increased neuroleptic side-effects and adversely affect compliance rate.

ANTIPSYCHOTIC METABOLISM AND PHARMACOKINETICS

Ethnicity has an influence on the pharmacokinetics of drugs. In general, potential ethnic differences exist with drugs that undergo gut and hepatic first-pass metabolism and which bind highly to plasma proteins [9]. Most antipsychotic drugs fall into this category. The cytochrome P-450 (CYP) system of isoenzymes is involved in the metabolism of antipsychotics. Genetic polymorphism exists with several CYP isoenzymes. For example, individuals with an abnormal functional form of CYP2D6 are called poor or slow metabolizers. It has been estimated that 1.9% of the African Americans are poor metabolizers and up to one-third are considered slow metabolizers [6, 10]. Such conditions could lead to accumulation of drugs and higher incidence of adverse effects. Antipsychotics with active metabolites, such as halo-peridol or risperidone, are predicted to have even more potential for ethnic variation in metabolism. African Americans seem to exhibit a higher level of reduced haloperidol (an active metabolite of haloperidol) than Caucasian patients under steady-state conditions [11]. However, no differences are found between African Americans and Caucasians in the plasma concentration of fluphenazine following a single dose [12]. Also, a single-dose pharmacokinetics study of trifluoperazine found no significant difference between Canadian Blacks and Caucasians [13].

ETHNIC DIFFERENCES IN ANTIPSYCHOTIC SIDE-EFFECTS

Most of the studies comparing the incidence of adverse effects of antipsychotic drugs among patients of different ethnic backgrounds have been conducted in Asians and Caucasians [10]. African-American patients have a 60% chance of developing acute extrapyramidal symptoms during the first 2 weeks of haloperidol treatment; the rate is 75% in Caucasian patients [14]. Tardive dyskinesia is a troublesome and debilitating adverse effect of neuroleptics. A study in patients hospitalized for at least 1 year found a slightly lower rate of tardive dyskinesia among African Americans (17%) than Caucasians (18.9%) [15]. However, when more stringent research criteria for defining treatment emergent tardive dyskinesia were used, the rate among the African Americans was higher than that of the Caucasian patients [16] and seems to have been independent of neuroleptic doses and treatment duration [17].

LIMITATIONS OF CONVENTIONAL NEUROLEPTICS AND RECENT ADVANCES IN ANTIPSYCHOTIC THERAPY

Despite the paucity of well controlled clinical trials of antipsychotics in African-American patients, it is generally accepted that antipsychotics are effective in this group. However, the limitations of the conventional neuroleptics are likely to also apply in African Americans. While conventional neuroleptics are mostly effective against psychotic symptoms, they have limited efficacy against negative symptoms and against many comorbid symptoms found with psychotic disorders such as depression, anxiety, and cognitive impairment. However, even in psychotic symptoms, as many as half of the patients with schizophrenia derive only partial benefit, or no benefit at all, from conventional agents. Conventional neuroleptics also cause many undesirable adverse effects, including acute extrapyramidal symptoms, tardive dyskinesia, and hyperprolactinemia. The troublesome adverse effects of conventional neuroleptics limit their use in many patients, contribute to non-compliance and frequent relapses, and serve as an impetus for the research of improved therapies.

In the last decade, antipsychotic research programs have successfully introduced a number of second-generation antipsychotic agents with differing pharmacology and side-effect profiles. Given that African Americans with mental illness are more likely to be prescribed with antipsychotics, to develop tardive dyskinesia, and to experience non-compliance with antipsychotic medications, these patients in particular should benefit from antipsychotic drugs with improved efficacy and minimal neurological side-effects. However, although the availability of more antipsychotic agents means that there are more treatment options, it also renders optimization of each individual antipsychotic regimen more complex. Ideally, clinical decisions should be guided by information derived from high-quality scientific research. A review of the efficacy and safety of each of the major second generation antipsychotic agent with relevant information pertaining to African Americans, when available, should provide a useful resource for clinicians who treat such patients.

Clozapine

Clozapine is the world's first novel and atypical antipsychotic agent. Clozapine was first introduced in the 1970s in Europe for the treatment of schizophrenia but was later withdrawn from the market when a number of patients developed fatal agranulocytosis. Scientific research resumed in the 1980s and clozapine was introduced in the USA in 1990 for the treatment of refractory schizophrenia; however, its use requires mandatory blood monitoring. The usefulness of clozapine in treatment-refractory schizophrenia was demonstrated in a landmark clinical trial comparing it with chlorpromazine [18]. Patients who failed to respond to at least three different neuroleptics and a prospective single-blind haloperidol lead-in period were randomized to receive either double-blind clozapine (up to 900 mg/day) or chlorpromazine (up to 1800 mg/day) for 6 weeks. After 6 weeks of double-blind therapy, 30% of the clozapine-treated patients and only 4% of chlorpromazine-treated patients ($p < 0.001$) had improved based on an *a priori* definition of response. Clozapine-treated patients showed significant improvement from baseline scores on the Simpson Angus Scale, suggesting low extrapyramidal symptoms. With a total of 319 patients entered into the study, close to one-fifth (74 of 319; 23%) were African Americans. However, because the results are presented as a group, it is not possible to determine the effect of clozapine in African-American patients.

A brief report from a group in the UK suggests that the stringent criteria of the mandatory Clozaril Patient Monitoring Program may be a barrier for the initiation of clozapine therapy in patients of African descent [19]. Hospital records in a British hospital show that Black African and African Caribbean patients usually have low white cell counts that prevent them from meeting the minimum level ($> 3.5 \times 10^9/l$) required for receiving clozapine. Because of the life-threatening nature of agranulocytosis and the need for protection of all patients receiving clozapine, the manufacturer of clozapine will not consider relaxation of the treatment criteria. Another study conducted among 805 patients treated with clozapine at 96 Department of Veterans' Affairs hospitals finds that African-American patients are more likely than non-African Americans to stop clozapine treatment, possibly due to low baseline white blood cell counts [20]. This hematological condition prevents many African-American patients from receiving clozapine.

In summary, African-American patients who are resistant to conventional neuroleptic agents may benefit from treatment with clozapine. Additional benefits of clozapine include its low potential to induce acute EPS and treatment-emergent dyskinesia [21]. Unfortunately, these benefits are mitigated by potential life-threatening adverse effects, a complex dosing regimen, and a costly and troublesome blood monitoring program. As safer novel antipsychotics become available, clozapine should be increasingly used as a back-up antipsychotic.

Risperidone

Risperidone was introduced in the USA in 1994. Its clinical development was supported by two placebo-controlled trials in North America [22, 23] and a large multinational trial [24]. In the two North-American studies, fixed doses of 2, 6, 12, and 16 mg/day of risperidone were compared with a fixed dose of 20 mg/day of haloperidol, or placebo. After 8 weeks, doses of risperidone above 2 mg (6, 12, and 16 mg) were more efficacious than placebo in improving overall psychotic symptoms. In the multinational study, fixed doses of 1, 4, 8, 12, and 16 mg/day of risperidone were compared with a fixed daily dose of 10 mg of haloperidol. After 8 weeks of therapy, the maximum efficacy against overall psychotic symptoms was achieved with 4 and 8 mg and the maximum efficacy against positive symptoms found with 16 mg of risperidone. All three studies reported dose-dependent treatment-emergent acute EPS in the subjects receiving risperidone. A review of the incidence of EPS in the two combined North-American studies concluded that there is a linear relationship between dose of risperidone and severity of EPS. This relationship translates into a dose-response curve that seems to mimic some of the conventional neuroleptics [25]. The North-American studies suggested an optimal dose of 6 mg/day; the multinational study suggested a range of 4–8 mg as an optimal range.

These three major risperidone trials contain no information of whether patients of African descent participated. In the absence of pertinent clinical trial data in African Americans, the usefulness of risperidone in patients of African origin can only be extrapolated from overall trial results. The antipsychotic advantage of the drug may be limited by the dose-dependent EPS seen in its entire spectrum of effectiveness (4–16 mg). Risperidone therapy should therefore be initiated by a period of slow upward titration before reaching the efficacious dose range. Individuals who are more susceptible to acute EPS may need to receive low or suboptimal doses of risperidone. These precautions and limitations may be seen as a disadvantage in managing African-American patients, who tend to experience more prominent first-rank symptoms. Also, the absence of well controlled long-term studies of risperidone in treatment-emergent tardive dyskinesia limits the usefulness of the drug in African-American patients who are prone to develop this condition. The risk of developing tardive dyskinesia has been linked to earlier treatment-related experiences of EPS [26, 27].

Olanzapine

Olanzapine is a novel atypical antipsychotic with a broad pharmacological profile similar to that of clozapine. Olanzapine has been available in the USA since October 1996. Results from four large, multicenter, double-blind studies suggest that the agent is effective against overall psychotic symptoms and negative symptoms in a dose range of 10–20 mg/day [28–31]. A placebo-controlled dose finding study shows that olanzapine has low EPS potential (comparable to that of placebo) and is not associated with dose-dependent EPS over even a wide therapeutic dose range [29]. Path analysis shows that the improvement in negative symptoms is mainly due to a direct effect of olanzapine on (presumably) primary negative symptoms [32]. Treatment with olanzapine is associated with a greater improvement in depressive symptoms than haloperidol, suggesting that olanzapine possesses antidepressant properties [33]. In a direct head-to-head comparative double-blind study between olanzapine (10–20 mg) and risperidone (4–12 mg), treatment with olanzapine has a better effect on response rates (>40% in PANSS total), negative symptoms (SANS summary, mean change from baseline), depressive symptoms (PANSS depression), and maintenance therapy, than treatment with risperidone, with significantly less treatment-emergent pseudoparkinsonism, akathisia, dyskinesia, sexual dysfunction, hyperprolactinemia, and fewer suicide attempts [34]. Additionally, long-term, double-blind treatment with olanzapine results in significantly fewer treatment-emergent dyskinesia reports than haloperidol, suggesting a low potential to induce tardive dyskinesia [35]. Finally, the dosing schedule of olanzapine is simple: the starting dose is generally an effective dose (10 mg) given once a day with no need for initial titration.

Many of the studies of olanzapine enrolled patients of African descent. The largest of these studies, an international multicenter, double-blind, collaborative study, enrolled a total of 1996 patients and compared olanzapine (5–20 mg) with haloperidol (5–20 mg) [31]. A total of 219 patients were of African descent (138 taking olanzapine, 81 taking haloperidol). When spontaneous treatment-emergent adverse events suggesting pseudoparkinsonism (akinesia, cogwheel rigidity, extrapyramidal syndrome, hypertonia, hypokinesia, masked facies, tremor, and parkinsonism) are examined, treatment with olanzapine results in significantly fewer such events (4.32%) than treatment with haloperidol (22.22%; $p<0.001$). These preliminary results, along with the overall clinical profile, suggest that olanzapine offers significant advantages over many existing antipsychotics in improving treatment outcome and compliance among African-American patients.

CONCLUSION

African-American patients suffering from schizophrenia represent an important group of minority patients. Advances in antipsychotic therapy with innovative agents such as olanzapine should benefit these patients as well as those in other ethnic groups. However, research examining potential ethnic differences in both the response and tolerability to these newer agents remains limited. Such research should be encouraged to help clinicians improve their prescription skills for optimal treatment outcome.

REFERENCES

1. Bennett CE, DeBarros KA. US Census Bureau, the Official Statistics.
2. Carter JH. 1974. Recognizing psychiatric symptoms in black Americans. *Geriatrics* **29**: 95–9.
3. Jones BE, Gray BA. 1986. Problems in diagnosing schizophrenia and affective disorders among blacks. *Hosp Community Psychiatry* **37**: 61–5.

4. Neighbors HW, Jackson JS, Campbell L, William D. 1989. The influence of racial factors on psychiatric diagnosis: a review and suggestions for research. *Community Ment Health J* **25**(4): 301–11.

5. Strakowski SM, Flaum M, Amador X, Bracha HS, Pandurangi AK, Robinson D, Tohen M. 1996. Racial differences in the diagnosis of psychosis. *Schizophr Res* **21**(2): 117–24.

6. Lawson WB. 1996. Clinical issues in the pharmacotherapy of African-Americans. *Psychopharmacol Bull* **32**(2): 275–81.

7. Strickland TL, Ranganath V, Lin KM, Poland RE, Mendoza R, Smith MW. 1991. Psychopharmacologic considerations in the treatment of Black American populations. *Psychopharmacol Bull* **27**(4): 441–8.

8. Segal SP, Bola JR, Watson MA. 1996. Race, quality of care, and antipsychotic prescribing. *Psychiatr Serv* **47**(3): 282–6.

9. Johnson JA. 1997. Influence of race or ethnicity on pharmacokinetics of drugs. *J Pharm Sci* **86**(12): 1328–33.

10. Frackiewicz EJ, Sramek JJ, Herrera JM, Kurtz NM, Cutler NR. 1997. Ethnicity and antipsychotic response. *Ann Pharmacother* **31**: 1360–9.

11. Jann MW, Chang WH, Lam FYW, Hwu HG, Lin HN, Chen H *et al*. 1992. Comparison of haloperidol and reduced haloperidol plasma levels in four different ethnic populations. *Progr Neuropsychopharmacol Biol Psychiatry* **16**: 193–202.

12. Midha KK, Hawes EM, Hubbard JW, Korchinski ED, McKay G. 1988. Variation in the single dose pharmacokinetics of fluphenazine in psychiatric patients. *Psychopharmacology* **96**(2): 206–11.

13. Midha KK, Hawes EM, Hubbard JW, Korchinski ED, McKay G. 1988. A pharmacokinetic study of trifluoperazine in two ethnic populations. *Psychopharmacology* **95**(3): 333–8.

14. Binder RL, Levy R. 1981. Extrapyramidal reactions in Asians. *Am J Psychiatry* **138**(9): 1243–4.

15. Sramek JJ, Roy S, Ahrens T, Pinanong P, Cutler NR, Pi E. 1991. Prevalence of tardive dyskinesia among three ethnic groups of chronic psychiatric patients. *Hosp Community Psychiatry* **42**: 590–2.

16. Glazer WM, Morgenstern H, Doucette J. 1994. Race and tardive dyskinesia among outpatients at a CMHC. *Hosp Community Psychiatry* **45**(1): 38–42.

17. Jeste DV, Lindamer LA, Evans J, Lacro JP. 1996. Relationship of ethnicity and gender to schizophrenia and pharmacology of neuroleptics. *Psychopharmacol Bull* **32**(2): 243–51.

18. Kane J, Honigfeld G, Singer J, Meltzer H and the Clozaril Collaborative Study Group. 1988. Clozapine for the treatment-resistant schizophrenic: A double-blind comparison with chlorpromazine. *Arch Gen Psychiatry* **45**: 789–96.

19. Fisher N, Baigent B. 1996. Treatment with clozapine. Black patients' low white cell counts currently mean that they cannot be treated. *BMJ* **313**: 1262.

20. Moeller FG, Chen YW, Steinberg JL, Petty F, Ripper GW, Shah N, Garver DL. ND Risk factors for clozapine discontinuation among 805 patients in the VA hospital system. *Ann Clin Psychiatry* **7**(4): 167–73.

21. Johnson CG, Littrell KH, Magil AMH. 1994. Starting patients on clozapine in a partial hospitalization program. *Hosp Community Psychiatry* **45**: 264–8.

22. Chouinard G, Jones B, Remington G, Bloom D, Addington D, MacEwan GW *et al*. 1993. A Canadian multicenter placebo-controlled study of fixed-doses of risperidone and haloperidol in the treatment of chronic schizophrenic patients. *J Clin Psychopharmacol* **13**: 25–40.

23. Marder SR, Meibach RC. 1994. Risperidone in the treatment of schizophrenia. *Am J Psychiatry* **151**(6): 825–35.

24. Peuskens J, on behalf of the Risperidone Study Group. 1995. Risperidone in the

treatment of patients with chronic schizophrenia: a multi-national, multi-centre, double-blind, parallel-group study versus haloperidol. *Br J Psychiatry* **166**: 712–26.

25. Simpson GM, Lindenmeyer JP. 1997. Extrapyramidal symptoms in patients treated with risperidone. *J Clin Psychopharmacol* **17**(3): 194–201.

26. Annable L, Chouinard G, Ross-Chouinard A *et al.* 1991. The relationship between neuroleptic-induced parkinsonism and tardive dyskinesia. *Biol Psychiatry* **29**(Suppl. 11S): 210S–226S.

27. Barnes TRE, Braude WM. 1985. Akathisia variants and tardive dyskinesia. *Arch Gen Psychiatry* **42**: 874–8.

28. Beasley CM, Sanger T, Satterlee W, Tollefson G, Tran P, Hamilton S, and the olanzapine HGAP study group. 1996. Olanzapine versus placebo: Results of a double-blind, fixed-dose olanzapine trial. *Psychopharmacology* **124**: 159–67.

29. Beasley CM, Tollefson G, Tran P, Satterlee W, Sanger T, Hamilton S, and the Olanzapine HGAD Study Group. 1996. Olanzapine versus placebo and haloperidol. Acute-phase results of the North American double-blind olanzapine trial. *Neuropsychopharmacology* **14**(2): 111–23.

30. Beasley CM, Hamilton S, Crawford AM, Dellva MA, Tollefson GD, Tran PV *et al.* 1997. Olanzapine versus haloperidol: Acute phase results of the international double-blind olanzapine trial. *Eur Neuropsychopharmacol* **7**: 125–37.

31. Tollefson GD, Beasley CM, Tran VP, Street JS, Krueger JA, Tamura RN *et al.* 1997. Olanzapine versus haloperidol in the treatment of schizophrenia and schizoaffective and schizophreniform disorders: Results of an international collaborative trial. *Am J Psychiatry* **154**(4): 457–65.

32. Tollefson GD, Sanger TM. 1997. Negative symptoms: A path analytic approach to a double-blind, placebo- and haloperidol-controlled clinical trial with olanzapine. *Am J Psychiatry* **154**(4): 466–74.

33. Tollefson GD, Sanger TM, Lu Y, Thieme ME. 1988. Depressive signs and symptoms in schizophrenia. A prospective blinded trial of olanzapine and haloperidol. *Arch Gen Psychiatry* **55**: 250–8.

34. Tran VP, Hamilton SH, Kuntz AJ, Potvin JH, Andersen SW, Beasley CM Jr, Tollefson GD. 1997 Double-blind comparison of olanzapine versus risperidone in the treatment of schizophrenia and other psychotic disorders. *J Clin Psychopharmacol* **17**(5): 407–18.

35. Tollefson GD, Beasley CM, Tamura RN, Tran PV, Potvin JH. 1997 Blind, controlled, long-term study of the comparative incidence of treatment-emergent tardive dyskinesia with olanzapine or haloperidol. *Am J Psychiatry* **154**(9): 1248–54.

13

Schizophrenia Among Hispanics

**Albana M. Dassori, Alexander L. Miller
and Delia Saldaña**
University of Texas Health Science Center, San Antonio, TX, USA

INTRODUCTION

A number of studies point to the influence of culture and ethnicity on the presentation and course of schizophrenia. The goals of this chapter are to review the literature on schizophrenia among Hispanics in the USA and to use the results of this review as a basis for identifying areas for future research into cultural and ethnic factors that affect the presentation and course of schizophrenia in this group.

The underlying premise of this work is that culture and ethnicity can influence the presentation and course of schizophrenia in a variety of ways [1]. Much of the support for this premise comes from two related studies: the International Pilot Study of Schizophrenia (IPSS) and the Determinants of Outcome of Severe Mental Disorders (DOSMD) [2, 3]. These studies examined the prevalence and course of schizophrenia in a number of developing and developed countries. Some of the most important findings were that (1) the prevalence of schizophrenia did not differ significantly across sites and (2) the course of schizophrenia, from the vantage points of hospitalization and a wide range of measures of social functioning, was more benign in developing countries. Among the developing countries there was one Hispanic site: Cali, Colombia.

The finding of similar prevalence across widely divergent cultures and ethnic groups according to the International Classification of Diseases criteria (ICD-9) [4] is partial evidence that the phenomenology of schizophrenia is not grossly altered by the cultural and ethnic background of the patient. One must recognize, however, that there is a certain tautology in the IPSS study in that only patients who met certain phenomenological criteria were diagnosed with schizophrenia. There was (and is) no test for schizophrenia that is independent of phenomenological criteria. Thus, some aspects of schizophrenic psychopathology could differ substantially among groups in ways that significantly influence the applicability of diagnostic criteria while having little influence on gross measures of

Cross Cultural Psychiatry. Edited by John M. Herrera, William B. Lawson and John J. Sramek.
© 1999 John Wiley & Sons Ltd.

prevalence. Even more likely, cultural and ethnic backgrounds may influence the degree, form, and recognition of manifest psychopathology. Further, the cultural and ethnic backgrounds of the interviewers could also influence the recognition of overt psychopathology. It should be noted that the IPSS used raters of the same ethnic and cultural backgrounds as the interviewees. Consequently, the interactive effects of differing interviewer–interviewee backgrounds on the identification of psychopathology, a common reality in the USA, were not explored.

The differences in the course of schizophrenia among countries are particularly intriguing. They suggest a powerful influence of environmental factors and imply the need for research into their nature and their ability to be modified for therapeutic purposes. Because the range of sociocultural environments in the countries of the IPSS was so great, it has been difficult to identify specific environmental factors that may have contributed to the differences in the course of schizophrenia among countries. The study of Hispanic groups within the USA has the potential for identifying and measuring a more manageable number of variables that may affect the phenomenology and course of schizophrenia. Further, since there is variation in generation and immigrant status within members of each ethnic group, studying Hispanics in the USA could also allow for evaluating the relationship between cultural change and psychopathology. Moreover, there are coexisting comparison groups of different ethnicities, and they can be matched sociodemographically (e.g. income, rural versus urban population) in order to assess the influences of culture and ethnicity independent of other sociodemographic factors.

REVIEW

Our review of the literature is divided into three major areas: epidemiology, phenomenology, and illness course and outcome. It is important to note that the term *Hispanic*, when applied to the US population, includes four major groups by area of family origin: Mexican, Puerto Rican, Central American, and Caribbean. As there is considerable cultural heterogeneity across these groups, this review specifies the group examined in the discussion of each study.

Epidemiology

Jaco [5] conducted the first major psychiatric epidemiological study of Mexican Americans, assessing the rate of new-onset psychosis in Texas over a 2-year period. He reported that the rate for Mexican Americans in Texas was the lowest of three cultural groups (Anglo Americans, African Americans, and Mexican Americans). Two major issues should be considered in evaluating this study. First, it focused on treated psychotic illness and consequently patients who were not in contact with mainstream health services were not included. Second, diagnostic criteria were not standardized; therefore, there may have been individual variations among clinicians' perceptions of the clinical picture.

In contrast to Jaco's study, the Los Angeles Epidemiologic Catchment Area (LAECA) study [6] used a standardized instrument, the Diagnostic Interview Schedule (DIS) [7], to assess the lifetime prevalence of specific DSM-III-defined psychiatric disorders [8] in a community sample in Los Angeles. The results of the LAECA study indicated that, although the lifetime prevalence of schizophrenia was not significantly different between Mexican Americans (0.4%) and non-Hispanic Whites (0.8%), there was a low rate among Hispanic males. Specifically, virtually no Hispanic males aged 30 and over were included in the 1-year prevalence category [9].

Although the use of standardized instruments and well-defined diagnostic criteria represents important methodological improvement, some issues are still problematic.

1. First, prevalence estimates can be affected by respondents' language, which can influence how symptoms are reported. In this regard, results have been conflicting. For example, Marcos et al. [10] indicated that patients with schizophrenia who spoke primarily Spanish could appear more disturbed when interviewed in English. On the other hand, del Castillo [11] and Segovia-Price and Cuellar [12] reported that bilingual schizophrenics tended to express more psychopathology when interviewed in Spanish.

2. Second, response styles may differ across ethnic groups. For example, Randolph et al. [13] compared 81 Anglo and Hispanic subjects with schizophrenia in their responses to the DIS, the Brief Psychiatric Rating Scale (BPRS) [14], the Clinical Global Impression (CGI) [15], and the Hopkins Symptom Checklist 90 (SCL-90) [16]. The proportion of patients who 'denied' lifetime schizophrenic symptoms in the DIS (DIS-negative subjects) was very similar in both ethnic groups. Responses by DIS-negative subjects to the SCL-90 were significantly different, however. While a subgroup of Anglo subjects volunteered symptoms in the SCL-90, Hispanics continued to deny symptomatology, which suggests that Hispanics may underreport symptomatology even when using self-report instruments. These results conflict with a previous study of applicants to outpatient psychotherapy [17], in which Hispanic patients reported the highest symptom levels on 8 of 11 measures of the SCL-90. Differences in the stigma experienced by the two patient populations (psychotic patients versus candidates for outpatient psychotherapy) might explain the inconsistency.

3. Third, diagnostic categories are based on the prevailing definition of mental disorders as conceptualized by 'Euro–American' psychiatry; cultural variations in the construction and definition of psychiatric syndromes have not been fully addressed, because most of the literature has focused on the so-called culture-bound syndromes.

In summary, no statistically significant differences in prevalence rates were reported. The very low prevalence rate among Mexican-American males is worth noting and warrants further investigation. The influences of the diagnostic criteria used, the language of the interview and the response style of the subjects under study also need to be evaluated.

Phenomenology

Several attempts have been made to evaluate the phenomenology of schizophrenia among Hispanics. The studies are quite diverse in terms of the population assessed and the methodology and criteria used. Fabrega *et al.* [18, 19] compared the clinical profiles of Mexican-American, Anglo-American, and African-American patients in the Texas State mental hospital system. Their findings indicate the importance of controlling for social class variables and point to a trend toward greater impairment or pathology within Mexican-American patients with schizophrenia. The possibility of a more debilitating illness presentation among Hispanics (mainly Mexican Americans) and African Americans was also postulated by Velazquez and Callahan [20] on the basis of the Minnesota Multiphasic Personality Inventory (MMPI) [21] profiles of the sample. In contrast, Cuellar [22], using the Psychotic Inpatient Profile (PIP) [23], concluded that Mexican-American psychotic patients (DSM-II) [24] displayed behaviors very similar to those of other psychotic groups.

Primary symptoms of schizophrenia were also very similar among a group of Hispanic and Anglo veterans [25]. The Hispanic sample was relatively well acculturated, and more than two-thirds of the subjects were at least second-generation Americans. Symptoms were elicited by means of the DIS and a battery of rating instruments including the BPRS, the Global Assessment Scale (GAS) [26], and the SCL-90. Major differences were found between Anglo and Hispanic subjects in age at onset and use of services. Hispanics reported a later age at onset and less overall use of inpatient services. In addition, in DIS interviews Hispanics had a greater number of lifetime DSM-III diagnoses, including substance abuse and affective and somatization disorders. The existence of ethnic differences even in a fairly well acculturated sample of Hispanic veterans supports the concept of ethnic (cultural or biological) factors influencing the clinical presentation of schizophrenia.

The complexity of the diagnostic process among Hispanics is also suggested by Chen *et al.* [27], who evaluated the association of demographic factors with change in diagnosis from schizophrenia to other disorders and from other disorders to schizophrenia, as well as the time elapsed before diagnostic change. The authors conducted a retrospective longitudinal study of inpatient data from a public psychiatric hospital from a 7-year period. Results indicate that Hispanics had a significantly higher rate of diagnostic change from schizophrenia to another disorder (odds ratio 2.79) than Caucasians, and had average time between the initial diagnosis and a change in diagnosis of 31 months. Potential explanations for this finding include interviewer biases and ethnic variation in the prominence of psychotic symptomatology within the context of mental disorders other than schizophrenia.

Ethnic differences between Hispanic groups in the DIS profile of psychotic disorder have also been reported. Rubio-Stipec *et al.* [28] compared the psychotic disorder factor structure obtained in a Puerto Rican sample with an Anglo-American sample and a Mexican-American sample. They reported a lower level of concordance (0.66) between the Puerto Ricans and the Mexican Americans than between the Puerto Ricans and the Anglo Americans (0.92).

Two other developments in the study of schizophrenia have also contributed to the growing interest in the understanding of its phenomenology. First, schizophrenia has gradually been recognized as phenomenologically diverse. Second, the clinical significance of positive and negative symptoms as markers of separable aspects of the illness in terms of etiology and prognostic significance is being increasingly recognized. These developments have raised important questions regarding the diagnosis of the different syndromes included under the term *schizophrenia*, and difficulties in conceptualizing these syndromes are still significant.

Using the Positive and Negative Syndrome Scale (PANSS) [29], Ramirez *et al.* [30] reported on ethnic differences in the total score of negative symptoms as well as in the scores of some of the subscales (passive–apathetic social withdrawal, lack of spontaneity in the flow of conversation), with Puerto Ricans showing fewer negative symptoms than Anglo patients. In addition, Puerto Ricans spent less time in the hospital and reported a later age at onset. The authors discussed various cultural explanations for these differences, including the placing of more emphasis on social interaction by Puerto Ricans than by Anglos.

In contrast, our own work has found that Mexican Americans exhibited more withdrawal on the social activity factor and more impairment on the cognition factor of the Negative Symptoms Scale (NSA) [31] than Anglo Americans [32]. These measures were obtained both at admission to the hospital and at the end of 1–2 weeks off antipsychotic drugs. Ethnic groups did not differ on any of the factors of the BPRS. Although these results are preliminary, they provide support for the hypothesis of ethnic differences in the presentation of negative, but not positive, symptoms in schizophrenia. Alternatively, they may indicate that cognition has not been assessed in a culturally sensitive manner, particularly because the assessment of certain items (abstraction, temporal orientation) included in the cognition subscale may be influenced by the respondents' culture. In this regard, investigators at our program have examined the utility of another measurement of cognitive functioning in different ethnic groups: the Allen Cognitive Level (ACL) Assessment [33]. The ACL measures the patient's ability to follow instructions in performing a simple stitching task. In their triethnic comparison (non-Hispanic Whites, Mexican Americans and African Americans), Velligan *et al.* [34] found that the ACL is a valid and culturally unbiased measure of cognitive functioning that can help determine how a patient is likely to perform activities of daily living.

In summary, several studies suggest the existence of ethnic differences in the clinical presentation of schizophrenia. Moreover, differences in phenomenology appear to exist among certain subgroups of Hispanics. Inferences should be made with caution, because studies vary in the diagnostic groups assessed (psychosis, schizophrenia), in the criteria used to select subjects (clinicians' diagnoses, DSM-II, DSM-III, DSM-III-R [35]), in the samples included (hospital samples versus community samples, new-onset versus chronic patients), and in the instruments employed for the evaluation of psychopathology (DIS, BPRS, CGI, SCL-90, MMPI, PIP, GAS, PANSS, NSA). Therefore, the extent to which the reported differences are due to the method of assessment, the type of population evaluated, or the impact of cultural or socioeconomic factors is still unclear. Finally, most of these studies had a cross-sectional design and provide us with information on illness phenomenology at a single point in time. The extent to which symptoms vary over time across ethnic groups is not known.

ILLNESS COURSE AND OUTCOME

We have divided research done on the course and outcome of schizophrenia among Hispanics into four areas: (1) illness definition, (2) help-seeking behavior, (3) response to pharmacological treatment, and (4) post-treatment adjustment.

Illness Definition

The first area involves understanding how Hispanics conceptualize schizophrenia, since that concept partially determines their attitudes toward the sick member, their help-seeking behavior, and compliance with treatment. Jenkins [36] reported that relatively unacculturated Mexican-American families used the term *nervios* to refer to a wide range of distressing emotional experiences and illness phenomena, including depression, anxiety, panic, and schizophrenia. She suggested that preference for the use of the term *nervios* was linked to family efforts to reduce the stigma associated with mental illness, strengthening the bonds among the members. She postulated that its use could mediate the course and outcome of the schizophrenic disorder. In another ethnographic study of unacculturated Mexican origin families of severely mentally ill patients [37], the term *nervios* was used by 47% of the family members to describe the ailment of their sick relative, while the term *enfermedad mental* was used by only 18%.

The knowledge of the terminology used by patients and families is only one step toward improving the understanding of schizophrenia cross culturally. Further research is needed on identifying those symptoms that indicate the presence of an 'illness' and trigger help-seeking behavior. And, despite postulated interpretations of labels, further information from respondents on the meaningfulness of various terms would help to guide interventions addressing perceptions of stigma, tolerance, or prognostic expectations.

Help-seeking Behavior

Urdaneta et al. [37] report that 60% of the respondents attached importance to the patients' symptoms and tried to do something about them. Even when formal services were immediately consulted, almost one-quarter of the whole sample reported attempting to treat symptoms at home. These results conflict with earlier beliefs that Mexican Americans are fatalistically inclined and resigned to suffer whatever destiny brings them. In fact, Mexican Americans, as well as other Hispanics, may attempt to cope with the problem of mental illness within the solidarity of the family [38, 39].

A significantly more negative view of hospitalization among Mexican Americans than among European Americans was reported by Lawson et al. [40] and partially supported by Escobar and colleagues' [25] findings of less overall use of inpatient services in Hispanics. Yet underuse of inpatient mental health services by Hispanics may not be a uniform phenomenon, as indicated by Snowden and Cheung [41]: region, and type of institutions represented (public, private, and Veterans Affairs hospitals) in the data, are important qualifiers.

Although results are far from conclusive, they point to the possibility that illness course among Hispanics may be characterized by fewer hospitalizations. The cause may be differential access to care, differential availability of services, or cultural characteristics that discourage use of professional services.

Response to Pharmacological Treatment

Once patients are in treatment, ethnic differences in response to medication and in the prevalence of adverse effects can also be present. These factors have been identified as important in determining compliance, which in turn influences illness course.

Lu et al. [42] reviewed records of 158 admissions from four ethnic groups (Asians, Hispanics, African Americans, and Caucasians). They found no significant differences in prevalence of extrapyramidal symptoms (EPS) and neuroleptic dosage associated with EPS. However, immigrant Asians and Hispanics had significantly lower mean maximal dosages than the other Asian or Hispanic groups and also than the Caucasian and African-American groups. The authors propose that environmental and cultural factors (diet, alcohol and other substances, smoking, and exposure to toxins) could differentially affect the absorption and metabolism of neuroleptics [43]. Ruiz et al. [44] and Collazo et al. [45] report that Hispanics and Asians received significantly less neuroleptic medication than Anglos in both outpatient and inpatient settings.

Using a more general approach, Lawson *et al.* [40] evaluated ethnic differences in treatment response by assessing the changes in psychopathology exhibited by a group of Mexican-American and European-American patients at the time of discharge from hospital. There were no ethnic differences in degree of psychopathology at admission or in response to treatment. Both groups showed a high degree of improvement as measured by both MMPI and clinical judgment.

Post-treatment Adjustment

The post-treatment adjustment of Hispanic patients with schizophrenia has been evaluated in terms of employment status, rehospitalization rates, and social functioning. This literature is scarce and tends to include patients with various psychiatric diagnoses within a single group. For example, Gonzalez and Cuellar [46] reported on the readmission rates of Mexican-American patients discharged from the San Antonio State Hospital. More than 60% of the patients carried a diagnosis of schizophrenia; the remaining patients had diagnoses of bipolar disorder and psychotic depression. Mexican Americans were found to have readmission rates similar to those of other ethnic groups.

The post-treatment adjustment of the sample appeared to be bleak, because none of the non-readmitted patients were employed full time after discharge. However, owing to the severity and chronicity of the illness, it is very likely that employment after discharge may not have been a useful criterion for measuring rehabilitation in this sample. Further, rates of employment after leaving hospital may reflect community factors such as vocational rehabilitation opportunities, stigma of mental illness, and ethnic discrimination.

In terms of social functioning, Sue *et al.* [47] used the GAS as a measure of post-treatment adjustment and reported a better outcome for Mexican Americans using outpatient services in the Los Angeles County mental health system. Ethnic match between therapist and client was significantly related to a decreased probability of dropping out from treatment only for the Mexican-American group whose primary language was not English.

Family factors may be moderators of the illness course and outcome. An important contribution to this research has been the attempts of Jenkins and colleagues [48–51] to assess the cultural validity of the constructs under study. One of these constructs has been expressed emotion (EE), which assesses the family's extent of criticality/overinvolvement with the relative with schizophrenia. Karno *et al.* [6] reported a significantly lower level of EE among Mexican-American households than in Anglo-American households. In addition, high levels of household EE, while significant, were slightly less predictive of relapse among Mexican Americans than among Anglo Americans and British patients. A tentative explanation given by the authors is the buffering of the high levels of EE by the larger size of Mexican-American households.

Research on the relationship between EE and relapse has led to the development of psychosocial interventions targeted at reducing relapse by lowering levels of EE [52]. The applicability of these interventions to a culturally diverse population remains unclear. In fact, Telles *et al.* [53] assessed the effectiveness and cross cultural applicability of one of these psychosocial interventions, Behavioral Family Management (BFM) [52] to a low-income Spanish-speaking population. The authors report that unacculturated patients who were treated with the BFM program had a significantly poorer course and 1-year outcome than those who received case management. The authors suggest that a highly structured intervention program such as the BFM might be experienced as intrusive and stressful by unacculturated families.

In summary, studies suggest that culture affects various aspects of the illness process and that family may have a central role in the course of illness. Nevertheless, the effect of inequalities in access to care, or type of assessment tools and outcome measures, on the differences observed is still unclear. Furthermore, the interplay among illness definition, help-seeking behavior, response to treatment, type of psychosocial interventions, and post-treatment adjustment requires further investigation.

DIRECTIONS FOR FUTURE RESEARCH

While research on schizophrenia among Hispanics in the USA has not been extensive, some intriguing findings have emerged. In fact, ethnic differences in phenomenology, clinical picture, and illness course and outcome have been reported. These results indicate the need for more research on the influence of ethnicity, on the various stages of illness, and on the context in which the illness process unfolds.

Some guidelines follow that can be used to direct future research ventures.

Delineation of the Sociocultural Attributes of the Group Under Study

To address the heterogeneity of the Hispanic population, investigators should focus on specific ethnic groups (Mexican Americans, Cuban Americans, Puerto Ricans, etc.), because regional variations in the extent of Indian, African, or European influences and differences in the social and historical realities of these groups can determine the way in which schizophrenia is experienced. Regional comparisons within a group (rural versus urban, southern Texas versus southern California, etc.) could be attempted. Further, comparisons of Hispanic patients with their counterparts in other ethnic groups within a limited geographic area could also yield important results that could be used to extend the conclusions of the IPSS and DOSMD studies.

Investigators need to evaluate how the process of cultural change influences the illness experience. As a first step towards achieving this goal, the concepts and operationalizations of acculturation should be refined. It is important to develop instruments that are inclusive enough to assess a wide array of cultural elements (values, behaviors, attitudes). At the same time, instruments should be succinct to allow efficient research applications. A possible approach could be to design an instrument in which investigators can select the number and nature of the cultural elements to be included on the basis of the problem under study. For example, some investigators may be interested in pursuing a detailed description of the cultural characteristics of a specific group: in this case, the assessment instrument should be as inclusive as possible. On the other hand, other investigators may be interested in evaluating the relationship between acculturation and compliance: in this case, the focus could be on the specific values (e.g. fatalism, religiosity) that the investigator conceptually identifies as influential for the behavior under study.

Finally, given that education and socioeconomic status can influence attitudes, values, and behaviors, investigators need to evaluate the variation of these cultural elements across social strata within the same ethnic group. Socioeconomic status and education levels should also be considered when illness process is compared across ethnic groups, particularly since ethnicity and lower social status often overlap in the USA [54]. Diverse approaches can be used (e.g. matching, stratification) in the study design and data analyses to help to separate the influences of socioeconomic status and education from the influence of culture. Some authors have proposed the use of a triethnic design [55], suggesting that if the differences between ethnic groups persist after controlling for the impact of minority status cultural factors need to be further explored. However, these approaches may be insufficient: for example, belonging to a specific social class or achieving a certain educational level may have very different implications in different ethnic groups. To address some of these biases, investigators have proposed the use of 'culture-neutral' measures as covariates, but there is little agreement on how to define these measures.

Validation of Assessment Instruments Across Ethnic Groups

The applicability of commonly used instruments to subjects from different cultural backgrounds needs to be examined. In general, investigators have addressed this issue by restricting their samples to English-speaking subjects, limiting the generalizability of results to other segments of the population. Recently, steps have been undertaken to develop methodologically sound translations, although few instruments have actually undergone this process [56]; in fact, little attention has been directed at regional language variations (local idioms, bilingual flexibility). Furthermore, the psychometric properties of the translated instruments have rarely been evaluated. To address this issue, investigators must examine the internal consistency of instruments as well as the distribution of scores in the population. As a complement to these validation studies, it would be important to evaluate the effects of the ethnic and cultural match between interviewer and interviewee on expression and perception of psychopathology.

Use of Innovative Approaches to Assess the Incidence and Prevalence of Illness in the Various Hispanic Groups and Regions

For example, the incidence and prevalence rates of schizophrenia could be initially examined by using a single set of diagnostic criteria. Subsequently, the effects on incidence and prevalence rates under broader and narrower definitions of schizophrenia in different ethnic cultural groups could be assessed.

Incorporation of a Qualitative Approach to Research Methodology

Although the strategies discussed above represent important steps, the applicability of the constructs under study to cultural groups other than non-Hispanic Whites remains elusive. Determining that applicability is a difficult process that implies the identification of universal versus group-specific concepts and requires qualitative analyses. A qualitative research approach focuses more on understanding the subject's perspective (emic) than on understanding the investigators' perspective (etic). Investigators, in turn, function primarily as witnesses to minimize artificial influences on the data collection process. This approach allows identification of indigenous categories, semantic expressions, attitudes, values, and norms. A qualitative analytic approach is also useful for theory building, as it can provide information to identify potentially important variables, point to possible causal networks, and generate hypotheses [57]. Likewise, as process is essential for this research strategy, a qualitative approach offers a good opportunity to investigate dynamic processes such as decision-making, interactions with healthcare providers, and so on [58].

Many investigators have been reluctant to apply a qualitative approach because of concerns with generalizability, subjectivity, and validity. Recent work has addressed these concerns, providing a systematic methodology for using these techniques [59, 60].

Use of Specific Illness Behavior Models

The use of specific models can benefit researchers by providing them with a conceptual paradigm to better understand the illness as a process. Through the use of a general model, investigators can conceptualize schizophrenia at various stages.

For example, by following the Suchman model [61], studies can focus on the prepatient phase or on the patient phase. The former includes the study of areas such as problem onset, recognition and identification, and response (lay consultation, lay referral, self-medication); the latter comprises the study of the patient–practitioner encounter and relationship, treatment compliance, and rehabilitation. Investigators can focus on specific aspects of the model, or can apply longitudinal research strategies to assess the unfolding of the illness process through the various phases, to identify help-seeking pathways [62] and to delineate the relationships among phenomenology, context (e.g. culture, family, socioeconomic factors), and course (prepatient and patient phases). A longitudinal approach, in which the assessment of use patterns across the whole array of services (e.g. day hospital, case management, outpatient clinic, emergency room, substance abuse) could be included, can also be applied to the study of ethnic/cultural differences in treatment careers.

Integration of Cross Cultural and Biological Studies

Biological measures (plasma/cerebrospinal fluid, 3-methoxy-4-hydroxyphenylglycol (MHPG), homovanillic acid (HVA)) and new, advanced diagnostic techniques such as positron emission tomography scanning should be applied to cross cultural studies for better insight into the biological substratum of the illness. For example, studies could evaluate the relationship between phenomenology and specific biological measures across ethnic groups. In doing so, investigators could start to comprehend whether ethnic differences are the result of cultural or biological variations.

Research on the relationship between schizophrenia and culture should not be understood as the result of an ethnocentric interest of a few investigators and as a product with limited practical applications. The growing number of culturally diverse patients demands an understanding of cultural influences if diagnosis and treatment are to be optimized.

REFERENCES

1. Kleinman, A. 1988. *Rethinking Psychiatry*. New York, NY: Free Press.
2. Sartorius N, Jablensky A, Shapiro R. 1977. Two-year follow-up of the patients included in the WHO International Pilot Study of Schizophrenia. *Psychol Med* **7**: 529–41.
3. Sartorius N, Jablensky A, Korten A, Ernberg, G *et al.* 1986. Early manifestations and first-contact incidence of schizophrenia in different cultures. *Psychol Med* **16**: 909–28.
4. World Health Organization. 1978. *ICD-9: International Classification of Diseases*. 9th ed. Geneva: WHO.
5. Jaco, EG. 1959. Mental health of the Spanish American in Texas. In: Opler MK, ed. *Culture and Mental Health: Cross-Cultural Studies*. New York: Macmillan, pp. 467–85.

6. Karno MJ, Hough RL, Burnam MA *et al.* 1987. Lifetime prevalence of specific psychiatric disorders among Mexican Americans and non-Hispanic whites in Los Angeles. *Arch Gen Psychiatry* **44**: 695–701.
7. Robins LN, Helzer JE, Weissman MM *et al.* 1984. Lifetime prevalence of specific psychiatric disorders in three sites. *Arch Gen Psychiatry* **41**: 949–58.
8. American Psychiatric Association. 1980. *DSM-III: Diagnostic and Statistical Manual of Mental Disorders.* 3rd ed. Washington, DC: APA.
9. Keith SM, Regier DA, Rae DS. 1991. Schizophrenic disorders. In: Robins LN, Regier DA, eds. *Psychiatric Disorders in America.* New York: Free Press, pp. 33–52.
10. Marcos LR, Albert M, Urcuyo L, Kesselman M. 1973. The effect of interview language on the evaluation of psychopathology in Spanish-American schizophrenic patients. *Am J Psychiatry* **130**: 549–53.
11. del Castillo JC. 1970. The influence of language upon symptomatology in foreign-born patients. *Am J Psychiatry* **127**: 242–4.
12. Segovia-Price C, Cuellar I. 1981. Effects of language and related variables on the expression of psychopathology in Mexican American psychiatric patients. *Hispanic J Behav Sci* **3**: 145–60.
13. Randolph ET, Escobar JI, Paz DH, Forsythe AB. 1985. Ethnicity and reporting of schizophrenic symptoms. *J Nerv Ment Dis* **173**: 332–40.
14. Overall JE, Gorham DR. 1962. The Brief Psychiatric Rating Scale. *Psychol Rep* **10**: 799–812.
15. Guy W. 1976. Clinical global impressions. In: Guy W, ed. *ECDEU Assessment Manual for Psychopharmacology.* Washington, DC: US Department of Health, Education, and Welfare, pp. 218–22.
16. Derogatis LD, Lipman RS, Rickels K. 1974. The Hopkins Symptom Checklist (HSCL): A self-report symptom inventory. *Behav Sci* **19**: 1–15.
17. Skilbeck WM, Acosta FX, Yamamoto J, Evans LA. 1984. Self-reported psychiatric symptoms among Black, Hispanic and White outpatients. *J Clin Psychol* **40**: 1184–9.
18. Fabrega H, Swartz JD, Wallace CA. 1968. Ethnic differences in psychopathology: 1. Clinical correlates under varying conditions. *Arch Gen Psychiatry* **19**: 218–26.
19. Fabrega H, Swartz JD, Wallace CA. 1968. Ethnic differences in psychopathology: II. Specific differences with emphasis on a Mexican American group. *J Psychiatry Res* **6**: 221–35.
20. Velazquez RJ, Callahan WJ. 1990. MMPI's of Hispanic, Black, and White DSM-III schizophrenics. *Psychol Rep* **66**: 819–22.
21. Hathaway SR, McKinley JC. 1943. *The Minnesota Multiphasic Personality Schedule.* Minneapolis: University of Minnesota Press.
22. Cuellar I. 1982. The diagnosis and evaluation of schizophrenic disorders among Mexican Americans. In: Becerra RM, Kamo M, Escobar JI, eds. *Mental Health and Hispanic Americans.* New York: Grune & Stratton, pp. 66–8.
23. Lorr M, Vestre ND. 1969. The Psychotic Inpatient Profile: A nurse's observation scale. *J Clin Psychol* **25**: 137–40.
24. American Psychiatric Association. 1968. *DSM-II: Diagnostic and Statistical Manual of Mental Disorders.* 2nd ed. Washington, DC: APA.
25. Escobar JI, Randolph ET, Hill M. 1986. Symptoms of schizophrenia in Hispanic and Anglo veterans. *Cult Med Psychiatry* **10**: 259–76.
26. Endicott J, Spitzer RL, Fleiss JL, Cohen J. 1976. The Global Assessment Scale: a procedure for measuring overall severity of psychiatric disturbance. *Arch Gen Psychiatry* **33**: 766–71.
27. Chen YR, Swann, AC, Burt DB. 1996. Stability of diagnosis in schizophrenia. *Am J Psychiatry* **153**: 682–6.
28. Rubio-Stipec M, Shrout P, Bird P, Canino G, Bravo M. 1989. Symptom scales of the

Diagnostic Interview Schedule: Factor results in Hispanic and Anglo samples. *Psychol Assessment* **1**: 30–4.

29. Kay SR, Opler LA, Fiszbein A. 1986. Significance of positive and negative syndromes in chronic schizophrenia. *Br J Psychiatry* **149**: 439–48.

30. Ramirez PM, Johnson PB, Opler LA. 1992. Ethnicity as a modifier of negative symptoms. Presented at the Annual meeting of the American Psychiatric Association; May 1992; Washington DC.

31. Alphs LD, Summerfelt A, Lann H, Muller RJ. 1989. The Negative Symptom Assessment: A new instrument to assess negative symptoms of schizophrenia. *Psychopharmacol Bull* **25**(2):159–63.

32. Dassori AM, Miller AL, Velligan DI, Saldana D, Mahurin R. 1993. Negative symptoms in Anglo-American and Mexican-American schizophrenics (abstract). *Schizophr Res* **9**: 97.

33. Allen CK. 1987. Occupational therapy: measuring the severity of mental disorders. *Hosp Community Psychiatry* **38**: 140–2.

34. Velligan DI, True JE, Lefton RS, Moore TC, Flores CV. 1995. Validity of the Allen Cognitive Levels Assessment: a tri-ethnic comparison. *Psychiatry Res* **56**: 101–9.

35. American Psychiatric Association. 1987. *DSM-III-R: Diagnostic and Statistical Manual of Mental Disorders*. 3rd ed., revised. Washington, DC: APA.

36. Jenkins J. 1988. Ethnopsychiatric interpretations of schizophrenic illness: the problem of nervios within Mexican-American families. *Cult Med Psychiatry* **12**: 301–29.

37. Urdaneta ML, Saldana DH, Winkler A. 1995. Mexican-American perceptions of severe mental illness. *Hum Org* **54**: 70–7.

38. Edgerton RB, Karno M. 1971. Mexican-American bilingualism and the perception of mental illness. *Arch Gen Psychiatry* **24**: 286–90.

39. Guarnaccia PJ, Parra P, Deschamps A, Milstein G. 1992. Si Dios quiere: Hispanic families' experiences of caring for a seriously mentally ill family member. *Cult Med Psychiatry* **16**: 187–215.

40. Lawson HH, Kahn MW, Heiman EM. 1982. Psychopathology, treatment outcome and attitude toward mental illness in Mexican American and European patients. *Int J Soc Psychiatry* **28**: 20–6.

41. Snowden LR, Cheung FK. 1990. Use of inpatient mental health services by members of ethnic minority groups. *Am Psych* **45**: 347–55.

42. Lu EG, Chien CP, Heming G, Hinton L, Soussain D. 1987. Ethnicity and neuroleptic drug dosage. Presented at the 140th Annual Meeting of the American Psychiatric Association, May 1987; Chicago, IL.

43. Mendoza R, Smith MW, Polan RE, Lin K, Strickland TL. 1991. Ethnic psychopharmacology: The Hispanic and Native American perspective. *Psychopharmacol Bull* **27**: 449–61.

44. Ruiz S, Chu P, Sramek J, Rotavu E, Herrera J. 1996. Neuroleptic dosing in Asian and Hispanic outpatients with schizophrenia. *Mount Sinai J Med* **63**: 306–9.

45. Collazo Y, Tam R, Sramek J, Herrera J. 1996. Neuroleptic dosing in Hispanic and Asian inpatients with schizophrenia. *Mount Sinai J Med* **63**: 310–13.

46. Gonzalez R, Cuellar I. 1983. Readmission and prognosis of Mexican American psychiatric inpatients. *Interam J Psychol* **17**: 81–96.

47. Sue S, Fujino DC, Hu L, Takeuchi DT, Zane N. 1991. Community mental health services for ethnic minority groups: A test of the cultural responsiveness hypothesis. *J Consult Clin Psychol* **59**: 533–40.

48. Jenkins JH, Karno M, de la Selva A, Santana F. 1986. Expressed emotion in cross-cultural context: Familial responses to schizophrenic illness among Mexican Americans. In: Goldstein M, Hand K, Hahlweg K, eds. *Treatment of Schizophrenia*. New York: Springer-Verlag, pp. 35–49.

49. Jenkins JH. 1991. Anthropology, expressed emotion and schizophrenia. *Ethos* **19**: 387–431.

50. Jenkins JH. 1992. Too close for comfort: schizophrenia and emotional overinvolvement among Mexican families. In: Gaines AD, ed. *Ethnopsychiatry: The Cultural Construction of Professional and Folk Psychiatries.* Stony Brook, NY: State University of New York Press, pp. 203–21.

51. Jenkins JH, Karno M. 1992. The meaning of expressed emotion: theoretical issues raised by cross cultural research. *Am J Psychiatry* **149**: 9–21.

52. Falloon IR, Boyd JLT, McGill CW *et al.* 1982. Family management in the prevention of exacerbation of schizophrenia: a controlled study. *N Engl J Med* **306**: 1437–40.

53. Telles C, Karno M, Mintz J *et al.* 1995. Immigrant families coping with schizophrenia. Behavioral family intervention v. case management with a low-income Spanish-speaking population. *Br J Psychiatry* **167**: 473–9.

54. Brekke JS, Barrio C. 1997. Cross-ethnic symptom differences in schizophrenia: the influence of culture and minority status. *Schizophr Bull* **23**: 305–16.

55. Neff JA, Hoppe SK. 1993. Race/ethnicity, acculturation and psychological distress: fatalism and religiosity as cultural resources. *J Community Psychol* **21**: 3–20.

56. Bravo M, Canino GJ, Rubio-Stipec M, Woodbury-Farina M. 1991. A cross-cultural adaptation of a psychiatric epidemiologic instrument: The Diagnostic Interview Schedule's adaptation in Puerto Rico. *Cult Med Psychiatry* **15**: 1–18.

57. Strauss A, Corbin J. 1990. *Basics of Qualitative Research. Grounded Theory Procedures and Techniques.* Newbury Park, CA: Sage Publications.

58. Marshall C, Rossman GB. 1989. *Designing Qualitative Research.* Newbury Park, CA: Sage Publications.

59. Eisenhart MA, Howe KR. 1992. Validity in educational research. In: LeCompte M, ed. *The Handbook of Qualitative Research in Education.* New York, NY: Academic Press.

60. Denzin NK, Lincoln YS. 1994. *Handbook of Qualitative Research.* Thousand Oaks, CA: Sage Publications.

61. Suchman E. 1972. Stages of illness and medical care. In: Jaco E, ed. *Patients, Physicians and Illness.* New York: Free Press, pp. 155–71.

62. Rogler LH, Cortes DE. 1993. Help-seeking pathways: a unifying concept in mental health care. *Am J Psychiatry* **150**: 554–61.

14

Neuroleptic Dosing in Hispanics and Asian Patients with Schizophrenia

Sigfried Ruiz[a], Peter Chu[a], Yasmine Collazo[a], Raymond Tam[a], John J. Sramek[b] and John M. Herrera[c]

[a]*Mount Sinai School of Medicine, Elmhurst, NY, USA;*
[b]*California Clinical Trials, Beverly Hills, CA, USA;*
[c]*Eli Lilly and Company, Indianapolis, IN, USA*

INTRODUCTION

A great deal of literature has been published suggesting that Asian patients with schizophrenia need lower doses of neuroleptic drugs than other ethnic groups to achieve a clinical response. Many of the studies in this field have been retrospective reviews of inpatient populations [1–4], though they do not unanimously confirm the above finding [5]. Multiethnic *prospective* studies in patients with schizophrenia are scarce [6]. However, a closely related finding has emerged, proposing that Asian patients may require lower doses because they are more vulnerable to extrapyramidal reactions than their Caucasian counterparts. Recent studies have also examined the relationship between ethnicity, dose and extrapyramidal symptoms, both prospectively [7–9] and retrospectively [2, 5, 10–13]—even in healthy normal subjects [14]. A distinct theme is recurring, wherein the nutritional [15] and cultural [16] differences among ethnicities which were previously explored are giving way to the strong possibility of genetic variances in pharmacokinetic and pharmacodynamic factors between these groups. One issue is agreed upon by all: further investigation of these issues is imperative.

As previously stated, studies relevant to this topic have traditionally been conducted in inpatients whose condition is typically more severe than outpatients. The few previous outpatient studies have not offered inpatient subjects for comparison. This report is a retrospective survey of inpatient and outpatient neuroleptic treatment, comparing dosing in different ethnic groups from the same institution. The unique setting provides the added advantage of medical teams

Cross Cultural Psychiatry. Edited by John M. Herrera, William B. Lawson and John J. Sramek.
© 1999 John Wiley & Sons Ltd.

similar in ethnicity to the patients, which was thought to reduce potential stereo-types that may be held in cross cultural treatment [3]. A second objective of these studies was to determine whether Hispanic patients with schizophrenia, for whom there is a remarkable lack of data, had neuroleptic dosage requirements different from either Asian or another control group.

SITE

Both the inpatient and outpatient portions of this study were conducted in the Department of Psychiatry at Elmhurst Hospital Center (EHC, Elmhurst, NY), an academic affiliate of Mount Sinai School of Medicine (New York, NY). EHC is located in a large multiethnic community in the borough of Queens, NY, which includes roughly 40% Hispanic and 20% Asian residents. To serve this diverse clientele more adequately, the Department of Psychiatry (EHC) developed special-ized clinical facilities, such as Hispanic and Asian inpatient units and outpatient clinics. All are staffed respectively by Hispanic or Asian psychiatrists, psychologists, social workers, nursing and support staff. These specialized facilities served as the research site for this study.

PROCEDURES

Medical records (inpatient records for inpatient subjects, outpatient records for outpatient subjects) were reviewed in order to extract and quantify selected bio-demographic, psychiatric history, and neuroleptic dosing patterns. These variables included:

- sex
- height
- weight
- age
- birthplace
- years in residence (if applicable)
- confirmation of the diagnosis (discharge summary or treating psychiatrist's most current progress notes)
- secondary psychiatric diagnosis (i.e. substance abuse)
- previous psychiatric hospitalizations
- the number of years since the onset of psychosis
- type of neuroleptic used, the current dose, the maximum dose and the dose associated with first report of extrapyramidal symptoms
- treatment with other psychiatric medications (i.e. antidepressants)
- treatment with antiparkinson medications and whether this medication was started prophylactically or only after extrapyramidal symptoms were detected
- the presence of documented movement disorder.

All outpatients were stabilized on their neuroleptic dose for at least 60 days and no subjects (inpatient or outpatient) who were receiving either risperidone or clozapine were included. For purpose of comparison, the neuroleptic doses were converted to chlorpromazine equivalents [17] and corrected for body weight to a standard of 68 kg. Both the actual and standardized doses were used in subsequent analyses.

STUDY I

Outpatient Subjects

A computer search of all clients registered with the EHC Hispanic and Asian outpatient clinics yielded 27 Hispanic 'schizophrenia'-spectrum DSM III-R diagnosed patients (10 paranoid, 11 undifferentiated, 6 schizoaffective patients). Demographic characteristics of the resulting sample groups are listed in Table 14.1. All patients had been born outside the USA, and the mean (± SD) number of years in this country was 18 ± 8.44 (range 1–31). A total of 48 Asian schizophrenic subjects were identified, including 28 paranoid, 11 unidentified and 9 schizo-affective patients. Only three were born in the USA; among those remaining ($n = 45$), the mean number of years in this country was 13.8 ± 8.85 (range 1–42). A third, 'general' sample was selected from the non-minority (primarily Caucasian) clinic base. Initially 74 were selected to match the Hispanic and Asian subjects one-to-one; however, only 64 patients were found to have sufficient medical records for inclusion in the study. The group included 1 disorganized, 36 paranoid, 4 schizo-phreniform, 1 residual, 17 undifferentiated, and 5 schizoaffective patients. Of these subjects 30 were born in the USA; among the 34 born elsewhere the mean number of years in this country was 13.82 ± 8.03 (range 1–37).

Outpatient Results

χ^2 comparisons failed to reveal significant gender differences among the three outpatient schizophrenic samples (see Table 14.1). Similar comparisons did reveal large differences ($\chi^2 = 35.92$; $p < 0.0001$) between the number of Hispanic, Asian, and Caucasian patients born in the USA or elsewhere. Although approximately half of the Caucasian group had been born in the USA, most Hispanic and Asian patients were born elsewhere. However, one-way analysis of variance (ANOVA) procedures failed to yield significant differences among the three samples in the number of years in residence in the USA (only those Caucasian group patients born outside of the country were included in this analysis; $n = 33$). Similar procedures yielded no significant age differences among the three outpatient schizophrenic groups; nor were significant differences found in the number of years since the onset of psychosis. Significant differences were found in the number of previous psychiatric hospitalizations ($F = 5.64$; $p < 0.004$) and subsequent within-

TABLE 14.1 Biodemographic variables and psychiatric history: outpatients

	Hispanics	Asians	Caucasians	χ^2	F
Male	11	21	26		
Female	16	27	38	0.17	
US born	0	3	30		
Other	28	45	30	35.92[a]	
Mean years in residence	18.00	13.82	13.82		1.94
Mean age in years	42.82	39.08	38.17		1.65
Mean years since onset	13.00	10.58	11.30		1.65
Mean psychiatric hospitalizations	3.09	1.68	3.00		5.64[b]

[a] $p<0.001$; [b] $p<0.01$

sample comparisons revealed differences (see Table 14.1) between the Asian and Hispanic samples ($p<0.009$) and the Asian and Caucasian groups ($p<0.004$). Previous reports have noted that Asians tend to shun psychiatric treatment until late in the course of their disorder [18].

ANOVA procedures were used to compare both the actual and the standardized neuroleptic doses across the three samples. As seen in Table 14.2, these analyses revealed a significant main effect for both actual ($F = 5.68$; $p<0.004$) and standardized dose ($F = 4.79$; $p<0.009$). With regard to the former, secondary analysis yielded significant differences between the Caucasian group and the Hispanic ($p<0.029$) and Asian ($p<0.002$) samples, which did not differ significantly from each other. These results were similar to the standardized dose comparisons (see Table 14.2). Significant differences between the Caucasian group and the two ethnic minority samples were found ($p<0.029$ for Hispanics and $p<0.008$ for Asians), although neither differed significantly from each other. Examination of the direction of mean differences for both medication dosing variables revealed that the Caucasian group was prescribed significantly larger doses of antipsychotic medication than either of the two ethnic minority samples. χ^2 comparisons revealed no significant differences among the three samples in the prescription of other psychiatric medications nor any documented movement disorder. However, significant differences were found in the prescription of antiparkinson medication ($\chi^2 = 22.69$; $p<0.0001$). As seen in Table 14.2, Asian patients were prescribed antiparkinson medication significantly more often than subjects in either of the other samples. To further understand these dosing differences, neuroleptics were differentiated on the basis of potency (high versus low) and χ^2 tests revealed significant differences among the three samples ($p<0.035$). Both ethnic minority groups were prescribed more low-potency medications than the Caucasian group.

Outpatient Summary

The outpatient study revealed that for both actual and weight-standardized dosing, members of the Caucasian group received significantly larger doses of neuroleptic

TABLE 14.2   Mean actual and standardized dose of chlorpromazine, psychiatric medication, movement disorder, and antiparkinson medication: outpatients

	Hispanics	Asians	Caucasians	F	χ^2
Mean actual dose	223.67	194.89	347.33	5.68[a]	
Mean standard dose	211.53	212.26	339.60	4.79[b]	
Other psychiatric medication	yes 8; no 18	yes 9; no 39	yes 16; no 48		1.76
Movement disorder	yes 1; no 25	yes 2; no 46	yes 1; no 62		0.74
Antiparkinson medication	yes 11; no 15	yes 42; no 6	yes 33; no 30		22.69[c]
Other psychiatric medication	high 20; low 6	high 37; low 9	high 56; low 3		6.72[b]

[a] $p<0.001$; [b] $p<0.01$; [c] $p<0.0001$

TABLE 14.3   Biodemographic variables and psychiatric history: inpatients

	Hispanics	Asians	Caucasians	χ^2	F
Male	4	0	18		
Female	23	10	16	15.44[a]	
United States	3	0	24		
Other	24	10	10	28.43[a]	
Mean years in residence	13.65	8.60	18.01		
Mean age in years	36.07	38.4	45.45		4.04[b]
Mean years since onset	7.28	9.3	17.05		8.28[a]
Mean psychiatric hospitalizations	3.50	2.20	4.55		

[a] $p<0.001$; [b] $p<0.01$

agents than Hispanics or Asians. These minority groups did not differ significantly from each other. There was no significant discrepancy among the three sample groups in the prescribing of other psychiatric medications or the occurrence of movement disorders; Asians did, however, receive more antiparkinson medication. Finally, both Hispanic and Asian subjects were prescribed more low-potency medications than the Caucasian group.

STUDY II

Inpatient Subjects

Inpatients were selected using a method similar to the selection process for outpatients; a computer search of EHC hospital records was conducted to identify all 'schizophrenia'-spectrum DSM III-R diagnosis patients (discharge diagnosis) treated during a 1-year period in the inpatient Hispanic and Asian psychiatric units: 27 Hispanic and 14 Asian patients were identified. For the purpose of comparison, a second computer search was completed to identify a matched (by admission date) sample of 41 Anglo patients from the EHC inpatient psychiatry services. Six of these patients were excluded from data analysis due to misidentification or insufficient chart information. The Asian sample included 10 Chinese and 4 Korean subjects; only the Chinese patients were included in this study as the Korean patients will be included in a subsequent (ongoing) report. The resulting study group consisted of 27 Hispanic, 10 Asian (Chinese) and 35 Anglo subjects. Demographic characteristics are listed in Table 14.3. Among the Hispanic subjects, there were 1 disorganized, 14 paranoid, 2 schizophreniform, 1 residual, 5 schizoaffective and 4 undifferentiated types. All but three were born outside the USA, and the mean ± SD number of years in this country was 13.65 ± 11.2 (range 1–41). The inpatient Asian schizophrenic sample included 3 paranoid, 1 schizophreniform, 3 residual, 2 schizoaffective and 1 disorganized type. All were born outside of the USA; mean number of years in this country was 8.6 ± 7.0 (range 1–24). The inpatient Anglo schizophrenic sample included 19 paranoid, 7 residual, 5 schizoaffective, and 4 undifferentiated types. Of these, 24 were born in the USA; among those born elsewhere the mean number of years of residence was 18.01 ± 12.4 (range 4–38).

Inpatient Results

χ^2 comparisons revealed significant gender differences among the three samples ($p < 0.01$); as seen in Table 14.3, both ethnic minority samples were predominantly female. One-way analysis of variance (ANOVA) procedures revealed significant age differences ($F = 4.05$; $p < 0.021$); however, secondary comparisons yielded significant differences ($p < 0.007$) only between the Hispanic and Anglo samples (see Table 14.1). The χ^2 comparisons also revealed large differences ($\chi^2 = 28.44$; $p < 0.0001$) in the number of Hispanic, Asian, and Anglo patients born in the USA or elsewhere. Although approximately two-thirds of the Anglo sample had been born in the USA, most Hispanic and Asian patients were born elsewhere. However, ANOVA procedures did not yield significant differences among the three samples in the number of years in residence in the country (only those Anglo patients born outside of the USA were included in this analysis; $n = 11$). Similar ANOVA calculations yielded no significant differences in the number of previous psychiatric hospitalizations among the three samples; however, significant differences were revealed in years since the onset of psychosis ($F = 8.28$; $p < 0.006$). Subsequent within-sample comparisons yielded significant differences between the Anglo sample and the Hispanic and Asian samples ($p < 0.026$ and $p < 0.002$, respectively), which did not differ significantly from each other.

ANOVA procedures were used to compare both actual and standardized neuroleptic chlorpromazine doses across the three groups, for both maximum and stabilized doses. As may be seen in Table 14.4, the analysis with maximum dose revealed a significant main effect for both actual ($F = 6.74$; $p < 0.002$) and standardized dose ($F = 3.18$; $p < 0.047$). Similar results were also found for stabilized

TABLE 14.4 Mean actual and standardized chlorpromazine dose, psychiatric medication, movement disorder, and antiparkinson medication: inpatients

	Hispanics	Asians	Caucasians	F	χ^2
Mean maximum actual dose	527.59	392.50	726.00	6.74[a]	
Mean maximum standard dose	535.44	487.19	712.23	3.18[b]	
Mean stabilized actual dose	396.56	257.50	599.14	5.92[a]	
Mean stabilized standard dose	411.78	317.89	593.00	3.26[a]	
Other psychiatric medication	yes 21; no 6	yes 5; no 5	yes 17; no 18		5.86[b]
Movement disorder	yes 12; no 15	yes 0; no 10	yes 3; no 32		14.94[a]
Antiparkinson medication	yes 24; no 3	yes 8; no 2	yes 32; no 2		

[a] $p<0.001$; [b] $p<0.01$

doses with both actual ($F = 5.92$; $p = 0.004$) and 68-kg standardized chlorpromazine doses ($F = 3.26$; $p = 0.044$). Secondary analysis yielded significant differences in maximum and actual dose between the Anglo sample and the Hispanic and Asian samples ($p<0.009$ and $p<0.002$, respectively), which did not differ significantly from each other. The results of maximum dose and 68-kg standardized chlorpromazine comparisons were similar (see Table 14.4); significant differences between the Anglo sample and the two ethnic minority samples were found (Hispanic versus Anglo, $p<0.036$; Asian versus Anglo, $p<0.056$), although neither minority differed significantly from the other. Secondary analysis with actual and stabilized doses of chlorpromazine also yielded significant differences between the Anglo sample and the Hispanic and Asian samples ($p<0.017$ and $p<0.003$, respectively), which did not differ significantly from each other. These results were similar to those found in 68-kg standardized and stabilized dose comparisons (see Table 14.4: Hispanic versus Anglo, $p<0.057$; Asian versus Anglo, $p<0.033$). Examination of the direction of mean differences for both medication dosing variables (maximum and stabilized dose) using both chlorpromazine comparisons (actual and standardized) revealed that significantly larger doses of antipsychotic medication were prescribed for patients in the Anglo sample than in either of the two ethnic minority samples.

χ^2 comparisons (see Table 14.4) revealed significant differences among the three samples in the prescription of other psychiatric medications ($\chi^2 = 5.86$; $p<0.053$); however, differentiating these medications by type (antidepressant, anxiolytic, antiseizure, lithium, hypnotic) did not yield significant differences (because of the number of subsequent cells and the small sample sizes). χ^2 examination of the use of antiparkinson medications failed to reveal significant differences among the three samples, and there were no differences in the use of these medications prophylactically or only after extrapyramidal side-effects had been detected. With few exceptions, subjects in all samples had been treated prophylactically with anti-parkinson medication. Highly significant differences were found in the diagnosis of movement disorders ($\chi^2 = 14.94$; $p < 0.0006$); as shown in Table 14.3 these resulted from the presence of movement disorders in approximately half of the Hispanic sample. Subsequent examination of the neuroleptic dosage (actual and standardized) at discharge (stabilized dose) of those patients with documented movement disorder (i.e. EPS, tardive dyskinesia) did not reveal significant differences within any of the ethnic groups.

Inpatient Summary

Significant differences were found among the Anglo, Asian and Hispanic sample groups in terms of age, male/female ratio, number of patients born in the USA, and years since onset of psychosis. Nevertheless, consistent results were found. Anglos were prescribed higher doses of neuroleptic medication than Hispanics and Asians, even when dose was standardized for weight, and dosing in the two minority groups did not differ significantly from each other. Of note, there was a significant difference in the prescription of other psychiatric medications among the three groups, though further analysis of drug type and use circumstances yielded no significant findings. The excessive number of movement disorders in Hispanics was highly significant. Analysis of dosing in patients with and without movement disorders revealed no significant differences within each ethnic group. This finding, however, warrants further investigation.

DISCUSSION

Our retrospective survey of neuroleptic dosing practices with outpatients who have schizophrenia confirmed previous reports that Asians may require lower dosages. Although inpatient subjects at our institution were treated by different clinicians, the inpatient survey produced similar results. One concern in the study design was the lumping of American-born and foreign-born Asians into one category. However, a study by Lin et al. [14] showed no significant difference between the pharmacokinetic responses to haloperidol in healthy subjects from these two groups, although both differed significantly from Caucasians. In addition, our study grouped patients from different origins in Asia. Previous studies have independently observed lower dosing or higher sensitivity to neuroleptics in exclusively Chinese [6, 19] and Japanese [12] populations but, for the sake of future treatment standards, a prospective comparison of the prominent Asian peoples (Chinese, Japanese, Korean, Vietnamese) should be conducted to verify that this genetic factor is shared.

An unexpected finding of both portions of our study was that Hispanic patients with schizophrenia also received significantly lower doses than the

Caucasian group at this institution. The overall similar use of low-potency neuroleptic medications in both ethnic minority groups in this study contrasts with the lower use in the Caucasian group and suggests that Hispanics may be more sensitive to extrapyramidal symptoms than others. Unfortunately, Hispanics have not been studied systematically to the extent that Asians have with regard to their neuroleptic dosing requirements and sensitivity to extrapyramidal symptoms. One study on the treatment of mental illness in general among Hispanic patients in public facilities [13] found antipsychotic dosing to be lower but not significantly different from that of Caucasians. In a study of tardive dyskinesia prevalence by Sramek *et al.* [7] inpatient Hispanic psychiatric patients having various diagnoses (including schizophrenia, mania, and depression) received neuroleptic dosages no different from those received by Caucasian or African American patients. Clearly the inconsistency between new and previous findings warrants additional research.

Significant biodemographic differences in age, sex distribution, and duration of illness between the ethnic minority and Anglo patients limit confidence in the results of our study, but do suggest as an independent indicator that both ethnic groups deserve further study. Additional criticisms can be aimed at the retrospective methods used in this report as well as other retrospective surveys published previously. These include a lack of patients from different ethnic groups matched for severity of illness, treatment time period, prior history (in particular previous use of neuroleptics), and differing prescribing practices by clinicians. Surveys must be confirmed by carefully conducted prospective studies which control as many of these factors as possible and which ideally randomize patients to fixed dosages of neuroleptics and prospectively rate patients for improvement and appearance of extrapyramidal symptoms. Pharmacokinetic assessments would also be highly desirable in such studies to investigate potential differences in drug metabolism among ethnic groups.

One of the greatest barriers to further transcultural psychopharmacology research is that the minimum effective dose of neuroleptic drugs remains unknown, despite the availability of these drugs for nearly four decades [20, 21]. In an early elegant study by Wode-Helgodt *et al.* [8], improvement was positively related to a dose range of chlorpromazine which encompasses the chlorpromazine equivalent dose spectrum found in this study. Thus, an alternative hypothesis is that Anglos may also respond to the lower neuroleptic doses found effective with Asians and Hispanics. Use of fixed doses of an antipsychotic agent with a well demonstrated dose–response relationship is crucial for future cross cultural psychopharmacology research.

Our findings support recent cross cultural research that advocates tailoring the therapeutic environment to be more 'culturally responsive' to ethnic minorities. In a brief overview of the importance of a multiethnic approach to medicine, Lin [22] reminds us that historical antecedents should not dissuade us from recognizing that, as with all living organisms, the human species possesses remarkable biological diversity that is worthy of scientific attention.

REFERENCES

1. Okuma T. 1981. Differential sensitivity to the effects of psychotropic drugs: psychotics vs. normals; Asians vs. Western populations. *Folia Psychiatr Neurol Jpn* 35: 79–82.
2. Lin K, Finder E. 1983. Neuroleptic dosage for Asians. *Am J Psychiatry* 140: 490–1.
3. Rosenblat R, Tang S. 1987. Do Oriental psychiatric patients receive different dosages of psychotropic medication when compared with Occidentals? *Can J Psychiatry* 32: 270–4.
4. Chiu H, Lee S, Leung CM, Wing YK. 1992. Neuroleptic prescription for Chinese schizophrenics in Hong Kong. *Aust NZ J Psychiatry* 26(2): 262–4.
5. Sramek J, Sayles M, Simpson G. 1986. Neuroleptic dosage for Asians: a failure to replicate. *Am J Psychiatry* 143: 535–6.
6. Potkin S, Shen Y, Pardes H *et al.* 1984. Haloperidol concentrations elevated in Chinese patients. *Psychiatry Res* 12: 167–72.
7. Sramek J, Roy S, Ahrens T, Pinanong P, Cutler NR, Pi E. 1991. Prevalence of tardive dyskinesia among three ethnic groups of chronic psychiatric patients. *Hosp Community Psychiatry* 42: 590–2.
8. Wode-Helgodt B, Borg S, Fyro B, Sedvall G. 1978. Clinical effects and drug concentrations in plasma and cerebrospinal fluid in psychotic patients treated with fixed doses of chlorpromazine. *Acta Psychiatr Scand* 58(2): 149–73.
9. Lin SK, Chang WH, Chien CP, Lam YWF, Jann MW. 1996. Disposition of remoxipride in Chinese schizophrenic patients. *Int J Clin Pharmacol Ther* 34(1): 17–20.
10. Binder R, Levy R. 1981. Extrapyramidal reactions in Asians. *Am J Psychiatry* 38: 1243–4.
11. Glazer WM, Morgenstern H, Doucette J. 1994. Race and tardive dyskinesia among outpatients at a CMH. *Hosp Community Psychiatry* 45(1): 38–42.
12. Binder RL, Kazamatsure H, Nishimura T, McNiel DE. 1987. Tardive dyskinesia and neuroleptic-induced Parkinsonism in Japan. *Am J Psychiatry* 144(11): 1494–6.
13. Adams GL, Dworkin RJ, Rosenberg SD. 1984. Diagnosis and pharmacotherapy issues in the care of Hispanics in the public sector. *Am J Psychiatry* 141(8): 970–4.
14. Lin KM, Poland RE, Lau JK, Rubin RT. 1988. Haloperidol and prolactin concentrations in Asians and Caucasians. *J Clin Psychopharmacol* 8: 195–201.
15. Olatawara M. 1978. The effects of psychotropic drugs in different populations. *Bull WHPP* 56: 519–23.
16. Yamamoto J, Fung D, Lo S *et al.* 1979. Psychopharmacology for Asian Americans and Pacific Islanders. *Psychopharmacol Bull* 5: 29–31.
17. Davis J. 1974. Dose equivalence of the antipsychotic drugs. *J Psychiatr Res* 11: 65–9.
18. Lin K, Poland R, Nuccio I *et al.* 1989. A longitudinal assessment of haloperidol doses and serum concentrations in Asian and Caucasian schizophrenic patients. *Am J Psychiatry* 146: 1307–11.
19. Chiu H, Lee S, Leung CM, Wing YK. 1992. Neuroleptic prescription for Chinese schizophrenics in Hong Kong. *Aust NZ J Psychiatry* 26(2): 262–4.
20. Janicak P, Javaid R, Sharma A *et al.* 1994. Random assignment to three haloperidol plasma levels for acute psychosis. *Biol Psychiatry* 35: 666.
21. Stone C, Garver D, Griffith J *et al.* 1995. Further evidence of a dose-response threshold for haloperidol in psychosis. *Am J Psychiatry* 152: 1210–12.
22. Lin KM. 1996. Psychopharmacology in Cross-cultural psychiatry. *Mt Sinai J Med* 5/6(63): 283–4.

Treatment-Resistant Schizophrenia in African Americans

David C. Henderson

Erich Lindemann Mental Health Center, Boston, MA, USA

INTRODUCTION

Schizophrenia is a chronic syndrome which typically follows a deteriorating course over time. With the exception of about 10% of patients who may achieve relative remission, schizophrenia rarely responds fully to treatment and so 'treatment resistance' tends to be the rule rather than the exception [1]. Approximately 30% of patients with schizophrenia derive little or no benefit from conventional antipsychotic agents. The wide variability in response and the generally poor long-term treatment outcome have led to several different definitions of 'treatment resistance' for schizophrenic patients. An international study group convened for this purpose recently defined treatment-resistant schizophrenia as the presence of continuing psychotic symptoms with substantial functional disability for at least two years despite adequate pharmacological and psychological treatment [2]. In contrast, Meltzer has argued for a more inclusive clinical definition, suggesting that any patient who does not recover his or her premorbid level of functioning should be considered treatment resistant [3]. For the purposes of this review, which focuses on the psychopharmacological treatment of African Americans, treatment resistance will refer to the persistence of clinically significant symptoms of schizophrenia despite adequate trials of conventional antipsychotic agents.

Schizophrenia was thought to be more prevalent among African Americans, Hispanics, and Asians. However, when standardized diagnostic systems are used these populations do not differ from Whites in the prevalence of most psychiatric disorders, including schizophrenia [4–7]. More recent studies have suggested that, while the prevalence does not differ, differences may occur between Blacks and Whites in symptoms or expression of illness [8]. Fabrega and colleagues [9] found differences between African-American and White patients in the symptoms of schizophrenia and depression, which were attributed to alternative forms of expression of psychopathology.

Cross Cultural Psychiatry. Edited by John M. Herrera, William B. Lawson and John J. Sramek.

Much of the available research on psychotropic medications in the USA has focused primarily on White males. Therefore, information concerning specific pharmacokinetic and pharmacodynamic profiles of various medications in other populations is not readily available. The importance of such knowledge is apparent when one considers the potential side-effects, morbidity and mortality related to particular medications. Understanding ethnicity and psychopharmacology is essential in order to provide high-quality care for African Americans.

DIAGNOSTIC ASSESSMENT

The first step in approaching a patient with persistent symptoms of schizophrenia is to reassess the diagnosis and degree of compliance with treatment. The diagnosis of schizophrenia is not made solely on the basis of a cross-sectional view of active symptoms, but rather requires careful review of the course of illness, and consideration of exclusionary criteria. Smith and colleagues [10] examined 50 consecutive admissions with treatment-resistant psychosis and concluded that 46% were incorrectly diagnosed. In most cases patients previously diagnosed with schizophrenia were rediagnosed with bipolar disorder or psychotic depression. These patients were given mood-stabilizing agents and tended to show more improvement than patients whose diagnosis was not changed.

Recently, there has been considerable debate as to whether there are differences in response to medications as well as side-effect profiles in African Americans. In the USA, race has a significant effect on psychiatric diagnosis and treatment. African Americans are frequently misdiagnosed as having a more severe psychiatric illness than their White counterparts [11]. African-American patients with bipolar disorder or psychotic depression are frequently diagnosed as having schizophrenia and committed to lifelong treatment with antipsychotic medications [12, 13]. They receive higher doses of antipsychotic medications, continue to have a higher rate of involuntary committal to psychiatric hospital, even in the managed care environment, and have a significantly higher rate of seclusion–restraint in psychiatric hospitals [14].

It should be noted, however, that schizophrenic patients often present with superimposed depressive episodes, which may not always benefit from the addition of tricyclic antidepressants [15, 16]. Kramer and colleagues [17] found that addition of amitriptyline or desipramine during the early stages of treatment of a psychotic exacerbation did not improve depressive symptoms and appeared to delay response of psychotic symptoms. However, addition of an antidepressant to an antipsychotic agent in depressed schizophrenic patients with stable psychotic symptoms may be helpful for depressive symptoms [18].

In addition to assessing for an underlying psychotic mood disorder, patients should be carefully evaluated for the presence of substance abuse. Approximately 40–60% of schizophrenic patients actively abuse drugs, most commonly alcohol and stimulants [19]. These drugs may produce persistent psychotic symptoms and will further impair level of functioning [20, 21]. It is important to observe patients with active substance abuse during a period of abstinence: distinguishing between primary psychiatric disorder with comorbid substance and primary substance abuse with psychiatric symptoms is critical for appropriate treatment [22]. Wilkins and colleagues [23] found that schizophrenic patients are less likely than other psychiatric patients to acknowledge substance abuse, so direct questioning may not adequately assess this important factor. When possible, urine and blood screens, as well as interviews with family and residential staff, should be pursued.

Tobacco is also widely used by schizophrenic patients, possibly in part to self-medicate neuroleptic side-effects, dysphoric mood, and attentional deficits [24]. Because tobacco smoking may significantly lower neuroleptic blood levels [25], assessment of patients in a smoke-free environment may further complicate decisions about the adequacy of neuroleptic dose and the presence of adverse drug effects. It is not clear whether the effects of cigarette smoking on drug levels and medication effects result from a pharmacokinetic interaction with nicotine or from one of the more than 1000 other constituents of cigarette smoke. More appropriate dosing of conventional neuroleptics and the use of atypical neuroleptics may reduce nicotine use in African American schizophrenic patients.

Patients should also be assessed for other potential causes of psychosis including drug-induced, delirium, medical or neurologic disorders, or other psychiatric disorders. Most can be ruled out by history, physical examination, and routine laboratory screening. Although the yield from brain imaging tends to be quite low in the absence of any focal neurological signs, it is generally recommended that a brain scan (CT or MRI) is performed at least once in any patient with atypical or non-responsive psychotic symptoms [26].

ASSESSING COMPLIANCE WITH TREATMENT

An equally important step in the assessment of treatment-resistant patients is to determine the level of compliance with pharmacotherapy. It has been estimated that 30–50% of schizophrenic patients do not take their medication as prescribed [27, 28]. Adverse effects are a major reason for this very high rate of non-compliance and need to be carefully assessed and managed. Switching the patient to haloperidol and monitoring plasma haloperidol concentrations, or switching to a depot preparation may help to rule out compliance as a factor in the treatment-resistant patient. In addition to removing the question of compliance, depot neuroleptics also reduce interindividual variability in steady-state plasma drug concentrations because first-pass hepatic metabolism is bypassed [29]. The newer atypical antipsychotic agents with a lower extrapyramidal symptom profile may significantly improve compliance in some patients.

Another important area of attention with an impact on compliance is a patient's cultural background and beliefs. Culturally shared beliefs play a major role in determining whether an explanation and treatment will make sense to a patient.

An understanding of how a culture treats a person with particular symptoms as well as how they respond to such treatments is important. A patient's expectations about treatment and outcome may also affect compliance. For instance, some Asian and Hispanic populations often expect a rapid response to treatment. With the slow onset of action with many psychotropic medications, compliance with appointments and medications may suffer. It is important to explore a patient's 'world view' and their explanatory model as to their illness. A clinician can develop a more acceptable model that integrates Western medicine with a patient's cultural beliefs.

Concern about the addictive quality of medications and side-effects may also reduce the chance that a patient takes a medication for an extended period of time. Attention should be given as to how medications work and the importance of taking them as prescribed. African Americans show particular concerns about the addictiveness of psychotropic medications or whether they will be considered a 'drug addict'.

Finally, it is estimated that up to one in three Americans use traditional and alternative methods of healing [30]. African Americans and Blacks in the USA continue to use traditional medical treatments that have their origins in the slave culture in the South or from other traditional cultures (e.g. Haiti). This has been labeled rootwork, conjure medicine, hoodoo and voodoo [31]. A belief in magically induced illness and the natural causation of illness leads to the belief in cures with herbs and other natural substances. People will frequently seek traditional healing methods before they turn to Western medicine or after initial failure in the Western medical system.

HERBAL MEDICINES

It is important to inquire whether a person is currently taking, or has been treated in the past with, traditional or alternative medicines. Herbal medicines are naturally occurring substances—but this does not mean that they are free of side-effects or interactions with other medications or substances. Many herbal medicines have not been well studied though there is a current movement towards this.

The Japanese herbs *Swertia japonica* and kamikihi-to or Cuban *Datura candida* have anticholinergic properties that may interact with tricyclic antidepressants, low-potency neuroleptics, and clozapine [32–34]. Elderly people are particularly sensitive to this interaction, which could lead to blurred vision, constipation, urinary retention, confusion, psychosis and delirium. The South American holly *Ilex guayusa* has a high caffeine content and may worsen anxiety and akathisia caused by neuroleptics and selective serotonin reuptake inhibitors (SSRIs) [35]. The Nigerian root extract of *Schumanniophyton problematicum*, used to treat psychosis, is a sedative and may interact with benzodiazepines and neuroleptics [36].

A number of herbs are potent stimulators of cytochrome P-450 enzymes including *Schizandrae fructus*, *Corydalis bungeane* diels, *Kopsia officinalis*, *Clausena lansium*, muscone, ginseng, and glycyrrhiza. These agents may increase the rate of metabolism of many psychotropic agents including antidepressants, anticonvulsants, and antipsychotic agents. Oleanolic acid inhibits the cytochrome P-450 enzymes, which could lead to higher blood levels, increase in adverse effects and toxicity [37]. Recently, a herbal weight loss supplement containing *E. sinica* (Ma-Huang) was reported to cause mania in a patient who did not have a previous psychiatric history [38]. *E. sinica* is the main plant source of ephedrine, which has been reported to cause mania and delusional disorders [38]. Many of these agents, found in preparations at natural food stores and major pharmacies, are readily available.

OPTIMIZING THE ANTIPSYCHOTIC DOSE

After the diagnosis has been reassessed, along with issues of compliance and psychosocial stressors, the next step is to optimize the dose of conventional neuroleptics. Studies using PET scanning have indicated that approximately 60–75% occupancy of dopamine D_2 receptors is necessary for antipsychotic efficacy, regardless of which conventional agent is used [39]. Once an antipsychotic effect is achieved, the dose–response curve tends to plateau, meaning that further increases in plasma drug concentrations generally do not produce substantial increases in efficacy [40]. Extrapyramidal symptoms, particularly parkinsonism, are associated with D_2 receptor blockade of approximately 80% or greater [41]. In most cases, inadequate dosing is not the primary cause of treatment resistance, although adjustment of the dose may minimize side-effects while optimizing therapeutic response.

The decision whether to increase or decrease the dose of neuroleptic can usually be based on clinical assessment, although use of neuroleptic blood levels may be helpful, particularly in cases of potential drug–drug interactions [42]. Unfortunately, attempts to correlate clinical response with plasma drug concentrations have been complicated by the great interindividual variability in potential drug responsiveness characteristic of schizophrenia. It is unclear to what extent plasma drug levels reflect concentrations in the brain. There is evidence of a 'therapeutic window' for haloperidol, suggesting that some patients may experience clinical worsening if plasma concentrations fall above or below an optimal range. Patients have been described who develop agitation or worsening of psychotic symptoms at high plasma concentrations, which then improve with dose reduction [43]. African-American patients with schizophrenia may benefit from this clinical intervention as the trend of overprescribing in this population persists. Of all antipsychotic agents, haloperidol blood levels are best studied and probably are most clinically relevant because haloperidol metabolism is least complicated by active metabolites.

The presence of akathisia (a sensation of motor restlessness in the lower extremities) or parkinsonism (rigidity, tremor, stooped posture, slowed gait, and reduced affective display) suggest that the dose of the neuroleptic should be tapered downwards. The absence of extrapyramidal symptoms should lead to upward titration of dose in partial or non-responders. This process of dose adjustment is intended to identify the most effective antipsychotic dose with the least level of adverse effects. Additional agents, such as beta-blockers for akathisia and anticholinergics or amantadine for parkinsonism, may be added if antipsychotic efficacy continues to improve in conjunction with the emergence of side-effects as the dose is increased. Significant effort must be made to find the lowest effective antipsychotic dose for African-American patients as they appear to have a greater risk of neuroleptic-induced tardive dyskinesia, which is not necessarily dose related [44].

The overlap of an optimal antipsychotic dose with extrapyramidal side-effects may necessitate switching to a lower-potency agent or an atypical agent. If increasing the antipsychotic dose does not result in clear clinical benefit within 4–6 weeks, one should return to the lowest effective dose. Again, this process should be guided by clinical response and an appreciation of the wide variability between patients in degree of potential response and range of optimal doses. For example, some patients exhibit complete remission of psychotic symptoms at a daily dose of haloperidol 1–2 mg, whereas others improve when the dose is raised to 40–60 mg of haloperidol.

PHARMACOKINETICS OF PSYCHOTROPIC MEDICATIONS IN AFRICAN AMERICANS

Pharmacokinetics of medications deal with metabolism and blood levels, absorption, distribution, and excretion. Most psychotropic medications are metabolized in the liver, and the mitochondrial enzymes in the cytochrome P-450 (CYP) system are most studied. There are a number of other pharmacokinetic variables such as conjugation, plasma protein binding, as well as oxidation by the CYP isoenzymes [45, 46]. Drug-binding proteins in the plasma play a major role as only the unbound fraction of the drug is active. Ethnic variations in quantity and structure of drug-binding proteins have been reported [47, 48].

The activity of liver enzymes is controlled genetically, although environmental factors can alter their activity. These factors include medications, drugs, herbal medicines, steroids, sex hormones, constituents of tobacco, caffeine, alcohol, and dietary factors.

Understanding how a medication is metabolized will help to predict side-effects, blood levels, and potential drug–drug interactions. Many of the antidepressants, including the tricyclic and heterocyclic antidepressants, and the SSRIs, are partly metabolized in the CYP2D6 isoenzyme system. The SSRIs play a major role in that they can inhibit the activity of the CYP2D6 isoenzymes, thereby raising blood levels of other medications and substances. The CYP2D6 isoenzymes also play a role in metabolizing antipsychotic agents including clozapine, haloperidol perphenazine, risperidone, thioridazine and sertindole.

The incidence of poor metabolizers at the CYP2D6 system ranges from 3 to 10% of Caucasians, 0.5 to 2.4% of Asians, and approximately 1.9% of African Americans. Lin and colleagues have discovered individuals with a genetic variation that decreases activity at this enzyme, the 'slow metabolizers' [45]. This 'slow metabolizer' group have enzyme activity levels that are intermediate between poor and extensive metabolizers. Approximately 33% of Asians and African Americans have this gene variation. This may partly explain ethnic differences in the pharmacokinetics of neuroleptics and antidepressants.

The P-450 2C9 isoenzyme is involved in the metabolism of ibuprofen, naproxen, phenytoin, warfarin, and tolbutamide. Approximately 18–22% Asians and African Americans are poor metabolizers of these drugs [49, 50].

Isoenzyme CYP2C19 is involved in the metabolism of diazepam, clomipramine, imipramine, and propranolol and is inhibited by fluoxetine and sertraline. The rates of poor metabolizers at this enzyme system are approximately 3% for Caucasians and 18–22% for Asians. Studies of African Americans found 3.8% of people between the ages of 18 and 41 and 18.5% of elderly people to be poor metabolizers [51, 52]. This may explain slower metabolism of benzodiazepines and a build-up of metabolites in this population. Attention must be given to active metabolites as they can be metabolized by different pathways than the parent compound.

AFTER FAILURE OF A FIRST ANTIPSYCHOTIC DRUG TRIAL

If symptoms persist after optimizing the dose of a first antipsychotic agent, the next step involves a switch to a second conventional agent or an atypical agent, or addition of an adjuvant. To meet the current definition of treatment resistance required for eligibility for clozapine, patients must complete at least two trials of antipsychotic agents lasting a minimum of 6 weeks. Although there are anecdotal accounts of patients responding dramatically to a second conventional agent after failing to respond to a first, this is probably an uncommon occurrence. In theory, all conventional agents act by the same mechanism, blockade of D_2 receptors, so that an optimal dose of one agent should have therapeutic effects roughly comparable to those of any other conventional agent.

Whereas the evidence for efficacy of clozapine in treatment-resistant schizophrenic patients is quite compelling, evidence supporting the use of other agents in combination with conventional neuroleptics is scant and generally inconsistent [53]. The growing clinical trend is to switch to one of the newer atypical antipsychotic agents such as risperidone, olanzapine, or quetiapine.

NEW ATYPICAL ANTIPSYCHOTIC AGENTS

Risperidone

In a recent multicenter trial, patients were randomly assigned to one of four doses of risperidone, ranging from 2 to 16 mg/day, or haloperidol 20 mg/day. Only the group receiving risperidone 6 mg/day displayed significantly greater therapeutic effect than the haloperidol group [54]. Additional trials are needed to assess whether superior efficacy is consistently achieved and is restricted to a narrow dose range. A recent double-blind randomized study showed that risperidone and clozapine were equally effective for psychotic symptoms in chronic schizophrenics [55]. However, the patients chosen were not treatment resistant and the question remains unanswered whether risperidone is as effective as clozapine in this population. No drug has yet been demonstrated to equal the efficacy of clozapine in treatment-resistant patients.

Olanzapine

Olanzapine has high affinity for dopamine $D_{1,2,3,4}$, serotonin $5HT_{2,3,6}$, alpha 1-adrenergic, muscarinic M_1, and histaminic H_1 receptors, and most resembles clozapine structurally [56, 57]. Double-blind trials comparing olanzapine 2.5–17.5 mg with haloperidol 10–20 mg showed that intermediate and high doses of olanzapine were superior to placebo and comparable to haloperidol for positive symptoms. The studies also showed that olanzapine was superior to both placebo and haloperidol for negative symptoms. Olanzapine appears to be effective at doses of 7.5–20 mg and well tolerated [56, 57]. The most common adverse effects reported during the trials included drowsiness, anxiety, nausea, tremor, dizziness, dry mouth, orthostatic hypotension, and insomnia. Titration of olanzapine appears to be rather easy and well tolerated.

Quetiapine

Quetiapine has high affinity for serotonin $5TH_2$, alpha 1 and alpha 2-adrenergic, and histaminic receptors, and moderate affinity for dopamine D_2 receptors [58]. Higher doses of quetiapine were better than placebo and equal to chlorpromazine for positive symptoms, although results for negative symptoms were less consistent. Quetiapine appears to be effective at doses of 150–750 mg [59]. The most common side-effects reported during the trials included dyspepsia, weight gain, abdominal pain, orthostatic hypotension, dizziness, drowsiness, headache, and dry mouth.

Sertindole

Sertindole has high affinity for serotonin $5HT_2$, dopamine D_2, and alpha 1-adrenergic; lower affinity for dopamine D_1, and minimum affinity for alpha 2-adrenergic, histaminic H_1, and muscarinic M_1 receptors [60]. Double-blind studies showed doses of 12–24 mg to be superior to placebo and comparable to haloperidol for positive symptoms. Doses of 20–24 mg were effective for negative symptoms compared with placebo but not haloperidol. During clinical trials, African Americans achieved twice the blood level of Caucasians with the same dose of medication. Common adverse effects of sertindole include tachycardia, mild prolongation of the QT interval, decreased ejaculatory volume, weight gain, nasal congestion, and nausea [60]. Sertindole appears to be effective at doses of 4–24 mg. The titration of sertindole should be slow as tachycardia is significant with rapid titration. The significance of the prolongation of the QT interval is still under debate. However, caution should be used in prescribing sertindole in combination with other medications that have similar cardiac effects or in patients with significant cardiac history. To date, risperidone, olanzapine, quetiapine, and sertindole have not shown any risk of agranulocytosis.

Lithium Augmentation

Addition of lithium to a conventional antipsychotic in treatment-resistant schizophrenic and schizoaffective patients has been studied in three small, controlled trials [61–63]. The results have been modestly encouraging, and suggest that one-third to one-half of patients will exhibit some improvement within four weeks. Augmentation of antipsychotic efficacy has been associated with lithium blood levels in the range of 0.8–1.2 mEq/l. Although patients with an affective component to their clinical presentation may be most likely to benefit from addition of lithium, the literature indicates that response may also occur in the absence of affective symptoms and may include improvement of psychotic symptoms and negative symptoms. It remains uncertain whether addition of lithium to neuroleptic places a patient at greater risk for neurotoxic reactions, including neuroleptic malignant syndrome [64]. Clinicians should monitor carefully for extrapyramidal symptoms, confusion, or fever when this combination is employed.

Studies have shown that the erythrocyte lithium-sodium pathway operates at a slower rate in African Americans [65, 66]. In one study the erythrocyte lithium concentration levels were identical in Caucasians and African Americans immediately after the first dose of lithium; however, at 25 h the levels were significantly higher in the African Americans [67]. There is some evidence that lithium may be excreted more slowly in African Americans. As a result, the risk of neurotoxicity, fatigue, dizziness, loss of initiative, and urinary frequency in this population is a major concern [66]. The differences in lithium ratios suggest that African Americans may need less lithium than is currently recommended.

African Americans with hypertension deserve special attention when treated with lithium. Salt restriction or diuretics that lower sodium levels may alter lithium plasma levels and increase the risk of adverse effects and neurotoxicity. Thiazide diuretics are frequently used to treat hypertension in African Americans and are known to reduce lithium excretion, leading to elevated blood levels. Lithium blood levels should be monitored regularly in this setting.

Benzodiazepines

Addition of benzodiazepines may improve agitation, psychotic symptoms and social withdrawal in a subgroup of treatment-resistant schizophrenic patients, although controlled trials have produced inconsistent results [53, 68]. Benzodiazepines are probably most effective for patients with high levels of psychotic symptoms and anxiety. A typical dose of adjunctive lorazepam is 0.5–1.0 mg three times daily. Because abuse and disinhibition may develop, benzodiazepines should be tapered and discontinued if no benefit is apparent after 2–3 weeks. Some patients may even display worsening of psychosis following addition of benzodiazepines [69]. Withdrawal of the short-acting benzodiazepine alprazolam has been associated with worsening of psychotic symptoms in some patients [70]. Although controlled trials have not been conducted, Goff and colleagues [71] have observed encouraging results with the atypical anxiolytic buspirone at doses of 15–40 mg daily, particularly in agitated patients.

Care must be taken when prescribing benzodiazepines because of the risk of reduced metabolism, particularly in elderly patients. CYP2C19 is responsible for metabolizing diazepam, and other benzodiazepines have diazepam as an active metabolite. There is some evidence to suggest that African Americans may experience a larger drug effect when benzodiazepines are present: one study of adinazalom, an anxiolytic, in African Americans showed an increased clearance of parent compound and a longer half-life of the metabolites. The active metabolite concentrations were much higher in African Americans and they exhibited greater drug effect on psychomotor performance [45].

Anticonvulsants

Carbamazepine is the best studied anticonvulsant for augmentation of conventional antipsychotics. At doses producing typical anticonvulsant plasma levels (7–12 ng/ml), carbamazepine has produced moderate improvement of tension, excitement, manic symptoms and suspiciousness in a series of small trials [53]. Carbamazepine may be most effective for patients with abnormalities on the electroencephalogram (EEG), manic symptoms, or episodic violence, although cases have been reported of clinical improvement in the absence of any of these characteristics [72, 73]. Addition of carbamazepine to neuroleptic agents is complicated by a potential pharmacokinetic interaction, because carbamazepine increases hepatic microsomal enzyme metabolism and so can substantially lower plasma concentrations of antipsychotic agents [64]. When added to low-dose haloperidol this drug–drug interaction may produce clinical deterioration [74]. For this reason, clinicians should be prepared to increase the dose of neuroleptic, or possibly switch to haloperidol so that plasma concentrations can be more easily monitored. Carbamazepine should not be added to clozapine because of the risk of bone marrow suppression complicating clozapine's hematological adverse effects.

Valproate has also been reported to improve treatment-resistant psychosis when added to conventional neuroleptics, although not all trials have produced positive results and no controlled trials have been conducted [75]. Valproate is generally recommended as the most appropriate anticonvulsant for combination therapy with clozapine.

Beta Blockers

The beta blockers, particularly propranolol, have received considerable attention as augmentors of conventional neuroleptics [76, 77]. Used at high doses (up to 1200 mg/day), propranolol is reported to decrease agitation, psychotic symptoms and violence in some treatment-resistant patients, but results from controlled trials have generally been disappointing. It has been suggested that the inconsistent therapeutic effect of propranolol may result in some cases from either its potential to elevate plasma concentrations of antipsychotic agents or its beneficial effect on akathisia [78]. Because the evidence for efficacy remains unconvincing, and the potential adverse effects upon cardiovascular and pulmonary function are considerable, high-dose propranolol augmentation should be utilized only when other approaches fail.

Clozapine

Currently, the most effective intervention for treatment resistant or intolerant patients is the atypical agent, clozapine. When rigorously defined treatment-resistant patients were treated with clozapine for 6 weeks in the Clozapine Collaborative Trial, 30% exhibited a clinically significant improvement, defined by a reduction of at least 20% in the Brief Psychiatric Rating Scale (BPRS) score [79]. Response to clozapine was superior to response to chlorpromazine in most items of the BPRS, including psychotic symptoms, negative symptoms, depression, anxiety and hostility. Subsequently, open trials have suggested that the response rate may reach 50–60% if trials are extended to 6 months [80]. In general, because it is not possible to predict response to clozapine with any reasonable degree of specificity, a trial of clozapine should be attempted in all seriously ill patients who have failed at least two trials of conventional agents. Depending on results from trials in treatment-resistant patients, risperidone, olanzapine, or quetiapine may be considered appropriate intermediate steps before proceeding to a clozapine trial.

The considerable expense of clozapine has limited its availability to many populations, including African Americans [81, 82]. However, several studies have indicated that clozapine can be quite cost-effective because it typically reduces the annual number of days patients spend in the hospital [83]. The 1–2% risk of agranulocytosis has also limited use of the drug and has greatly complicated its administration because of the mandatory hematological monitoring system. However, this monitoring system has successfully reduced mortality from agranulocytosis. Benign leukopenia [84, 85], prevalent in the African-American population, is not a contraindication for clozapine trial and does not appear to increase the risk of agranulocytosis.

I routinely start clozapine at 12.5 mg by adding it to conventional high-potency neuroleptics in our outpatient clinic. Dose increases of 25 mg can be made every 2–3 days, as tolerated, during the first week. Once the clozapine dose has reached 100 mg/day, the conventional neuroleptic can gradually be tapered and discontinued as the clozapine dose is increased, usually in increments of 50 mg as tolerated. Combining clozapine with low-potency agents, such as thioridazine, should be avoided, because cardiovascular, anticholinergic and sedative side-effects of the two drugs can be additive. Benzodiazepines should be tapered to the lowest possible dose to minimize the additive sedative effects with clozapine. The gradual transition from conventional antipsychotic to an optimal dose of clozapine may require up to 2 months to achieve under outpatient conditions.

There are no clear guidelines for determining the optimal dose of clozapine. European clinicians have tended to use clozapine in a range of 200–300 mg/day, whereas average doses in the USA generally run in the range of 400–600 mg, with a maximum allowed dose of 900 mg/day. In a clinician-determined dose optimization study, Pickar and colleagues [86] reported a mean optimal clozapine dose of 550 mg/day. Ethnic differences in the CYP microsomal enzyme system may effect clozapine blood levels and response. Clozapine is metabolized, in part, in the CYPIID6 and CYP1A2 microsomal enzyme system. In a recent study, Korean Americans treated with clozapine had a greater response, lower doses and blood levels than Caucasians [87]. To date, no study has examined dosing, side-effects, and blood levels in African-American patients treated with clozapine.

Titration of clozapine is often complicated by a considerable delay in the emergence of therapeutic effects: as many as 50% of patients do not exhibit therapeutic improvement until after 4–6 months of treatment, thus necessitating at least a 6-month trial to identify potential responders [80]. The rate and ultimate endpoint of upward titration of clozapine is usually determined by adverse effects, particularly sedation, orthostatic hypotension, and sialorrhea. If tolerated, a dose of 400–500 mg/day is probably adequate for most patients. The dose can be kept at this level while awaiting evidence of clinical effect. If a patient has not responded by 4 months, the dose may be gradually increased up to 900 mg/day, guided by adverse effects. Because seizure risk is related to both the absolute dose and rate of dose increase, dose titration should be performed gradually and prophylactic treatment with valproate should be considered for patients receiving doses above 600 mg/day [88]. Once an adequate response has been achieved, the dose can be decreased gradually, particularly if side-effects are present. Preliminary work with clozapine blood levels suggests that plasma concentrations above 350 ng/ml are associated with better outcome, although further research is needed before clozapine blood levels become a standard clinical tool [89].

CLOZAPINE PARTIAL RESPONDERS OR NON-RESPONDERS

No information from systematic research is available to guide treatment options for the 40–60% of patients who fail to respond to clozapine. If psychotic symptoms persist despite increasing the dose to 900 mg/day, it may be useful to try lowering the dose. Preliminary data suggest a possible 'therapeutic window' for clozapine in some patients [89, 90]. Addition of a high-potency neuroleptic may also improve antipsychotic response, although patients should be carefully monitored for emergence of extrapyramidal symptoms. Buspirone, 10–40 mg/day, is helpful for anxiety and agitation in combination with clozapine. Some clozapine-resistant patients also appear to benefit from addition of valproate or an SSRI. The SSRIs fluoxetine, sertraline, and paroxetine may inhibit hepatic metabolism of clozapine and thus elevate blood levels. These drugs may improve depressive and negative symptoms in some patients and rarely exacerbate psychotic symptoms. Also, the addition of 2–4 mg of risperidone to clozapine may improve positive, negative, and depressive symptoms in some patients [91]. This combination, if clinically effective, can lead to a reduction in the clozapine dose and clozapine-related side-effects.

Finally, the impact of the newer atypical antipsychotic agents, such as risperidone, olanzapine, quetiapine, and sertindole, on the treatment-resistant population is unclear at this time. At a minimum, these medications have more favorable side-effect profiles. Historically, advances in medicine have been slow to reach the African-American population. Clinicians must quickly familiarize themselves with these newer agents and aggressively seek appropriate funding and formulary approval to make these drugs available to their patients.

CONCLUSION

Treatment resistance in schizophrenic African-American patients should prompt a careful review of diagnosis, compliance and psychosocial stressors. The dose of conventional antipsychotic can be optimized by titrating antipsychotic efficacy against the emergence of extrapyramidal symptoms. Careful consideration of differences in metabolism and response to psychotropic medications is vital.

Preliminary evidence suggests that the newer atypical agents risperidone, olanzapine and quetiapine may represent a reasonable second step. Although some patients may benefit from augmentation of conventional antipsychotic agents with lithium, benzodiazepines or buspirone, the information supporting these approaches remains somewhat sparse and inconsistent. The alternative most likely to produce substantial improvement in patients resistant to or intolerant of conventional antipsychotic agents is clozapine. After two adequate trials of conventional or newer atypical antipsychotic agents have been completed, a clozapine trial lasting at least 6 months should be offered to patients who remain seriously impaired by their illness.

REFERENCES

1. Breier A, Schreiber J, Dyer J, Pickar D. 1991. National institute of mental health longitudinal study of chronic schizophrenia: Prognosis and predictors of outcome. *Arch Gen Psychiatry* **48**: 239–46.
2. Brenner HD, Sven DJ, Goldstein MJ, Hubbard JW, Keegan DL, Kruger G *et al.* 1990. Defining treatment refractoriness in schizophrenia. *Schizophr Bull* **16**: 551–61.
3. Meltzer HY. 1992. Treatment of the neuroleptic-nonresponsive patient. *Schizophr Bull* **18**: 515–42.
4. Lawson BL. 1986. Racial and ethnic factors in psychiatric research. *Hosp Community Psychiatry* **37**: 50–4.
5. Neighbors HW, Jackson JS, Campbell L, Williams D. 1989. The influence of racial factors on psychiatric diagnosis: A review and suggestions for research. *Community Ment Health J* **25**: 301–11.
6. Armstrong HE, Ishiki D, Heiman J *et al.* 1984. Service utilization by black and white clientele in an urban community mental health center: revised assessment of an old problem. *Community Ment Health J* **20**: 269–81.
7. Somervell PD, Leaf PJ, Weissman MM *et al.* 1989. The prevalence of major depression in black and white adults in five United States communities. *Am J Epidemiol* **130**: 725–35.
8. Griffith J. 1985. A community survey of psychological impairment among Anglo- and Mexican-Americans and its relationship to service utilization. *Community Ment Health J* **21**: 28–41.
9. Fabrega H, Mezzich J, Ulrich RK. 1988. Black-white differences in psychopathology in an urban psychiatric population. *Compr Psychiatry* **29**: 285–97.
10. Smith GN, MacEwan GW, Ancill RJ, Honer WG, Ehmann TS. 1992. Diagnostic confusion in treatment-refractory psychotic patients. *J Clin Psychiatry* **53**: 197–200.
11. Adebimpe V. 1981. White norms and psychiatric diagnosis of black patients. *Am J Psychiatry* **138**: 279–85.
12. Bell C, Mehta H. 1979. The misdiagnosis of black patients with manic depressive illness. *J Natl Med Assoc* **72**: 141–5.
13. Mukherjee S, Shukla S *et al.* 1983. Misdiagnosis of schizophrenia in bipolar patients: a multicultural comparison. *Am J Psychiatry* **140**: 1571–6.
14. Lawson WB, Hepler N *et al.* 1994. Race as a factor in inpatient and outpatient admissions and diagnosis. *Hosp Community Psychiatry* **45**: 72–4.
15. Knights A, Hirsch SR. 1981. 'Revealed' depression and drug treatment for schizophrenia. *Arch Gen Psychiatry* **38**: 806–11.
16. Green MF, Nuechterlein KH, Ventura J, Mintz J. 1990. The temporal relationship between depressive and psychotic symptoms in recent-onset schizophrenia. *Am J Psychiatry* **147**: 179–82.
17. Kramer M, Vogel W, DiJohnson C, Dewey D, Sheves P, Cavicchia S *et al.* 1989. Antidepressants in 'depressed' schizophrenic inpatients: A controlled trial. *Arch Gen Psychiatry* **46**: 922–8.
18. Siris SG, Mason SE, Bermanzohn PC, Alvir JJ, McCorry TA. 1990. Adjunctive imipramine maintenance in post-psychotic depression/negative symptoms. *Schizophr Bull* **26**: 91–4.
19. Cuffel BJ. 1992. Prevalence estimates of substance abuse in schizophrenia and their correlates. *J Nerv Ment Dis* **180**: 589–92.
20. Bartels SJ, Teague GB, Drake RE, Clark RE, Bush PW, Noordsy DL. 1993. Substance abuse in schizophrenia: Service utilization and cost. *J Nerv Ment Dis* **181**: 227–32.
21. Bowers MBJ, Mazure CM, Nelson JC, Jatlow PI. 1990. Psychotogenic drug use and neuroleptic response. *Schizophr Bull* **16**: 81–5.

22. Cohen SI. 1995. Overdiagnosis of schizophrenia: Role of alcohol and drug misuse. *Lancet* **346**: 1541–2.
23. Wilkins JN, Shaner AL, Patterson CM, Setoda D, Gorelick D. 1991. Discrepancies between patient report, clinical assessment, and urine analysis in psychiatric patients during inpatient admission. *Psychopharmacol Bull* **27**: 149–54.
24. Goff DC, Henderson DC, Amico E. 1992. Cigarette smoking in schizophrenia: Relationship to psychopathology and medication side effects. *Am J Psychiatry* **149**: 1189–94.
25. Jann MW, Saklad SR, Ereshefsky L, Richards AL, Harrington CA, Davis CM. 1986. Effects of smoking on haloperidol and reduced haloperidol plasma concentrations and haloperidol clearance. *Psychopharmacology* **90**: 468–70.
26. Weinberger DR. 1984. Brain disease and psychiatric illness: When should a psychiatrist order a CAT scan? *Am J Psychiatry* **141**: 1521–7.
27. Buchanan A. 1992. A two-year prospective study of treatment compliance in patients with schizophrenia. *Psychol Med* **22**: 787–97.
28. Van Putten T. 1974. Why do schizophrenic patients refuse to take their drugs? *Arch Gen Psychiatry* **31**: 67–72.
29. Marder SR, Hubbard JW, Van Putten T, Midha KK. 1989. Pharmacokinetics of long-acting injectable neuroleptic drugs: Clinical implications. *Psychopharmacology* **98**: 433–9.
30. Marwick C. 1995. Growing use of medicinal botanical forces assessment by drug regulators [news]. *JAMA* **273**: 607–9.
31. Mathews HF. 1987. Rootwork: description of an ethnomedical system in the American south. *South Med J* **80**: 885–91.
32. Yamahara J, Kobayashi M *et al.* 1991. Anticholinergic action of *Swertia japonica* and an active constituent. *J Ethnopharmacol* **33**: 31–5.
33. Egashira T, Sudo S *et al.* 1991. Effect of kamikihi-to, a Chinese traditional medicine, on various cholinergic biochemical markers in the brain of aged rats. *Nippon Yakurigaku Zasshi* **98**: 273–81.
34. Carbajal D, Casaco A *et al.* 1991. Pharmacological screening of plant decoctions commonly used in Cuban folk medicine. *J Ethnopharmacol* **33**: 21–4.
35. Lewis WH, Kennelly EJ *et al.* 1991. Ritualistic use of the holly Ilex guayusa by Amazonian Jivro Indians. *J Ethnopharmacol* **33**: 25–30.
36. Amadi E, Offiah NV, Akah PA. 1991. Neuropsychopharmacologic properties of a Schumanniophyton problematicum root extract. *J Ethnopharmacol* **33**: 73–7.
37. Liu GT. 1991. Effects of some compounds isolated from Chinese medicinal herbs on hepatic microsomal cytochrome P-450 and their potential biological consequences. *Drug Metab Rev* **23**: 439–65.
38. Capwell R. 1995. Ephedrine-induced mania from a herbal diet supplement (letter). *Am J Psychiatry* **152**: 647.
39. Farde L, Wiesel F, Nordstrom AL, Sedvall G. 1989. D1- and D2-dopamine receptor occupancy during treatment with conventional and atypical neuroleptics. *Psychopharmacology* **99**: S28–S31.
40. Perry PJ, Pfohl BM, Kelly MW. 1988. The relationship of haloperidol concentrations to therapeutic response. *J Clin Psychopharmacol* **8**: 38–43.
41. Farde L, Nordstrom AL, Wiesel FA, Pauli S, Halldin C, Sedvall G. 1992. Positron emission tomographic analysis of central D1 and D2 dopamine receptor occupancy in patients treated with classical neuroleptics and clozapine: Relation to extrapyramidal side effects. *Arch Gen Psychiatry* **49**: 538–44.
42. Goff D, Midha K, Sarid-Segal O, Hubbard J, Amico E. 1993. A placebo-controlled trial of fluoxetine added to neuroleptic in patients with schizophrenia. *Am J Psychiatry* **13**: 57–67.
43. Van Putten T, Marder S, Wirshing W, Aravagiri M, Chabert N. 1991. Neuroleptic plasma levels. *Schizophr Bull* **17**: 197–216.

44. Glazer WM, Morgenstern H, Doucette J. 1994. Race and tardive dyskinesia among outpatients at a CMHC. *Hosp Community Psychiatry* **45**: 38–42.

45. Lin K, Anderson D, Poland RE. 1995. Ethnicity and psychopharmacology bridging the gap. *Psych Clin N Am* **18**: 635–47.

46. Lin K, Poland R, Nakasaki G. 1993. *Psychopharmacology and Psychobiology of Ethnicity*. Washington, DC: American Psychiatric Press.

47. Juneja RK, Weitkamp LR, Stratil A *et al.* 1988. Further studies of the plasma 1 B-glycoprotein polymorphism: two new alleles and allele frequencies in Caucasians and in American Blacks. *Hum Hered* **38**: 267–72.

48. Kumana CR, Lauder IJ, Chan M *et al.* 1987. Differences in diazepam pharmacokinetics in Chinese and White Caucasians-relation to body lipid stores. *Eur J Clin Pharmacol* **32**: 211–15.

49. Devane CL. 1994. Pharmacokinetics of the newer antidepressants: Clinical relevance. *Am J Med* **97**: 13S–23S.

50. Risby ED. 1996. Ethnic considerations in the pharmacotherapy of mood disorders. *Psychopharmacol Bull* **32**: 231–4.

51. Daniel HI, Edeki TI. 1996. Genetic polymorphism *S*-mephenytoin 4'-hydroxylation. *Psychopharmacol Bull* **32**: 219–30.

52. Pollock BG, Perel JM, Kirshner M *et al.* 1991. *S*-mephenytoin 4'-hydroxylation in older Americans. *Eur J Clin Pharmacol* **40**: 609–11.

53. Christison G, Kirch D, Wyatt R. 1991. When symptoms persist: Choosing among alternative somatic treatments. *Schizophr Bull* **17**: 217–45.

54. Chouinard G, Jones B, Remington G, Bloom D, Addington D, MacEwan GW *et al.* 1993. A Canadian multicenter placebo-controlled study of fixed doses of risperidone and haloperidol in the treatment of chronic schizophrenic patients. *J Clin Psychopharmacol* **13**: 25–40.

55. Kleiser E *et al.* 1995. Randomized, double-blind, controlled trial of risperidone versus clozapine in patients with chronic schizophrenia. *J Clin Psychopharmacol* **15**: 45S–51S.

56. Tollefson GD, Beasley CM, Tran PV *et al.* 1996. Olanzapine versus haloperidol: results of the multicenter, international trial. *Schizophr Res* **18**: 131.

57. Beasely CM, Tollefson G, Tran P *et al.* 1996. Olanzapine versus placebo and haloperidol: acute phase results of the North American double-blind olanzapine trial. *Neuropsychopharmacology* **14**: 111–23.

58. Small JG, Hirsch SR, Arvantis LA *et al.* 1997. Quetiapine and low-dose double-blind comparison with placebo. *Arch Gen Psychiatry* **54**: 549–57.

59. Arvanitis LA, Miller BG, and the Seroquel Trial 13 Study Group. 1997. Multiple fixed doses of Seroquel (quetiapine) in patients with acute exacerbation of schizophrenia: a comparison with haloperidol and placebo. *Biol Psychiatry* **42**: 233–46.

60. Schultz SC, Mack R, Zborowski J, Morris D, Sebree T, Wallin B. 1996. Efficacy, safety, and dose response of three doses of sertindole and three doses of haldol in schizophrenia patients. *Schizophr Res* **18**: 133.

61. Carmen JS, Bigelow LB, Wyatt RJ. 1981. Lithium combined with neuroleptics in chronic schizophrenic and schizoaffective patients. *J Clin Psychiatry* **42**: 124–8.

62. Growe GA, Crayton JW, Klass DB, Evans H, Stizich M. 1979. Lithium in chronic schizophrenia. *Am J Psychiatry* **7**: 178–82.

63. Small JG, Kellams JJ, Milstein V, Moore J. 1975. A placebo-controlled study of lithium combined with neuroleptics in chronic schizophrenic patients. *Am J Psychiatry* **132**: 1315–17.

64. Goff D, Baldessarini R. 1993. Drug interactions with antipsychotic agents. *J Clin Psychopharmacol* **13**: 57–67.

65. Trevisan M, Ostrow D *et al.* 1984. Sex and race differences in sodium-lithium countertransport and red cell sodium concentration. *Am J Epidemiol* **120**: 537–41.

66. Strickland TL, Lin KM, Fu P *et al.* 1995. Comparison of lithium ratio between African-American and Caucasian bipolar patients. *Biol Psychiatry* **37**: 325–30.

67. Okpaku S, Fraxer A, Mendels J. 1980. A pilot study of racial differences in erythrocyte lithium transport. *Am J Psychiatry* **137**: 120–1.

68. Arana G, Ornsteen ML, Kanter F, Friedman HL, Greenblatt DJ, Shader RI. 1986. The use of benzodiazepines for psychiatric disorders: A literature review and preliminary findings. *Psychopharmacol Bull* **22**: 77–87.

69. Dixon L, Weiden PJ, Frances AJ, Sweeney J. 1989. Alprazolam intolerance in stable schizophrenic outpatients. *Psychopharmacol Bull* **25**: 213–14.

70. Wolkowitz OM, Breier A, Doran A, Kelsoe J, Lucas P, Paul SM, Pickar D. 1988. Alprazolam augmentation of the antipsychotic effects of fluphenazine in schizophrenic patients. *Arch Gen Psychiatry* **143**: 664–71.

71. Goff D, Midha K, Brotman A, McCormick S, Waites M, Amico E. 1991. An open trial of buspirone added to neuroleptics in schizophrenic patients. *J Clin Psychopharmacol* **11**: 193.

72. Neppe VM. 1983. Carbamazepine as adjunctive treatment in nonepileptic chronic inpatients with EEG temporal lobe abnormalities. *J Clin Psychiatry* **44**: 326–31.

73. Sramek J, Herrera J, Costa J, Heh C, Tran-Johnson T, Simpson G. 1988. A carbamazepine trial in chronic treatment-refractory schizophrenia. *Am J Psychiatry* **145**: 748–50.

74. Arana GW, Goff DC, Friedman H, Ornsteen M, Greenblatt DJ, Black B, Shader RI. 1986. Does carbamazepine-induced reduction of plasma haloperidol levels worsen psychotic symptoms? *Am J Psychiatry* **143**: 650–1.

75. Wassef A, Waston DJ *et al.* 1989. Neuroleptic-valproic acid combination treatment of psychotic symptoms: A three-case report. *J Clin Psychopharmacol* **9**: 45–8.

76. Yorkston NJ, Zaki SA, Pitcher DR, Gruzelier JH, Hollander D, Sergeant HGS. 1977. Propranolol as an adjunct to the treatment of schizophrenia. *Lancet* **2**: 575–8.

77. Donaldson SR, Gelenberg AJ, Baldessarini RJ. 1986. *Alternative Treatments for Schizophrenic Psychoses. American Handbook of Psychiatry.* New York: Basic Books.

78. Adler L, Angrist B, Peselow E, Corwin J, Maslansky R, Rotrosen J. 1986. A controlled assessment of propranolol in the treatment of neuroleptic-induced akathisia. *Br J Psychiatry* **149**: 42–5.

79. Kane J, Honigfeld G, Singer J, Meltzer H. 1988. Clozapine for the treatment-resistant schizophrenic: A double-blind comparison with chlorpromazine. *Arch Gen Psychiatry* **45**: 789–96.

80. Meltzer HY, Burnett S, Bastani B, Ramierz LF. 1990. Effect of six months of clozapine treatment on the quality of life of chronic schizophrenic patients. *Hosp Community Psychiatry* **41**: 892–7.

81. Lawson WB. 1996. Clinical issues in the pharmacotherapy of African-Americans. *Psychopharmacol Bull* **32**: 275–81.

82. Henderson DC. 1993. The use of clozapine in minority schizophrenics in Massachusetts. In: *Proceedings of the First Annual Symposium for Mental Health Professionals of Color.* Boston: Massachusetts Department of Mental Health.

83. Frankenburg FR, Zanarini MC, Cole JO, McElroy SI. 1992. Hospitalization rates among clozapine-treated patients: A prospective cost-benefit analysis. *Ann Clin Psychiatry* **4**: 247–50.

84. Caramikat E, Karayalcin G, Aballi A, Lunzkowsky P. 1975. Leukocyte count differences in healthy white and black children 1–5 years of age. *J Pediatr* **86**: 252–4.

85. Karayalcin G, Rosner F, Sawitsky A. 1972. Pseudoneutropenia in Negroes: A normal phenomenon. *NY State J Med* **72**: 1815–17.

86. Pickar D, Owen RR, Litman RE, Konicki PE, Guitierrez R, Rapaport MH. 1992.

Clinical and biological response to clozapine in patients with schizophrenia. *Arch Gen Psychiatry* **49**: 345–53.

87. Matsuda KT, Cho MC, Lin KM, Smith MW, Young AS, Adams JA. 1996. Clozapine dosage, serum levels, efficacy, and side-effect profiles: A comparison of Korean-American and Caucasian patients. *Psychopharmacol Bull* **32**: 253–7.

88. Baldessarini RJ, Frankenburg R. 1991. Clozapine—a novel antipsychotic agent. *N Engl J Med* **324**: 746–54.

89. Perry PJ, Miller D, Arndt SV, Cadoret R. 1991. Clozapine and norclozapine plasma concentrations and clinical response of treatment refractory schizophrenic patients. *Am J Psychiatry* **148**: 231–5.

90. Spector PJ, Opler LA. 1993. Schizophrenia and clozapine therapy (letter). *Am J Psychiatry* **150**: 1269.

91. Henderson DC, Goff DC. 1996. Risperidone as an adjunct to clozapine in chronic schizophrenics. *J Clin Psychiatry* **57**: 395–7.

16

Risperidone in the Treatment of Hispanic Schizophrenic Patients

Edyta J. Frackiewicz[a], John J. Sramek[a], Yasmine Collazo[b], Ecaterina Rotaru[b] and John M. Herrera[c]

[a]California Clinical Trials, Beverly Hills, CA, USA;
[b]Mount Sinai School of Medicine, Elmhurst, NY, USA;
[c]Eli Lilly and Company, Indianapolis, IN, USA

INTRODUCTION

In the last few decades the field of cultural psychiatry has become increasingly relevant and influential due in part to a large migration of ethnically and racially diverse individuals. This migration has led to the development of multiethnic and pluralistic communities throughout the USA [1, 2], and the evolving diversity has spurred interest in the conduct of clinical research in order to improve the mental healthcare for these individuals.

Hispanics represent a rapidly growing percentage of the population of the USA, and make up the fastest growing ethnic minority group [1]. 1990 census figures state that Hispanics constituted 8% of the total population, and this figure is expected to rise to 11% by the year 2000 [3]. The largest Hispanic-American subgroup is Mexican American, comprising approximately 5.4% of the population. Puerto Ricans comprise the second largest subgroup and Cuban Americans the third largest. Hispanics are an important subpopulation, whose special needs and responses to medical treatment have unfortunately traditionally been ignored [4].

DIAGNOSIS AND PREVALENCE OF MENTAL DISORDERS IN HISPANICS

The prevalence rates for mental disorders in Hispanics are similar to the rates for mental disorders in the general population. However, greater diagnosis rates of schizophrenia have been reported in Hispanic Americans than in non-Hispanics

Cross Cultural Psychiatry. Edited by John M. Herrera, William B. Lawson and John J. Sramek.
© 1999 John Wiley & Sons Ltd.

even though Hispanics have the same, or even slightly lower, prevalence rates [5]. This has been attributed to cultural miscommunication, which causes providers to diagnose schizophrenia in a patient who may actually be suffering from hypomania or depression [6]. A condition known as 'the Puerto Rican syndrome' serves as an example; an acute episode of this syndrome is a specific form of hysteria, which consists of seizures of a bizarre nature at a time of acute tension and anxiety, and is commonly misdiagnosed as schizophrenia [7, 8]. Visions of ancestors, religious images, and recently deceased family members are also culturally accepted phenomena among Hispanics that can, to an inexperienced clinician, seem to be caused by a perceptual disorder symptomatic of schizophrenia or other psychosis [9]. In this regard clinicians treating Hispanics must become familiar with the Hispanic culture(s) in order to understand the diversity of cultural values that can be misunderstood or misdiagnosed [9].

Studies reporting rates of hospitalization among Hispanics are conflicting. Some studies have reported higher rates in this group [10, 11]. These higher rates of hospitalization are thought to be caused by a false perception of mental illness as a manifestation of weakness, particularly among males. Mentally ill Hispanics tend to reject the possibility of mental illness or need for psychiatric treatment, and these beliefs lead mentally ill Hispanics to seek treatment only when their illness is severe and requires hospitalization [1]. Those studies reporting lower use of inpatient psychiatric services attribute the lower rates to barriers to obtaining healthcare [12, 13].

BARRIERS TO MENTAL HEALTHCARE

Hispanics have a lower utilization rate of mental healthcare services [14, 15]. Factors that contribute to this lower utilization include low income and lack of health insurance [16, 17]. A study conducted in 1989 found that 78% of the Caucasian population had private third-party health insurance coverage, 54% of the African-American population had insurance coverage and 50% of Hispanic Americans had insurance coverage [18]. Cultural and other non-financial barriers also limit access to care; these include communication problems secondary to difficulty in comprehending English, a cultural heritage which uses different methods of treatment such as spiritual and folk healers, lack of transportation to healthcare services outside the community, and a lack of provider sensitivity caused by prejudices in treatment. Additionally, less acculturated Hispanic Americans are less likely to use mental heath professional services and more likely to receive their mental health services from a general medical provider [6].

Non-compliance is a trait that has been widely observed with Hispanic Americans, and is felt to be due to cultural factors. Many Hispanic Americans believe that medical/psychiatric illnesses result from supernatural conditions, and healthcare providers must be sensitive and respectful of these cultural explanations if they are to succeed in assuring treatment compliance [19]. This is especially important in mental illness, where the rapport between the patient and provider is essential [6]. A poor initial experience may have a deleterious effect by causing a patient to discontinue treatment or to avoid treatment in the event of a relapse.

CYTOCHROME P-450 GENETIC POLYMORPHISM

Subtle and overt differences in the treatment of Hispanic mental patients cannot be explained only on the basis of cultural and financial factors. Ethnic and racial differences in antipsychotic drug disposition and response have been demonstrated by several researchers [20–23]. Currently the factors in determining response to medication in different ethnic and racial groups are complex and have not been fully elucidated; however, research in the area of pharmacogenetics has revealed significant ethnic and racial differences in the metabolism, clinical effectiveness and side-effects of antipsychotics [24–28]. Interethnic/racial differences in response to medication are thought to be due to environmental factors such as diet, chronic alcohol ingestion, and cigarette smoking and, most importantly, to genetic factors such as cytochrome P-450 (CYP) polymorphism [29].

Most of the studies evaluating antipsychotic dosing requirements in ethnic groups have been conducted in Asian populations, and Hispanics have not been studied systematically regarding antipsychotic dosing requirement and sensitivity to extrapyramidal symptoms (EPS). Anecdotal reports from Latin American countries support the belief that Hispanic patients need less medication than Caucasian patients for the treatment of disorders such as major depression, panic, or schizophrenia [30]. Two studies evaluating antipsychotic dosing in Asian and Hispanic inpatients and outpatients found that Hispanic and Asian patients received significantly less medication than the general population [31, 32]. The researchers conducting these studies believe that these results suggest that Hispanics may also be more sensitive to EPS than other groups.

CHARACTERISTICS OF RISPERIDONE

Risperidone is a benzisoxazole derivative pharmacologically characterized as a potent serotonin $5\text{-}HT_2$ and central dopamine D_2 antagonist. The advantages of risperidone over haloperidol include a faster onset of activity, a lower incidence of EPS, and possibly greater efficacy against the negative symptoms of schizo-phrenia [33]. Owing to its more favorable side-effect profile and possibly greater efficacy, risperidone may be superior to typical antipsychotics such as haloperidol [34]. A number of studies [34–37] have reported that risperidone is efficacious in treating schizophrenia, with a clinical profile of less EPS, more rapid onset of action, and efficacy for negative symptoms of schizophrenia. The incidence of EPS with risperidone increases linearly with dose, and the incidence at therapeutic doses of 4–8 mg/day is comparable to that seen with placebo and significantly less than that seen with haloperidol [33]. Additionally, one study suggests that lower doses (for example, 4–6 mg/day) may be more effective in the treatment of negative symptoms [34].

RISPERIDONE IN THE TREATMENT OF HISPANICS

A recent meeting organized by Janssen Pharmaceuticals had psychiatrists from Colombia, Argentina, and Mexico reporting that dosages of risperidone used to treat their patients with schizophrenia was similar to the amounts recommended in the USA (6 mg/day); however, they reported a tendency for lower dosages in a large number of patients [30]. A study of ten Hispanic and eight non-Hispanic schizophrenic subjects who entered into a double-blind, parallel group, inpatient multicenter risperidone dosing trial (6 mg/day of once daily versus twice daily dosing) found that Hispanic patients demonstrated a more rapid rate of symptom improvement with risperidone treatment than non-Hispanic patients (Table 16.1) [38]. Whereas both groups demonstrated substantial improvement from baseline to week 4, Hispanics responded to risperidone at a significantly faster rate from weeks 2 through 4. Statistical analyses revealed significant clinical improvement in both Hispanic and non-Hispanic subjects for each Positive and Negative Syndrome Scale (PANSS) subscale, and a significant interaction effect ($p < 0.02$) was revealed for the PANSS general psychopathology subscale, indicative of a differential rate of improvement between the two subject groups. A higher incidence of adverse events including EPS was observed in the Hispanic patients [38]. The authors concluded that risperidone may be a preferred treatment for this population at lower doses (less than 6 mg/day) because it offers the benefits of reduced EPS, rapid onset of action and alleviation of positive and negative symptoms.

COST-EFFECTIVENESS OF RISPERIDONE

Schizophrenia, due to its early age of onset and chronicity, is the most costly of the mental illnesses. The introduction of premium-priced antipsychotic agents has stimulated cost control effort by formularies [39]. At an average daily dose of 6 mg, risperidone treatment for 1 year costs $2400 whereas generic haloperidol, at a daily dose of 10 mg, costs about $250. In assessing the cost-benefit of these agents in the treatment of schizophrenia, the total costs (direct and indirect) of the illness in relation to the cost of treatment must be taken into account [40]. New antipsychotic agents, such as risperidone, may prove highly cost-effective in treating schizophrenia by preventing relapse and reducing length of stay in hospital. A retrospective study conducted by Addington et al. [41] compared days of hospitalization in 27 patients maintained for 1 year on risperidone with the number in the preceding year and found that the mean number of days of inpatient care was reduced by 20%. This study adds to the knowledge that new atypical antipsychotics

TABLE 16.1 Mean PANSS (general psychopathology) scores from baseline to week 4

	Baseline	Week 1	Week 2	Week 3	Week 4	F-value
Hispanic	53.20	52.00	36.90	31.50	28.50	92.24[a]
Non-Hispanic	52.87	49.25	41.25	38.00	33.50	

[a] $p<0.001$

seem to be able to reduce costly inpatient days. A prospective study conducted by Lindstrom *et al.* [42] evaluated the long-term clinical outcomes and effect of risperidone use on resource utilization in patients with treatment-resistant chronic schizophrenia. With risperidone therapy patients had fewer positive and negative symptoms and showed clinical improvement. The number of patients requiring hospitalization declined as did the use of anticholinergic medication to treat adverse effects. Albright *et al.* [43], in a study of the cost-effectiveness of risperidone, found that risperidone treatment reduced hospital admissions by 60.3%, and the length of hospital stay by 58.2%. The total number of physician visits in three outpatient settings decreased by 27.3% and the number of schizophrenia-related visits fell by 29.4%. The annual cost of antipsychotic drug usage increased by $907—however, the overall cost decreased by $6134 per patient. Judging the cost of care solely on comparisons of the acquisition cost of antipsychotic drugs can be misleading: the costs of all the elements of healthcare must be considered in order to make valid comparisons between treatment regimens. Newer antipsychotic agents may actually be more cost-effective in the long term, and therefore could be used to effectively treat patients under financial constraint.

RECOMMENDATIONS FOR FUTURE RESEARCH

As mentioned earlier, few studies have been conducted to observe differences in antipsychotic response in Hispanic populations. Racial and ethnic minorities are less likely to be included in pharmaceutical trials [44], although major pharmaceutical companies are now making an effort to include African Americans, Hispanics and Asians in their clinical drug trials [4].

Future studies need to be carefully designed to account for differences in antipsychotic drug metabolism. Risperidone undergoes extensive metabolism by the CYP2D6 enzyme, and therefore its oxidative metabolism is subject to genetic polymorphism. The oral bioavailability of risperidone varies from 66% in extensive metabolizers to 82% in slow metabolizers. The plasma elimination half-lives of risperidone and its metabolite in extensive metabolizers are 2.8 and 20.5 h, respectively, whereas in poor metabolizers the elimination half life is 16 h (the half-life of the active metabolite is unchanged) [33]. Poor metabolizers may therefore accumulate higher plasma concentrations following standard doses [45]. These pharmacokinetic differences are significant because variations occur in the frequencies of extensive and poor metabolizers between different ethnic groups.

Studies estimate that 6–10% of Caucasians [46–49], 1% of Asians [50–54], 1–19% of Africans [55–57], and 4.5% of Hispanics [30] are poor metabolizers. Genetic polymorphism of CYP therefore plays a role in ethnic variability in drug response and may explain why a higher incidence of side-effects is observed in certain ethnic groups. Any future studies examining dosing in ethnic groups should consider CYP2D6 genotyping/phenotyping.

Future studies also need to provide homogeneous non-Hispanic and Hispanic groups. In studies conducted to date [31, 32, 38] Asians, Blacks, and Caucasians were grouped under the classification of non-Hispanic; however, extensive research has shown that these groups differ in their response to and metabolism of anti-psychotic agents [20, 22, 23]. The Hispanic-American population is culturally diverse and consist of individuals from Mexico, Puerto Rico, Cuba, countries in Central and South America, and the Caribbean. Studies often inappropriately generalize from one subpopulation, drawing conclusions for all Hispanics that may not be necessarily accurate [6]. Intraracial and intraethnic variability can confound the results of studies because differences exist even within a relatively well defined ethnic or racial group [50, 52, 58]. Cultural factors also play an important role because cultures differ in eating and food preparation habits, exposure to pesticides, smog and other toxins, and in caffeine, nicotine and medication use patterns [59]; all of these factors are known to affect drug metabolism, disposition and excretion to a certain extent. If groups are not homogeneous it is not possible to establish whether observed differences in the incidence of EPS are exclusively due to genetic polymorphism of the cytochrome P-450 enzymes. Future studies evaluating ethnic differences in drug response need to identify and evaluate homogeneous ethnic groups and pay special attention to including racial and ethnic groups in clinical trials where genetic polymorphism for that class of medication plays a significant role [4]. By focusing on the inclusion of individuals of differing ethnic and racial backgrounds in clinical trials, drug action and side-effects specific to a particular ethnic/racial group may be revealed; this may prompt the discovery of treatments that are advantageous to specific groups.

CONCLUSIONS

The Hispanic-American population faces barriers to access to mental healthcare, and healthcare professionals need to have an increased awareness of cultural and financial factors that play a role in access to the mental healthcare system for these patients. Researchers and clinicians are faced with the challenge of finding cost-effective agents for the treatment of schizophrenia in this group. Recent findings suggest that symptoms in Hispanic patients improve more rapidly with risperidone treatment than in non-Hispanic patients and that EPS is more frequent. Initiating risperidone treatment at lower doses (less than 6 mg/day) in Hispanic patients may offer the benefits of reduced EPS, rapid onset of action, and alleviation of positive and negative symptoms of schizophrenia. Risperidone may also prove to be more cost-effective than classical antipsychotics because it apparently reduces inpatient hospital days, facilitating the return of schizophrenic patients into the community. Further investigation of ethnic and racial differences in response to novel antipsychotic compounds is warranted to optimize the potential of the new atypical antipsychotic medications.

REFERENCES

1. Ruiz P. 1995. Assessing, diagnosing and treating culturally diverse individuals: An Hispanic perspective. *Psychiatr Q* **66**(4): 329–41.
2. Gaw AC (ed.) 1993. *Culture, Ethnicity and Mental Illness.* Washington, DC: American Psychiatric Press, Inc.
3. United States Department of Commerce, Bureau of the Census. 1986. Current Population Reports; Projections of the Hispanic Population: 1983 to 2080. In: Spencer G, ed. *Population Estimated and Projection,* Series P-25, No. 995. Washington, DC: Government Printing Office.
4. Levy RA. 1993. Ethnic and racial differences in response to medicines: preserving individualized therapy in managed pharmaceutical programmes. *Pharmaceut Med* **7**: 139–65.
5. Cheung FK, Snowden LR. 1990. Community mental health and ethnic minority populations. *Community Ment Health J* **26**: 277–91.
6. Woodward AM, Dwinell AD, Arons BS. 1992. Barriers to mental health care for Hispanic Americans: A literature review and discussion. *J Ment Health Admin* **19**(3): 224–36.
7. Rendon M. 1974. Transcultural aspects of Puerto Rican mental illness in New York. *Int J Soc Psychiatry* **20**: 18–24.
8. Rendon M. 1985. Myths and stereotypes in minority groups. *Int J Soc Psychiatry* **30**: 297–309.
9. Marcos LR. 1988. Understanding ethnicity in psychotherapy with Hispanic patients. *Am J Psychoanal* **48**(1): 35–42.
10. Ruiz P. 1979. Psychiatric research and Hispanic culture: needs and direction. *World J Psychosynth* **11**(1): 32–5.
11. Rubkin JG, Shriening EL. 1976. Ethnicity, social class and mental illness. New York. Institute of Pluralism and Group Identity. *Working Papers Series* **17**: 1–37.
12. Scheffler RM, Miller AB. 1989. Demand analysis of mental health service use among ethnic subpopulations. *Inquiry* **26**: 202–15.
13. Hu TW, Snowden LR, Jerrell JM *et al.* 1991. Ethnic populations in public mental health: services, choice, and level of use in Americans. *J Publ Health* **81**: 1429–34.
14. Burnam MA, Hough RL, Escobar JI *et al.* 1987. Six-month prevalence of specific psychiatric disorders among Mexican Americans and non-Hispanic whites in Los Angeles. *Arch Gen Psychiatry* **44**: 687–94.
15. Karno M, Hough RL, Burnam MA *et al.* 1987. Lifetime prevalence of specific psychiatric disorders among Mexican Americans and non-Hispanic whites in Los Angeles. *Arch Gen Psychiatry* **44**: 695–701.
16. Ginzberg E. 1991. Access to health care for Hispanics. *JAMA* **265**: 238–41.
17. Wilson KM. 1991. A register for chronic disease interventions for Hispanics: method and product. In: *Proceedings of the 1991 Public Health Conference on Records and Statistics.* HS Publication No. (PHS) 92–1214. Hyattsville, MD: US Public Health Service, National Center for Health Statistics.

18. Chelimsky E. 1991. Hispanic access to health care: significant gaps exist. GAO/T-PEMD-91-13, Washington, DC: IS General Accounting Office.
19. Ruiz P. 1985. Cultural barriers to effective medical care among Hispanic-American patients. *Annu Rev Med* **36**: 63–71.
20. Lin KM, Finder E. 1983. Antipsychotic dosage for Asians. *Am J Psychiatry* **140**(4): 490–1.
21. Lin KM, Poland RE, Lau JK, Rubin RT. 1988. Haloperidol and prolactin concentrations in Asians and Caucasians. *J Clin Psychopharmacol* **8**(3): 195–201.
22. Potkin SG, Shen Y, Pardes H, Phelps BH, Zhou D, Shu L et al. 1984. Haloperidol concentrations elevated in Chinese patients. *Psychiatry Res* **12**: 167–72.
23. Chiu H, Lee S, Leung CM, Wing YK. 1992. Antipsychotic prescription for Chinese schizophrenics in Hong Kong. *Aust NZ J Psychiatry* **26**(2): 262–4.
24. Binder RL, Levy R. 1981. Extrapyramidal reactions in Asians. *Am J Psychiatry* **138**(9): 1243–4.
25. Kalow W. 1982. Ethnic differences in drug metabolism. *Clin Pharmacokinet* **7**(5): 373–400.
26. Lin KM, Poland RE, Lesser IM. 1986. Ethnicity and psychopharmacology. *Cult Med Psychiatry* **10**(2): 151–65.
27. Jefferson JW, Greist JH. 1996. Brussels sprouts and psychopharmacology (understanding the cytochrome P450 enzyme system). In: Jefferson JW, Greist JH, eds. *Annual of Drug Therapy Volume 3* Philadelphia: WB Saunders, pp. 2–22.
28. Smith MW, Mendoza R. 1996. Ethnicity and pharmacogenetics. *Mt Sinai J Med* **63**(5&6): 285–90.
29. Frackiewicz EJ, Sramek JJ, Herrera J, Kurtz NM, Cutler NR. 1997. Ethnicity and antipsychotic response. *Ann Pharmacother* **31**: 1360–9.
30. Ramirez LF. 1996. Ethnicity and psychopharmacology in Latin America. *Mt Sinai J Med* **63**(5&6): 330–1.
31. Ruiz S, Chu P, Sramek JJ, Herrera J. 1996. Neuroleptic dosing in Asian and Hispanic outpatients with schizophrenia. *Mt Sinai J Med* **63**(5&6): 306–9.
32. Collazo J, Tam R, Sramek JJ, Herrera J. 1996. Neuroleptic dosing in Hispanic and Asian inpatients with schizophrenia. *Mt Sinai J Med* **63**(5&6): 285–90.
33. Grant S, Fitton A. 1994. Risperidone: A review of its pharmacology and therapeutic potential in the treatment of schizophrenia. *Drugs* **48**(2): 252–73.
34. Borison RL, Pathiraja AP, Diamond BI, Meibach RC. 1992. Risperidone: clinical safety and efficacy in schizophrenia. *Psychopharmacol Bull* **28**(2): 213–18.
35. Heylen SLE, Gelders YG. 1991. Risperidone: a clinical overview. In: Kane JM, ed. *Risperidone: Major progress in Antipsychotic Treatment.* Oxford: Oxford Clinical Communications, pp. 27–30.
36. Moller HJ, Pelzer E, Kissling W, Riehl T, Wernicke T. 1991. Efficacy and tolerability of a new antipsychotic compound (risperidone): results of a pilot study. *Pharmacopsychiatry* **24**(6): 185–9.
37. Marder SR, Meibach RC. 1994. Risperidone in the treatment of schizophrenia. *Am J Psychiatry* **151**(6): 825–35.
38. Frackiewicz EJ, Sramek JJ, Collazo Y, Rotavu E, Herrera JM. Risperidone in the treatment of Hispanic schizophrenic inpatients. *Cult Med Psychiatry* (submitted).
39. Hargreaves WA, Shumway M. 1996. Pharmacoeconomics of antipsychotic drug therapy. *J Clin Psychiatry* **57**(Suppl 9): 66–76.
40. Cardoni AA. 1995. Risperidone: review and assessment of its role in the treatment of schizophrenia. *Ann Pharmacother* **29**(6): 610–18.
41. Addington DE, Jones B, Bloom D, Chouinard G, Remington G, Albright P. 1993. Reduction of hospital days in chronic schizophrenic patients treated with risperidone: a retrospective study. *Clin Ther* **15**: 917–26.

42. Lindstrom E, Eriksson B, Hellgren A *et al.* 1995. Efficacy and safety of risperidone in the long-term treatment of patients with schizophrenia *Clin Ther* **17**: 402–12.

43. Albright PS, Livingstone S, Keegan DL *et al.* 1996. Reduction in healthcare resource utilization and costs following the use of risperidone for patients with schizophrenia previously treated with antipsychotic therapy. *Clin Drug Invest* **11**: 289–98.

44. Miranda J, Azocar F, Organista KC, Munoz RF, Lieberman A. 1996. Recruiting and retaining low-income Latinos in psychotherapy research. *J Consult Clin Psychol* **64**(5): 868–74.

45. Eichelbaum M, Gross AS. 1990. The genetic polymorphism of debrisoquine/sparteine metabolism: clinical aspects. *Pharmacol Ther* **46**: 377–94.

46. Mahgoub A, Idle JR, Dring LG, Gancaster R, Smithy RL. 1977. Polymorphic hydroxylation of debrisoquine in man. *Lancet* **2**: 584–6.

47. Wedlund PJ, Aslanian WS, McAllister CB, Wilkinson GR, Branch RA. 1984. Mephenytoin hydroxylation deficiency in Caucasians: frequency of a new oxidative drug metabolism polymorphism. *Clin Pharmacol Ther* **36**: 773–80.

48. Inaba T, Junma M, Nakano M, Kalow W. 1984. Mephenytoin and sparteine pharmacogenetics in Canadian Caucasians. *Clin Pharmacol Ther* **36**: 670–6.

49. Kroemer HK, Eichelbaum M. 1995. 'It's the genes, stupid'. Molecular basis and clinical consequences of genetic cytochrome P-450 2D6 polymorphism. *Life Sci* **56**(26): 2285–99.

50. Woolhouse NM, Andoh B, Mahgoub A, Sloan TP, Idle JR, Smith RL. 1979. Debrisoquin hydroxylation polymorphism among Ghanaians and Caucasians. *Clin Pharmacol Ther* **26**: 584–91.

51. Mbanefo D, Babbunkmi EA, Mahgoub A, Sloan TP, Idle JR, Smith RL *et al.* 1980. A study of the debrisoquine hydroxylation polymorphism in a Nigerian population. *Xenobiotica* **10**: 811–18.

52. Woolhouse N, Eichelbaum M, Oates NS, Idle JR., Smith, RL. 1985. Dissociation of coregulatory control of debrisoquin/phenformin and sparteine oxidation in Ghanaians. *Clin Pharmacol Ther* **37**: 512–21.

53. Iyun AO, Lennard MS, Tucker GT, Wood HJF. 1986. Metoprolol and debrisoquin metabolism in Nigerians: lack of evidence for polymorphic oxidation. *Clin Pharmacol Ther* **40**: 387–94.

54. Sommers K, Moncrieff J, Avenant J. 1988. Polymorphism of the 4-hydroxylation of debrisoquin in Bushmen of Southern Africa. *Hum Toxicol* **7**: 273–6.

55. Nakamura K, Goto F, Ray WA, McAllister CB, Jacqz E. 1985. Inter-ethnic differences in genetic polymorphism of debrisoquin and mephenytoin hydroxylation between Japanese and Caucasian populations. *Clin Pharmacol Ther* **38**: 402–8.

56. Lou YC, Ying L, Bertilsson L, Sjoqvist F. 1987. Low frequency of slow debrisoquine hydroxylation in a native Chinese population. *Lancet* **2**: 852–3.

57. Horai Y, Nakano M, Ishizaki T, Ishikawa K, Zhou HH, Zhou BJ *et al.* 1989. Metoprolol and mephenytoin oxidation polymorphisms in Far Eastern Oriental subjects: Japanese versus mainland Chinese. *Clin Pharmacol Ther* **46**: 198–207.

58. Lieberman JA, Yunis J, Egea E, Canoso RT, Kane JM, Yunis EJ. 1990. HLA-B38, DR4, Dqw3 and clozapine-induced agranulocytosis in Jewish patients with schizophrenia. *Arch Gen Psychiatry* **47**(1): 945–8.

59. Sramek JJ, Pi EH. 1996. Ethnicity and antidepressant response. *Mt Sinai J Med* **63**(5&6): 320–5.

17

Relationship of Ethnicity to the Effects of Antipsychotic Medications

Laurie Lindamer, Jonathan P. Lacro and Dilip V. Jeste
University of California, San Diego, La Jolla, CA, USA

INTRODUCTION

Considerable heterogeneity exists in the therapeutic response to and adverse events from antipsychotic medication. Although there is significant variability due to individual differences, some of the variation may be related to intergroup differences, such as ethnicity.

In this chapter we will briefly provide an overview of some of the published studies that have addressed the possible relationship between ethnicity and the effects of antipsychotic medications. Specifically, ethnic differences in: (1) the pharmacogenetics, pharmacokinetics and pharmacodynamics of antipsychotics, (2) the antipsychotic dosage prescribed, and (3) antipsychotic-induced tardive dyskinesia (TD) will be reviewed. We will also present findings from our own ongoing study on ethnicity and TD.

ETHNIC DIFFERENCES IN PHARMACOGENETICS, PHARMACOKINETICS AND PHARMACODYNAMICS

Pharmacogenetics

Drug-metabolizing enzymes are of paramount importance in drug detoxification [1]. Ethnic differences in the activity of these enzymes can influence the disposition of antipsychotic medication, and consequently the clinical response. Individual cytochrome P-450 (CYP) isoenzymes involved in the metabolism of psychiatric drugs include CYP1A2, CYP2C, CYP2D6, and CYP3A4, with the isoenzyme CYP2D6 metabolizing haloperidol, perphenazine, risperidone, and thioridazine

Cross Cultural Psychiatry. Edited by John M. Herrera, William B. Lawson and John J. Sramek.
© 1999 John Wiley & Sons Ltd.

[2–4]. Genetic polymorphism is complex and alterations at the DNA level may result in CYP2D6 enzyme activity that is absent (poor metabolizers), increased (ultrarapid metabolizers), or decreased (slow metabolizers) compared with that associated with the homozygous form of the enzyme [5]. Individuals possessing a mutation at the CYP2D6 locus lack a functional form of the CYP2D6 isoenzyme and are referred to as poor metabolizers, whereas individuals possessing a normally functioning enzyme are referred to as extensive metabolizers. Poor metabolizers may accumulate potentially toxic blood concentrations following the administration of standard doses of substrates dependent on CYP2D6, and the incidence of adverse effects is considerably higher in poor metabolizers [6]. To avoid increased adverse effects these patients will require a lower than usual dose, as deficient metabolism may lead to increased response.

Ethnic differences in the polymorphism of CYP2D6 have been reported. The rate of the poor metabolizers is approximately 6–10% among different Caucasian populations and has been extremely low (<1%) among Chinese and Japanese people [7, 8]. However, it has been estimated that 37% of Asians possess a mutation at the CYP2D6 gene that causes them to exhibit a lower metabolic capacity (slow metabolizers) than Caucasian extensive metabolizers [9]. However, methodological differences, such as the probe used, may explain some of the ethnic differences in the literature as it relates to the prevalence of CYP2D6 poor metabolizers. For example, the frequency of poor metabolizers in African Americans was 1.9% in one study [10] and 6.1% in another [11]. The frequency of CYP2D6 poor metabolizers has been estimated to be 4.5% in Hispanics [12].

Pharmacokinetics

The ethnic differences in the CYP2D6 isoenzyme system may partly explain some of the level:dose (pharmacokinetic) differences that have been reported in studies contrasting predominantly Asian and Caucasian groups. Potkin and colleagues found that Chinese patients with schizophrenia had 52% higher plasma haloperidol concentrations than a group of American (mostly Caucasian) patients matched for gender and body weight but not age [13]. Since the American patients were on average 7.4 years older than the Chinese patients, it is unlikely that age played a significant role in the higher plasma levels of the Chinese patients.

Significantly higher levels of serum haloperidol were observed in physically healthy normal volunteers of foreign-born and American-born people of Asian origin than in their Caucasian counterparts when they were randomly administered fixed doses of haloperidol on two separate days [14]. These findings remained statistically significant after controlling for body surface area, representing a pharmacokinetic difference. In a later study, however, Lin and colleagues re-examined these issues in 13 Caucasian and 16 Asian patients with schizophrenia and failed to observe any significant differences in haloperidol serum concentrations following 2 weeks of a fixed-dose (weight-adjusted) period of haloperidol treatment [15]. In neither of these studies was the CYP2D6 metabolizer status of the patients examined. Differences in the proportions of CYP2D6 metabolizers may have influenced the results of these studies, as poor metabolizers have been observed to have higher level:dose ratios of perphenazine than rapid metabolizers [6].

Few studies have compared pharmacokinetic parameters between African Americans and Caucasians. One study found no difference in maximum plasma concentrations (C_{max}), area under the curve (AUC), or time to maximum concentration (t_{max}), following a single dose of 10 mg fluphenazine in schizophrenia patients when diet, drug or alcohol, body weight and age were controlled [16]. The authors noted that there were 5–11-fold variations within groups, which probably would have obscured any between-group differences.

It should be noted, however, that factors other than metabolic isoenzymes may affect the disposition of antipsychotic medication. Smoking, alcohol intake, concurrent use of drugs which may interact with the CYP system (such as selective serotonin reuptake inhibitors), and exposure to environmental or occupational toxins may also influence the rate of drug metabolism. Whether or not these factors are influenced by ethnicity remains unanswered. Furthermore, the utility of antipsychotic blood levels in routine clinical practice is open to question.

Pharmacodynamics

Pharmacodynamic responses may differ among ethnic groups. After accounting for differences in plasma concentrations of haloperidol, Asians were found to have a more pronounced prolactin response [14] and were more likely to experience extrapyramidal symptoms and/or optimal reduction in psychopathology than their Caucasian counterparts at lower haloperidol levels [15].

ETHNICITY AND ANTIPSYCHOTIC DOSE

While some clinical investigators have suggested that Asian patients generally respond to substantially lower doses of neuroleptics than Caucasians [17], others have not found this to be the case [18]. Lin and Finder [17] compared the neuroleptic doses of 13 Asian and 13 White patients matched for age, sex, diagnosis, and time of discharge. Neuroleptic doses were converted to chlorpromazine-equivalent (CPZE) units for comparison and corrected for body weight. Significant differences in both the maximum and stabilized doses of CPZE were found for the Asian group (1066 and 827 mg/day, respectively) and for the Caucasians (2205 and 1568 mg/day, respectively). In contrast, Sramek and colleagues [18] failed to replicate these findings in 30 Asian patients and 30 matched Caucasian patients using similar methods: only small, statistically non-significant differences between Asians and Caucasians were found for either the maximum (1314 mg versus 1421 mg) or the stabilized neuroleptic doses (726 mg versus 966 mg).

When a sample of Hispanic outpatients was compared with Caucasians and African Americans, there was no significant difference in the mean daily dose of neuroleptic medication [19]. The mean (±SD) daily dose of antipsychotic medication, converted to CPZE units, given to Hispanics was 430 (±616) mg, to Caucasians was 431 (±611) mg, and to African Americans was 539.19 (±830) mg. Similarly, Sramek et al. [20] found no significant differences in the daily neuroleptic dosages prescribed to African Americans (2173 (±1954) mg), Hispanics (1785 (±1708) mg), or Caucasians (1701 (±1721) mg) in their multiethnicity study.

A recent retrospective survey [21] of neuroleptic treatment in schizophrenia outpatients belonging to Asian, Hispanic, or General (American-born and non-American-born) groups compared actual and standardized CPZE. The authors found a significant difference between the General sample and both the Asian and Hispanic groups, with the General sample receiving higher daily doses of neuroleptics using both the actual and standardized measures of CPZE. The General sample received 340 mg standardized CPZE/day, while the Asian and Hispanic groups received 212 mg and 211 mg, respectively. Furthermore, the authors noted that the two ethnic minority groups were more likely to be prescribed low-potency neuroleptics. A similar result was seen in a study of Asian, Hispanic, and Anglo inpatients with schizophrenia [22]. The Anglo group received a greater amount of neuroleptics than did the Asian and Hispanic groups in terms of both the maximum and stabilized doses.

Some of the controversy surrounding the relationship between ethnicity and the neuroleptic dose that is prescribed and required might be partly explained by clinical biases and misdiagnoses. In a review of the use of psychotropic medications in the African-American population, Strickland and colleagues [23–25] concluded that African-American patients tended to receive substantially higher daily doses of neuroleptics, although few studies of pharmacokinetic or pharmacodynamic differences support a biological mechanism for this finding. The authors concluded that clinical biases and misdiagnoses were at least partially responsible for those differences. Lawson [26] noted that African Americans were more likely to be hospitalized regardless of degree of psychopathology, to be treated later in the course of the illness, to be less compliant, to have more limited access to treatment, and to have different cultural beliefs about medication, all of which might influence prescribing of neuroleptic medications.

ETHNICITY AND ANTIPSYCHOTIC-INDUCED TD

Numerous investigators have contributed to studying the epidemiology of and risk factors for TD. In a review of 76 selected studies including 39 187 patients, Yassa and Jeste [27] noted TD prevalence rates ranging from 3% to 62% with an average prevalence of 24%. The wide variation in prevalence may be attributed to differences in methodology, the population sampled, the diagnostic criteria for TD and controlling for risk factors. Increasing age has been consistently associated with an increased risk of TD [28, 29].

Other factors less consistently associated with an increased risk of TD include female gender, psychiatric diagnosis with affective features, previous or early extrapyramidal symptoms, brain damage, and higher doses and longer duration of neuroleptic therapy [30]. Although considerable progress has been made in recent studies to provide better estimates of incidence and more meaningful data with regard to risk factors, only a few investigators have focused on the role of ethnicity as a risk factor.

There is limited evidence that there may be differences in the prevalence of TD among different ethnic groups. As noted earlier, Yassa and Jeste reviewed 76 selected TD studies published through 1989 [27]. The studies were also analyzed for potential cultural/environmental differences by grouping the prevalence rates from different countries into four continents: North America, Europe, Africa, and Asia. The patients from Asia (16.6%) seemed to have a lower prevalence of TD than those from North America (27.6%), Europe (21.5%), or Africa (25.5%). The reviewers speculated on likely reasons for this discrepancy including neuroleptic prescribing practices and ethnicity. The authors acknowledged that their findings were limited by their grouping of studies from various countries in a continent into a single group.

Several reports in the literature support a somewhat lower prevalence of TD in Asian (compared to Western) countries. Binder and colleagues found that the prevalence of TD in six psychiatric hospitals in Tokyo and Osaka, Japan was 20.6% [31]. In a multinational study of Asians in China (Beijing, Yanji, and Hong Kong), Korea (Seoul), and Japan (Tottori), Pi and colleagues found an overall prevalence of 17.2% [32, 33]. Interestingly, multiple logistic regression analysis revealed that the odds of being diagnosed as having TD were 1.9–2.9 times greater in patients outside of Beijing than those in Beijing. The prevalence rate of TD was 8.2% in Beijing, similar to those seen in the two studies conducted in Hong Kong [34] and Shanghai [35]. The prevalence of TD was 15.8% for the Koreans in Seoul, versus 20.3% for the Koreans in Yanji, and 19.4% for the Chinese in Hong Kong versus 18.6% for the Chinese in Yanji. Because of the significant differences in prevalence among different sites with the same ethnic group (e.g. Koreans in Korea versus those in China) and the similarities in the prevalence of TD among different ethnic groups at the same site (e.g. Chinese and Korean patients in Yanji), the authors concluded that environmental factors were more important predictors of TD risk than genetic factors.

Ko and colleagues investigated the prevalence of TD, as assessed using the Abnormal Involuntary Movement Scale (AIMS), at the Shanghai Psychiatric Hospital in the People's Republic of China [35]. Of the 866 neuroleptic-treated schizophrenia inpatients examined, only 73 (8.4%) were diagnosed as having TD. The authors suggested that the low prevalence rate may be related to the use of relatively low doses of neuroleptics. The (mean (±SD) daily neuroleptic dose for the entire patient sample was 311.3 (±254) mg CPZE. In another study, Chiu *et al.*

found a relatively low prevalence of TD (9.3%) when they surveyed 917 Chinese inpatients in Hong Kong with various psychiatric diagnoses [34]. When the analysis was restricted to the patients with schizophrenia, the prevalence rate was 8.5%. The mean daily neuroleptic dose (876.3 (±853.1) mg CPZE) was, however, two times greater than that observed in Ko's patient population.

Hayashi and colleagues compared the incidence of TD in an elderly Japanese sample admitted to a psychiatric hospital with a variety of diagnoses, including dementia (with psychotic or severe behavioral symptoms) treated with or without neuroleptics [36]. Although the mean dose in this sample was lower than that seen in Western countries, the incidence of dyskinesia over 20 months was 44% in neuroleptic-treated versus 14% in non-neuroleptic-treated patients. The authors also reported that polypharmacy might have been related to this high incidence of TD because 73% of the subjects were receiving three or more types of psychotropic medications.

Several multiethnicity studies conducted in the United States have examined the prevalence of TD. Sramek and colleagues [20] surveyed 491 chronic psychiatric patients at a large state psychiatric hospital and found no significant differences in the prevalence of TD among three ethnic groups: African Americans (17%), Caucasians (18.9%), and Hispanics (15.2%). On the other hand, Morgenstern and Glazer reported that non-White patients (mostly African American) in the Yale TD Study were nearly twice as likely to develop TD as Caucasian patients when controlling for age, years of previous neuroleptic use, and average dose of neuroleptic during the follow-up period (risk ratio estimate = 1.00 for Caucasians and 1.81 for African Americans) [37]. This result was confirmed in a study of new incidence of TD among outpatients treated with antipsychotics [38]: non-Caucasians (97% African American) were 1.83 times more likely to develop TD than Caucasians when controlling for age, years of previous neuroleptic use, and average dose of neuroleptic during the follow-up period. It may be noted, however, that significantly more of the non-Caucasian sample received over 500 mg/day of neuroleptic and were given high-potency neuroleptics.

TD RISK IN PATIENTS OVER 45 YEARS OF AGE

We have been studying the incidence of and risk factors for TD in psychiatric outpatients over the age of 45. In this section we report a comparison of the risk of antipsychotic-induced TD in terms of ethnicity (Caucasians versus African Americans).

Methods

The patients with various DSM-III-R [39, 40] or DSM-IV [41] psychiatric diagnoses who were being considered for (or were relatively early in the course of)

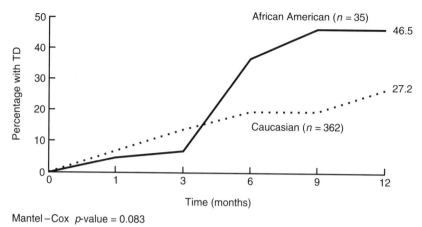

Mantel–Cox p-value = 0.083

FIGURE 17.1

treatment with antipsychotic medication were enrolled, and were treated with the lowest effective doses of neuroleptics (commonly haloperidol or thioridazine). All the patients received a comprehensive psychiatric, neurologic, other physical, and neuropsychological evaluation at study entry. Patients were assessed at study entry, at 1 and 3 months, and every 3 months thereafter for psychopathology, cognitive impairment, and TD (Figure 17.1). Details of the evaluation and treatment are described elsewhere [28].

Results

Of the 439 patients who entered the study and were included in the following analysis, 82.5% were Caucasian, 8.0% African American, and 77% were male. Forty-two percent of the sample had a diagnosis of a primary psychotic disorder, 10.4% had a mood disorder, 11.9% were diagnosed as having a diagnosis related to a general medical condition, 27.7% had a diagnosis of dementia, and 7.5% received other diagnoses. The mean age of our sample was 65.0 (standard deviation 12.5) years. To assess the role of ethnicity in the risk of TD in our study sample, we compared the Caucasians (n = 362) to the African Americans (n = 35). The cumulative proportion developing TD with 12 months of study treatment tended to be greater for the African Americans (46.5%) than Caucasians (27.2%) (Mantel-Cox = 3.00, df = 1, p = 0.083) (Figure 17.1). The groups were similar in terms of overall psychopathology (Brief Psychiatric Rating Scale, BPRS) [42], depressive symptoms (Hamilton Depression Rating Scale, HAM-D) [43], general cognitive functioning (Mini-Mental Status Examination, MMSE) [44], severity of TD (Abnormal Involuntary Movement Scale, AIMS) [45], and severity of extra-pyramidal symptoms (Simpson-Angus Total) [46], as well as average daily dose of

TABLE 17.1   Comparison of Caucasian and African-American patients in an ongoing study of TD

Variable	Caucasians (n = 362)	African Americans (n = 35)	p
Age (years)	65.7±12.6	59.3±11.4	0.005
Education (years)	12.8±3.2	11.4±3.7	0.012
Gender (percentage male)	75.6	88.2	0.0953
BPRS Total	32.3±8.0	31.5±9.7	NS
HAM-D Total	11.1±6.9	11.6±9.7	NS
MMSE Total	24.0±6.5	25.3±5.1	NS
Simpson-Angus EPS Scale Total	17.5±5.5	17.4±5.7	NS
AIMS Total	1.4±1.5	1.7±1.3	NS
Mean neuroleptic dose (mg CPZE /day) for all subjects	189.9±542.1	141.6±299.1	NS
Cumulative proportion of patients developing TD by 12 months	27.2	46.5	0.083

AIMS, Abnormal Involuntary Movement Scale; BPRS, Brief Psychiatric Rating Scale; CPZE, Chlorpromazine equivalents; EPS, extrapyramidal symptoms; HAM-D, Hamilton Depression Rating Scale; MMSE, Mini-Mental Status Examination.
The values for continuous variables represent means and standard deviations.
The rating scale scores represent values at the time of study entry.

neuroleptic (mg CPZE). The Caucasian group, however, was significantly older and had completed more years of formal education (Table 17.1).

Comment

Our unequally proportioned groups limit our ability to generalize the findings. Nevertheless, our finding that the risk of antipsychotic-induced TD tended to be greater among African Americans than among Caucasians has also been reported by others [26, 38]. In order to more appropriately address the role of ethnicity in determining the risk of TD, there is a need to study more African Americans and other ethnic minority patients in continuing TD investigations.

SUGGESTIONS FOR FUTURE RESEARCH

Ethnicity represents an important variable that may contribute to variations in drug response. In order to accurately assess the contribution of ethnicity towards antipsychotic response, investigators should address the influence of ethnicity in terms of antipsychotic dose prescribed, pharmacokinetics and pharmacodynamics. In a recent review of ethnicity and antipsychotic medication, Frackiewicz and colleagues [47] recommended that future research in this area 'should focus on homogenous ethnic groups, use recent advances in pharmacogenetic testing, and control for such variables as observer bias, gender, disease chronicity, dietary and environmental factors, and exposure to enzyme-inducing and -inhibiting agents.' We believe that this applies particularly to the problem of TD. Ethnic differences in the risk of TD have theoretical implications (in terms of neurotransmitter abnormalities; see ref. [48]), as well as clinical implications. Thus, higher risk of TD among African Americans would suggest increased caution in using neuroleptics (especially conventional ones) in this group.

ACKNOWLEDGMENTS

This work was supported, in part, by NIMH grants MH43693, MH45131, MH49671–01, MH01580, Department of Veterans Affairs, and the National Alliance for Research on Schizophrenia and Depression.

REFERENCES

1. Brosen K. 1996. Drug-metabolizing enzymes and therapeutic drug monitoring in psychiatry. *Ther Drug Monit* **18**: 393–6.
2. Eichelbaum M, Gross AS. 1990. The genetic polymorphism of debrisoquine/sparteine clinical aspects. *Pharmacol Ther* **46**: 377–95.
3. Llerena A, Dahl ML, Ekqvist B, Bertilsson L. 1992. Genetic factors in the metabolism of haloperidol. *Clin Neuropharmacol* **15**(Suppl 1, Pt A): 84A–85A.
4. Ereshefsky L. 1996. Pharmacokinetics and drug interactions: update for new antipsychotics. *J Clin Psychiatry* **57**: 12–25.
5. Edeki T. 1996. Clinical importance of genetic polymorphism of drug oxidation. *Mt Sinai J Med* **63**: 291–300.
6. Pollock BG, Mulsant BH, Sweet RA, Rosen J, Altieri LP, Perel JM. 1995. Prospective cytochrome P450 phenotyping for neuroleptic treatment in dementia. *Psychopharmacol Bull* **31**: 327–31.
7. Nakamura K, Goto F, Ray WA, McAllister CB, Jacqz E, Wilkinson GR, Branch RA. 1985. Interethnic differences in genetic polymorphism of debrisoquin and mephenytoin. *Clin Pharmacol Ther* **38**: 402–8.
8. Lou YC, Ying L, Bertilsson L, Sjoqvist F. 1987. Low frequency of slow debrisoquine hydroxylation in a native Chinese population. *Lancet* **2**: 852–3.
9. Johansson I, Yue QY, Dahl ML, Heim M, Sawe J, Bertilsson L et al. 1991. Genetic analysis of the interethnic differences between Chinese and Caucasians in the polymorphine of debrisoquin and codeine. *Eur Clin Pharmacol* **40**: 553–6.
10. Reling MV, Cherrie J, Schell MJ, Petros WP, Meyer WH, Evans WE. 1991. Lower prevalence of the debrisoquin oxidative poor metabolizer phenotype in African-American versus Caucasian subjects. *Clin Pharmacol Ther* **50**: 308–13.
11. Marinac JS, Foxworth JW, Willsie SK. 1995. Dextromethorphan polymorphic hepatic oxidation (CYP2D6) in healthy Black American adult subjects. *Ther Drug Monit* **17**: 120–4.
12. Ramirez LF. 1996. Ethnicity and psychopharmacology in Latin America. *Mt Sinai J Med* **63**: 330–1.
13. Potkin SG, Shen Y, Pardes H, Phelps BH, Zhou D, Shu L et al. 1984. Haloperidol concentrations elevated in Chinese patients. *Psychiatry Res* **12**: 167–72.
14. Lin K, Poland RE, Lau JK, Rubin RT. 1988. Haloperidol and prolactin concentrations in Asians and Caucasians. *J Clin Psychopharmacol* **8**: 195–201.

15. Lin K, Poland RE, Nuccio I, Matsuda K, Hathuc N, Su T, Fu P. 1989. A longitudinal assessment of haloperidol doses and serum concentrations in Asian and Caucasian schizophrenic patients. *Am J Psychiatry* **146**: 1307–11.

16. Midha KK, Hawes EM, Hubbard JW, Korchinski ED, McKay G, 1988. Variation in the single dose pharmacokinetics of fluphenazine in psychiatric patients. *Psychopharmacology* **96**: 206–11.

17. Lin K, Finder E. 1983. Neuroleptic dosage for Asians. *Am J Psychiatry* **140**: 490–1.

18. Sramek JJ, Sayles MA, Simpson GM. 1986. Neuroleptic dosage for Asians: A failure to replicate. *Am J Psychiatry* **143**: 535–6.

19. Adams GL, Dworkin RJ, Rosenberg SD. 1984. Diagnosis and pharmacotherapy issues in the care of Hispanics in the public sector. *Am J Psychiatry* **141**: 970–4.

20. Sramek J, Roy S, Ahrens T, Pinanong P, Cutler NR, Pi E. 1991. Prevalence of tardive dyskinesia among three ethnic groups of chronic psychiatric patients. *Hosp Community Psychiatry* **42**: 590–2.

21. Ruiz S, Chu P, Sramek J, Rotavu E, Herrera J. 1996. Neuroleptic dosing in Hispanic and Asian outpatients with schizophrenia. *Mt Sinai J Med* **63**: 306–9.

22. Collazo Y, Tam R, Sramek J, Herrera H. 1996. Neuroleptic dosing in Hispanic and Asian inpatients with schizophrenia. *Mt Sinai J Med* **63**: 310–13.

23. Bridge TP, Jeste DV, Wise CD, Potkin SG, Phelps BH, Wyatt RJ. 1981. Platelet monoamine oxidase in aged general population and elderly chronic schizophrenics. *Psychopharmacol Bull* **17**: 103–4.

24. Shah LP, Jeste DV. 1969. Hysteria and its management. *Indian J Med Sci* **23**: 273–82.

25. Vahia NS, Doongaji DR, Jeste DV. 1973. Psychological medicine. In: Vakil RJ, ed. *Textbook of Medicine*, 2nd ed. Bombay: Association of Physicians of India, pp. 1476–98.

26. Lawson WB 1996. The art and science of the psychopharmacology of African Americans. *Mt Sinai J Med* **63**: 301–5.

27. Yassa R, Jeste DV. 1992. Gender differences in tardive dyskinesia: a critical review of the literature. *Schizophr Bull* **18**(4): 701–15.

28. Jeste DV, Caligiuri MP, Paulsen JS, Heaton RK, Lacro JP, Harris MJ *et al.* 1995. Risk of tardive dyskinesia in older patients: A prospective longitudinal study of 266 patients. *Arch Gen Psychiatry* **52**: 756–65.

29. Saltz BL, Woerner MG, Kane JM, Lieberman JA, Alvir JM, Bergmann KJ *et al.* 1991. Prospective study of tardive dyskinesia incidence in the elderly. *JAMA* **266**: 2402–6.

30. Kane JM, Jeste DV, Barnes TRE, Casey DE, Cole JO, Davis JM *et al.* 1992. *Tardive Dyskinesia: A Task Force Report of the American Psychiatric Association.* Washington, DC: American Psychiatric Association.

31. Binder RL, Kazamatsuri H, Nishimura T, McNiel DE. 1987. Tardive dyskinesia and neuroleptic-induced parkinsonism in Japan. *Am J Psychiatry* **144**: 1494–6.

32. Pi EH, Gutierrez MA, Gray GE. 1993. Tardive dyskinesia: Cross-cultural perspectives. In: Lin K, Poland RE, Nakasaki G, eds. *Psychopharmacology and Psychobiology of Ethnicity.* Washington, DC: American Psychiatric Press.

33. Pi EH, Gray GE, Lee DG *et al.* 1990. Tardive dyskinesia in Asians: A multinational study. In: *New Research Abstracts, 143rd Annual Meeting of the American Psychiatric Association.* New York.

34. Chiu H, Shum P, Lau J, Lam L, Lee S. 1992. Prevalence of tardive dyskinesia, tardive dystonia, and respiratory dyskinesia among Chinese psychiatric patients in Hong Kong. *Am J Psychiatry* **149**: 1081–5.

35. Ko G, Zhang LD, Yan WW, Zhang MD, Buchner D, Xia ZY *et al.* 1989. The Shanghai 800: Tardive dyskinesia prevalence in China. *Am J Psychiatry* **146**: 387–9.

36. Hayashi T, Yamawaki S, Nishikawa T, Jeste DV. 1995. Usage and side effects of neuroleptics in elderly Japanese patients. *Am J Geriatr Psychiatry* **3**: 308–16.

37. Morgenstern H, Glazer WM. 1993. Identifying risk factors for tardive dyskinesia

among long-term outpatients maintained with neuroleptic medications: Results of the Yale Tardive Dyskinesia Study. *Arch Gen Psychiatry* **50**: 723–33.

38. Glazer WM, Morgenstern H, Doucette J. 1994. Race and tardive dyskinesia among outpatients at a CMHC. *Hosp Community Psychiatry* **45**(1): 38–42.

39. Jeste DV, Wyatt RJ. 1982. *Understanding and Treating Tardive Dyskinesia.* New York: Guilford Press, Inc.

40. Jeste DV, Grebb J, Wyatt RJ. 1985. Psychiatric aspects of movement disorders and demyelinating diseases. In Frances AJ, Hales RE, eds. *Psychiatry Update, Vol. 4.* Washington DC: American Psychiatric Press, pp. 159–89.

41. American Psychiatric Association. 1994. *Diagnostic and Statistical Manual of Mental Disorders,* 4th ed. Washington, DC: American Psychiatric Association.

42. Overall JE, Gorham DR. 1988. The Brief Psychiatric Rating Scale (BPRS): Recent developments in ascertainment and scaling. *Psychopharmacol Bull* **24**: 97–9.

43. Hamilton M. 1967. Development of a rating scale for primary depressive illness. *Br J Soc Clin Psychol* **6**: 278–96.

44. Folstein MF, Folstein SE, McHugh PR. 1975. Mini-Mental State: A practical method for grading the cognitive state of patients for the clinician. *J Psychiatr Res* **12**: 189–98.

45. National Institute of Mental Health. 1976. Abnormal Involuntary Movement Scale. In Rockville GW, ed. *ECDEU Assessment Manual for Psychopharmacology—Revised.* US Department of Health, Education, and Welfare Pub. No. (ADM)76–338, pp. 534–7. Washington, DC.

46. Simpson GM, Angus JW. 1970. A rating scale for extrapyramidal side effects. *Acta Psychiatr Scand Suppl* **212**: 11–19.

47. Frackiewicz EJ, Sramek JJ, Herrera JM, Kurtz NM, Cutler NR. 1996. Ethnicity and antipsychotic response. *Ann Pharmacother* **31**: 1360–9.

48. Eastham JH, Lacro JP, Jeste DV. 1996. Ethnicity and movement disorders. *Mt Sinai J Med* **63**(5&6): 314–19.

Affective Disorder

18

Antidepressant Response in Ethnic Populations

John J. Sramek[a] and Edmond H. Pi[b]

[a]*California Clinical Trials, Beverly Hills, CA, USA;*
[b]*University of Southern California Medical Center, Los Angeles, CA, USA*

INTRODUCTION

Advances in modern psychopharmacology have provided us with a number of effective antidepressant agents. However, treatment can often be hampered by adverse effects, delayed onset of action, and lack of response in a significant fraction (20–30%) of patients with depression [1]. Significant efforts have been made to develop agents that are more effective or have more rapid onset of action than the tricyclic antidepressant drugs; however, none yet is ideal [2]. One potential reason for the suboptimal performance of antidepressant compounds in some patients is the prevalence of interindividual differences in plasma concentrations observed with these drugs, which can vary 30–40-fold.

Increasing evidence suggests that ethnicity is an important factor in an individual's pharmacological response to antidepressant drugs [3]. Interest in this area has been fueled by the discovery of genetic polymorphism in enzyme systems responsible for metabolizing antidepressants. However, whilst the study of genetic polymorphism is an important area of transcultural psychopharmacology, there are several other factors which could potentially contribute to interethnic differences. Although the field of transcultural psychopharmacology is relatively young, researchers have undertaken efforts to determine the relative importance of society, culture, environment, genetics, and biophysiology on the prescribing practices, metabolism, and responses associated with psychotropic drugs. Unfortunately, cross cultural studies are notoriously difficult to interpret due to the many intercultural and intracultural variations in diagnostic criteria for mental illness, for therapeutic response, recommended dosages, attitudes toward healthcare, and incidence/severity of unpleasant side-effects.

Furthermore, some confusion can arise from the tendency of some researchers to group all members of a race together without regard to ethnic or cultural

Cross Cultural Psychiatry. Edited by John M. Herrera, William B. Lawson and John J. Sramek.
© 1999 John Wiley & Sons Ltd.

background. For example, Cambodian, Vietnamese, and Laotian Asians differ from Chinese, Japanese, Korean, and Polynesian Asians. 'Race' is a classification that groups individuals who share distinct genetic characteristics, while 'ethnic groups' are subpopulations that are set apart based on any number of traits which may include religion, language, appearance, ancestry, culture, or nationality. Some ethnic groups have a homogeneous gene pool; others do not. Cultural factors can further complicate the interpretation of cross cultural studies; for example, cultures can differ in their eating and food preparation habits, in exposures to pesticides, smog, and other toxins, and patterns of caffeine, nicotine, and other drug use. All of these factors can affect the processing of a drug and must be considered when trying to determine whether or not there are group differences in drug disposition. With these caveats in mind, we will review the literature on racial/ethnic responses to antidepressant medication and offer methodological suggestions for future studies.

BASIC PHARMACOLOGIC CONCEPTS

Pharmacogenetics can be defined as the study of the relationship between an individual's genotype and their ability to metabolize a particular pharmacological compound [4]. An individual's pharmacogenetic profile can influence both the pharmacokinetics (PK) and the pharmacodynamics (PD) of a given compound. While PK provides a physiological description of drug absorption, distribution, and elimination, PD refers to the response (efficacy, toxicity, etc.) which results from the drug's activity at the site of action. In other words, PK represents what the body does to a drug, and PD represents what the drug does to the body [5]. Together, pharmacogenetics, PK, and PD comprise our understanding of the pharmacology of a class of compounds. The magnitude of a compound's clinical effect is the product of these factors; however, it is also a product of individual and ethnic variances.

PHARMACOGENETIC DIFFERENCES BETWEEN ETHNIC GROUPS

Pharmacogenetic factors are believed to be a major source of interindividual variability in plasma concentrations following the administration of antidepressant compounds [6]. Specifically, differences in rates of antidepressant drug metabolism are believed to be associated with the genetic polymorphism and subsequent functional expression of the CYP2D6 and CYP2C19 subtypes of the cytochrome P-450 enzymes, with the more extreme variations resulting from the population classified as poor metabolizers [7–9].

We now recognize that there are substantial ethnic differences in the frequency distribution of CYP2D6- and CYP2C19-mediated poor metabolizers [6, 10]. For example, while only 2.9–10% of European Americans are estimated to be CYP2D6-mediated poor metabolizers [11], a recent study suggests that up to 33% of African Americans demonstrate an alteration of this enzyme resulting in lower metabolic rates [12]. Although a relatively low percentage of Asians have been designated poor metabolizers, lower overall average CYP2D6 activity has been noted in Chinese subjects than in Caucasians [13]. This difference could be due to the high frequency (approximately 50%) of an allele called CYP2D6Ch in Asian populations, which results in an unstable gene product with decreased CYP2D6 activity [6, 14, 15].

A higher percentage of CYP2C19-mediated poor metabolizers has also been documented in Japanese populations (18–23%) than in North American or European Caucasian populations (3–6%) [16–19]. Although less is known about the role of CYP2C19 in the metabolism of antidepressant compounds, evidence indicates the involvement of this enzyme in the N-demethylation of tricyclic antidepressants such as imipramine [20, 21]. This claim is supported by a recent study, in which Koyama *et al.* evaluated the steady-state plasma concentrations of imipramine and desipramine in 28 depressed Japanese patients, who had been phenotyped for CYP2C19 metabolizer status [22]. Patients received fixed doses of imipramine for a minimum of 2 weeks, and blood samples were collected 10–14 h after the last dose. These authors reported that the mean desipramine/imipramine concentration ratio (N-demethylation index) was significantly reduced in patients who were designated poor metabolizers, compared with those who were designated extensive metabolizers.

As the poor metabolism of antidepressants results in higher plasma drug levels, which can lead to a higher incidence of adverse events, these ethnic differences suggest that certain groups might require lower doses than others. The importance of studies in this area has been underscored by anecdotal reports and transcultural surveys of prescribing patterns, which indicate that antidepressant dosage requirements may indeed differ among racial groups [23–25].

PHARMACOKINETIC DIFFERENCES IN RESPONSE TO ANTIDEPRESSANTS

As early as two decades ago, researchers demonstrated that pharmacokinetic differences in response to antidepressants might exist between different ethnic groups. For example, a placebo-controlled, double-blind, randomized pilot study by Allen *et al.* reported on six East Asian (Indian/Pakistani) and eleven Caucasian (British) male volunteers who received single doses of 25 or 50 mg clomipramine [26]. There were no significant differences between the two groups with respect to mean age or body weight. At different time points up to 24 h post-treatment, the Asian subjects receiving 50 mg clomipramine attained significantly higher peak plasma and mean peak concentrations than the Caucasian subjects ($p < 0.01$). A later study, which expanded the Caucasian population to 25 volunteers, suggested that this was not an isolated finding [27]. In this report, the area under the curve values were significantly higher for Asian than for Caucasian subjects ($p < 0.005$) during the 24-h period following a single dose of 50 mg clomipramine. Like most of the studies reviewed here, however, these reports are limited by a small sample size, which increases the chance that an existing difference will not be found; interindividual variation can greatly affect statistical differences in pharmacokinetic parameters.

In a later open-label study, Rudorfer et al. examined the single-dose kinetics of 100 mg desipramine and its metabolite, 2-OH-DMI, in 14 Chinese and 16 Caucasian healthy volunteers [28]. Plasma samples were taken up to 96 h after dose administration, and serial urine samples were collected for 5 consecutive days following the dose. Mean plasma concentrations of desipramine and 2-OH-DMI were higher in the Chinese subjects at all time points, with statistically significant differences for desipramine sustained for up to 48 h ($p < 0.05$). The mean total clearance of desipramine from plasma was significantly higher ($p < 0.05$) in the Caucasian subjects than in the Chinese subjects. Although most of the volunteers had intermediate rates of clearance regardless of ethnicity, a few Chinese had slow clearances and a few Caucasians had fast clearances, leading investigators to propose the concept of a trimodal distribution, in which Chinese have slow or intermediate rates of clearance and Caucasians have intermediate or rapid rates. One potential limitation of this study is that, although the subjects were matched for age and gender, they were not matched for body weight. However, following an adjustment of the data for weight, total desipramine clearances remained significantly different.

In a subsequent related study, the same investigators looked for a similar pattern using single oral doses of 10 mg debrisoquine in 10 Chinese and 10 Caucasian volunteers, all but one of whom had participated in the previous study [29]. Compared with the Chinese subjects, the Caucasian subjects tended to excrete higher mean fractions of the dose as unchanged debrisoquine and its major metabolite, 4-hydroxydebrisoquine. However, due to the high intersubject variability, this difference did not reach statistical significance. Unlike desipramine, debrisoquine was cleared rapidly by every subject, including those who had shown slow clearance in the previous study. Contrary to expectations, debrisoquine hydroxylation did not correlate with total or hydroxylation clearance of desipramine in either ethnic group, and no trimodal distribution was observed. Because debrisoquine was thought to use the same primary metabolic pathway as desipramine, and was therefore predicted to behave in the same way, these results were difficult to explain. The finding that all subjects were rapid metabolizers of debrisoquine implies either that desipramine is metabolized by a different enzyme or that some other step in the metabolic pathway results in the trimodal distribution of desipramine clearance. Further research is necessary to evaluate the utility of debrisoquine as a biological marker for desipramine or tricyclic antidepressant metabolism in Asian and non-Asian populations [30].

One strength of these two studies is that they used an Asian group made up entirely of Chinese subjects, several of whom were genetically related. The use of more genetically homogeneous groups enhances the possibility of detecting differences caused by genetics rather than other outside factors. The use of a generic Caucasian population in the same studies, on the other hand, has a down side, because people descended from unrelated Caucasian peoples are likely to be genetically dissimilar. Additionally, potential confounding factors such as menopausal status and smoking were not controlled across groups in the first study.

Kishimoto and Hollister reported the results of a small open-label study of single doses of nortriptyline, designed to evaluate whether the lower doses of nortriptyline used in the Japanese population are related to body size or genetics [31]. Caucasian subjects in the USA (10 males) received 100 mg nortriptyline in capsule form, whereas Japanese subjects in Japan (10 males) received 50 mg in powdered suspension. Although the Japanese received half the dose taken by the Caucasians, they reached somewhat higher peak plasma concentrations and had a significantly higher mean area under the curve, a finding which investigators interpreted as a greater bioavailability of nortriptyline in Japanese. However, the differences in plasma concentration seem equally likely to be caused by formulation differences. Ideally, studies of this nature should use a single batch of study drug provided by the manufacturer. Furthermore, this study does not indicate whether or not a single laboratory was used in the PK analysis. Studies of populations in more than one location should strive to use a single laboratory to reduce variances arising from differences in analytical methods and techniques. Finally, Japanese subjects were younger and weighed significantly less than their Caucasian cohort. As body weight is a potential indicator of volume of distribution, values for clearance and bioavailability are difficult to compare.

In a similar report, Pi *et al.* compared the PK of single doses of 50 mg desipramine in 20 Asian volunteers with the results of a previous study in which 20 Caucasian volunteers had received 75 mg desipramine [32]. Asians were found to have a significantly earlier time to peak plasma concentration (4.0 h versus 6.9 h; $p<0.05$). No other significant differences in pharmacokinetic parameters between the two groups were noted. Despite having a relatively large sample size for research of this kind, the authors noted that statistical confidence remained low, limiting the generalizability of this finding to larger populations. The same investigators undertook a second study, similar to that of Rudorfer *et al.* [28], in which they looked at the clearance of 1 mg/kg desipramine in 18 Asians and 19 Caucasian volunteers [33]. Significant differences were found in time to peak plasma concentration (5.0 h for Asians; 3.0 h for Caucasians; $p<0.05$) and in desipramine and metabolite clearance, with Asians being slower than Caucasians in all cases. No other significant differences were found. Moreover, adjusting for body weight made clearance differences non-significant. Nevertheless, a visual analysis of the distribution of the clearance patterns spurred the investigators to suggest that a trimodal distribution does exist for desipramine clearance.

However, a more recent study evaluating the concentrations of clomipramine and its metabolites does not provide support for this conclusion. Shimoda *et al.* studied 108 Japanese psychiatric patients, more than 80% of whom were experiencing a major depressive episode [34]. Clomipramine was titrated up to doses ranging from 30 mg/day to 250 mg/day (average 112 mg/day, or 2.18 mg/kg body weight), and patients were maintained at the same dose for 14 days before blood sampling was performed. At the conclusion of the analysis, no poor desmethylators, hydroxylators, or glucoronidators were found, providing no evidence that Asians might metabolize clomipramine more slowly than people of other races.

Relatively little has been published regarding the pharmacokinetics of antidepressant drugs in Southeast Asian populations. In a study of imipramine treatment compliance in Vietnamese, Cambodian, and Mien patients with major affective disorder, plasma concentrations were evaluated in 19 patients [35]. Blood levels of imipramine were dose related, and indicated that patients require at least 150 mg/day to reach recommended therapeutic plasma concentrations. These preliminary results suggest that Southeast Asians need doses of imipramine similar to those required by Caucasian populations to obtain adequate blood levels. ·

One limitation of most of the studies discussed so far (three exceptions being those of Allen *et al.* [26], Lewis *et al.* [27], and Kishimoto and Hollister [31]) is that both female and male volunteers were used. Gender-related factors such as menopausal status, hormone replacement therapy, menstrual cycle changes, etc. could affect the absorption, distribution, or metabolism of drugs such that within-group variability would increase, making it more difficult to detect between-group differences. Furthermore, in some studies, both Asian and Caucasian groups were composed of more than one racial group. For example, in Pi's studies, Asians could be Vietnamese, Chinese, Korean, or Japanese, and Caucasians came from various European groups.

At this time, the question of cross cultural differences in the PK of anti-depressant drugs has largely centered around Caucasian and Asian populations. Much less in known about the PK of antidepressants in people of African or Hispanic descent. In an oft-cited study, Ziegler and Briggs treated 65 depressed patients with amitriptyline and nortriptyline in order to assess the influence of factors such as age, race, sex, and smoking behavior on steady-state plasma drug concentrations [36]. Black patients had significantly higher (50%) nortriptyline plasma levels than Caucasian patients, a finding which could explain why Black patients may respond more quickly to tricyclic antidepressant medications. The study remains difficult to interpret, however, because diagnostic criteria are unclear, no gender distribution was reported, and, most importantly, a fixed-dose protocol was not used. The correction for dose cited by the authors also resulted in further confounding of the drug plasma level data [37].

In a study of clomipramine treatment in Benin, West Africa, researchers com-pared plasma pharmacokinetics in an African Black population ($n = 29$) and a Caucasian population ($n = 29$) with major depression [38]. Patient groups were matched for age and sex. To control for the lower mean doses used in the African Black population, pharmacokinetic comparisons were based on a clomipramine/desmethylclomipramine level to weight-related daily dosage ratio. Although there was a trend toward higher values in the African Black sample, this difference did not reach statistical significance. As the method of investigating the ratio of clomipramine/desmethylclomipramine to weight-related doses may be limited by the non-linear pharmacokinetics of tricyclic antidepressants, further studies will be necessary to explain these findings.

In another area of research, although it has not been fully investigated, African American and African Black patients with bipolar disorder have been shown to have a higher erythrocyte/plasma lithium ratio than Caucasian patients with bipolar disorder, which suggests that people of African descent might require lower doses of lithium to achieve antidepressant and/or antimanic efficacy [39]. For example, in a study by Okpaku *et al.*, blood samples were drawn from healthy Black and Caucasian subjects, and erythrocytes were separated and loaded with lithium [40]. The erythrocyte lithium concentrations were then measured with spectrophotometry at 0 and 25 h after loading. While the concentrations were similar immediately after loading, the lithium concentrations were significantly higher in the Black subjects after 25 h. These results indicate that the efflux of lithium was lower in the erythrocytes of the Black subjects. In a later study, Chang *et al.* demonstrated a statistically significantly longer plasma lithium half-life in African Americans than in Caucasians and Chinese [41]. However, this study was limited by the fact that the estimation of half-life was based on only two time points (12 and 25 h post-dose).

In a comparison of Hispanic and Caucasian non-depressed volunteers, no significant differences were found between groups in PK parameters following a single oral dose of 75 mg nortriptyline [42]. However, this study might have been hindered by the use of a non-depressed population; investigators speculated that because depression itself may alter PK, healthy volunteers may not be a sufficiently representative group.

PHARMACODYNAMIC DIFFERENCES IN RESPONSE TO ANTIDEPRESSANTS

Although no attempts have been made to systematically assess differences in PD factors in response to antidepressants among different ethnic groups, several reports have noted that such differences may exist. For example, Asian patients hospitalized with severe depression appear to respond clinically to lower combined concentrations of imipramine and desipramine (130 mg/ml) than those that are generally reported in North American and European studies (180–200 ng/ml), suggesting that tricyclic dosage requirements may be governed by variances in brain receptor responsivity among different ethnic groups [24, 43]. Furthermore, anecdotal reports suggest that Asians also have a lower threshold for experiencing adverse drug reactions [23, 24]. In the studies of Allen *et al.* [26] and Lewis *et al.* [27], East Asian subjects experienced significantly more drug-related side-effects, and their reaction times on studies of response time, hand/eye coordination, and time required for new learning and decision-making were more affected by the medication than were the reaction times of Caucasians. However, the interpretation of these results is somewhat limited due to potential learning effects from repeated use of the tests.

The belief that Asians require lower doses of therapeutic medication to achieve positive response is also supported by several studies of lithium treatment in bipolar depression. For example, Yang studied 101 Taiwanese patients with bipolar depression treated over 2 years with clinically determined doses of lithium, and found that plasma lithium levels for the majority of good responders ranged between 0.5 and 0.79 mEq/l [44]. Similarly, Chang et al. reported optimal therapeutic lithium concentrations of 0.71 and 0.73 mEq/l for Chinese patients with bipolar depression living in Shanghai and Taipei, respectively, compared with a mean level of 0.98 mEq/l for matched Caucasian-American patients [41, 45]. These values are also lower than the 0.8–1.2 mEq/l generally thought to be standard in Europe and North America [46].

Black patients also appear to require lower doses of antidepressant medication than Caucasian patients to achieve a therapeutic response. For example, in a study of indigenous African outpatients from Tanzania, patients were reported to respond to much lower doses of clomipramine than the recommended doses in Western textbooks [47]. In another study of 159 Black and 555 Caucasian patients with depression, Raskin and Crook assessed responses to chlorpromazine, imipramine, and placebo on a number of standard psychometric scales [48]. Black patients showed greater improvement at 1 week regardless of treatment, suggesting that they might be more sensitive to antidepressant effects. However, a number of methodological concerns contribute to a difficulty in the interpretation of this study [49]. First, the percentage of patients diagnosed with schizophrenia was notable higher among the Black (particularly male) patients than the Caucasian sample. Additionally, the Black patients were younger and significantly more economically and educationally disadvantaged than their Caucasian counterparts. Nevertheless, this study is not alone in its findings. Previous large, multicenter studies have also noted similar differences in response [50, 51].

Black patients also appear to be more sensitive to the adverse effects of antidepressants than Caucasian patients. A chart review study of 125 inpatients with depression (102 Caucasians and 23 Blacks) found that delirium was significantly more common in Black patients, older patients, and those with higher tricyclic antidepressant levels [52]. In this study, Black patients comprised only 18% of the sample, but comprised 50% of the patients who experienced delirium. Unfortunately, it is unclear how race was related to the incidence of delirium independent of age and plasma concentrations in this study. The study conducted by Kilonzo et al. reported that notable drowsiness and tremulousness were observed in the African Black sample at what was considered to be a low-to-moderate dose of clomipramine hydrochloride (125 mg) [47]. In another retrospective investigation involving 19 patients who had overdosed on amitriptyline, plasma concentrations were shown to be significantly higher in the 6 Black patients (all female) than in the Caucasian patients (5 males and 13 females) [53]. Although both these studies are limited by the small numbers of Black patients or small size in general, and a lack of rigorous controls, they do suggest that African Americans are more susceptible to the central nervous system side-effects of tricyclic anti-depressant medications than are Caucasians. Whether or not this is caused by PD mechanisms is an issue which remains largely unexplored.

There is also some indication that differences in response to antidepressants exist between Hispanic and Caucasian patients. In a retrospective study, Marcos and Cancro studied 41 Hispanic (predominantly Puerto Rican) and 21 Caucasian females who were diagnosed with major depression and were receiving tricyclic antidepressant medications (amitriptyline, imipramine, or doxepin) [54]. The authors assessed the maximum daily dosage taken by each patient for at least 1 week, the type and occurrence of side-effects, and the outcome of treatment. The Hispanic patients used approximately half the dosage given to Caucasian patients, but had similar treatment outcomes. Furthermore, Hispanic patients complained of adverse effects, and had their medications discontinued because of adverse effects, significantly more often than Caucasians. Unfortunately, no PK data were collected in this study. Cultural factors relating to the significance of somatic complaints as depressive equivalents in the Hispanic population were thought to play an important role in the response to treatment.

RECOMMENDATIONS FOR FUTURE RESEARCH

Differences in antidepressant drug disposition among different ethnic/racial groups could have significant implications for the optimal treatment of diverse populations, particularly in countries with heterogeneous populations such as the USA. To date, however, most transcultural psychopharmacology studies have been limited by their small and often inadequately characterized samples. Future studies should use larger populations to permit detection of between-group differences with statistical confidence. Populations need to be extremely well characterized to maximize the ability to control for other variables such as gender, age, lean and actual body weight, birthplace, place of residence, concomitant illness and/or medications, diet, alcohol/nicotine/caffeine intake patterns, menopausal status, menstrual cycle effects, and (of course) diagnosis and severity of depression [30]. If a sample encompasses patients of several races residing in different countries, it may become easier to separate the influences of culture, race, and ethnicity.

However, there are also several methodological issues involved in conducting studies with larger populations, requiring careful monitoring to avoid the problems inherent in multicenter studies. To the greatest extent possible, diagnostic criteria and rating and diagnostic techniques should be standardized and confirmed (that is, by use of the SCID and frequent inter-rater training sessions). Furthermore, medication to be tested should be from a single source and given in a single-dosage form to minimize variances that arise from product formulations. Future research into the PK of antidepressant medications among ethnic groups should also be expanded to include study of the serotonin selective reuptake inhibitors (SSRIs). This class of drugs is widely prescribed for the treatment of depression, but the possibility of ethnic variations in response has not been systematically considered. As many SSRIs are metabolized by or inhibit the cytochrome P-450 isoenzymes, there are reasonable grounds to suspect that ethnic variations in response may exist for these compounds. Anecdotal clinical observations have suggested that African-American female patients experience significant adverse events while taking the recommended dose (20 mg) of SSRIs such as paroxetine and fluoxetine, and demonstrate adequate therapeutic response at lower doses [11]. At this time, the anecdotal evidence for PK and PD differences in various ethnic groups has gained limited support at best, and more research should be performed.

The systematic exploration of biological markers for depression in different populations is highly recommended. By examining patient responses on the dexamethasone suppression test, Escobar found significant differences in cortisol suppression across groups of outpatients with depression at a Veterans Administration hospital: 58% of Anglo patients with a major depressive disorder were non-suppressors compared with only 25% of Blacks and 0% of Hispanics [55]. However, as this study was retrospective, various factors such as age and psychiatric diagnosis were not controlled across groups. A later study of 553 non-medicated Mexican outpatients [56] concluded that there is little evidence to suggest differences among groups on the dexamethasone suppression test, although the 36% proportion of dexamethasone suppression test non-suppression among the 30 patients in the sample with major depressive disorders is still significantly different from the 58% figure for Anglo patients cited by Escobar. Clearly, elucidation of causes of differing values among different groups, if such differences are shown to exist, could be valuable.

In recent years, several other biochemical factors have been developed as surrogate markers of antidepressant function. Future studies in patients with depression should examine levels of these factors, including serotonin, norepinephrine, and dopamine metabolites in cerebrospinal fluid, plasma adrenocorticotrophic hormone, and growth hormone. Platelet imipramine binding could also be compared across ethnic groups. In addition, more direct imaging methods such as positron emission tomography may enable investigators to look at specifically targeted areas of the brain. Systematic investigation of the potential effects of ethnicity on the biological correlates of depression may help to improve our understanding and treatment of depression and other mental disorders. Furthermore, efforts should be made to determine the relative influence of genetic and environmental factors on cross cultural differences in antidepressant response. Although we devote significant efforts to the research of biological markers, we must also establish that clinically significant variations in response to antidepressants do indeed exist between different ethnic groups with respect to efficacy or adverse effects, and attempts should be made to identify factors contributing to these differences.

REFERENCES

1. Dawkins K, Manji HK, Potter WZ. 1994. Pharmacodynamics of antidepressants. In: Cutler NR, Sramek JJ, Narang PK, eds. *Pharmacodynamics of Drug Development: Perspectives in Clinical Pharmacology.* Chichester: John Wiley & Sons Ltd., pp. 157–80.

2. Katz MM, Koslow SH, Maas JW *et al.* 1987. The timing, specificity, and clinical prediction of tricyclic drug effects in depression. *Psychiatry Med* **17**: 297–309.

3. Sramek JJ, Pi EH. 1996. Ethnicity and antidepressant response. *Mt Sinai J Med* **63**(5–6): 320–5.

4. Linder MW, Prough RA, Valdes R Jr. 1997. Pharmacogenetics: a laboratory tool for optimizing therapeutic efficiency. *Clin Chem* **43**(2): 254–6.

5. Benet LA. 1994. Foreword. In: Cutler NR, Sramek JJ, Narang PK, eds. *Pharmacodynamics and Drug Development: Perspectives in Clinical Pharmacology.* Chichester: John Wiley & Sons Ltd., pp. xiii–xv.

6. Bertilsson L, Dahl M-L, Tybring G. 1997. Pharmacogenetics of antidepressants: clinical aspects. *Acta Psychiatr Scand* **96**(Suppl 391): 14–21.

7. Bertilsson L, Mellström B, Nordin C *et al.* 1983. Clinical Pharmacology in Psychiatry: Bridging the Experimental–Therapeutic Gap. In: Gram LF, Usdin E, Dahl SG *et al.* eds. *Frontiers in Neuropsychiatric Research: Proceedings of a Symposium held in Orfu, Greece, 28–30 June, 1982.* London: Macmillan Press, pp. 217–26.

8. Brisen K, Otton SV, Gram LF. 1985. Sparteine oxidation polymorphism in Denmark. *Acta Pharmacol Toxicol* **57**: 357–60.

9. Breyer-Pfaff U, Pfandl B, Nill K, Nusser E, Monney C, Jonzier-Perey M *et al.* 1992. Enantioselective amitriptyline metabolism in patients phenotyped for two cytochrome P450 isoenzymes. *Clin Pharmacol Ther* **52**: 350–8.

10. Meyer OA. 1992. Molecular genetics and the future of pharmacokinetics. In: Kalow W, ed. *Pharmacogenetics of Drug Metabolism.* New York: Pergamon Press.

11. Strickland TL, Stein R, Lin K, Risby E, Fong R. 1997. The pharmacologic treatment of anxiety and depression in African Americans. Considerations for the general practitioner. *Arch Fam Med* **6**: 371–5.

12. Kalow W. 1993. Pharmacogenetics: its biologic roots and the medical challenge. *Clin Pharmacol Ther* **54**: 235–41.

13. Bertilsson L, Lou YQ, Du YL, Liu Y, Kuang TY, Liao XM *et al.* 1992. Pronounced differences between native Chinese and Swedish populations in the polymorphic hydroxylations of debrisoquine and S-mephenytoin. *Clin Pharmacol Ther* **51**(4): 388–97.

14. Johansson I, Oscarson M, Yue QY, Bertilsson L, Sjoqvist F, Ingelman-Sundberg M. 1994. Genetic analysis of the Chinese cytochrome P4502D locus: characterization of variant CYP2D6 genes present in subjects with diminished capacity for debrisoquine hydroxylation. *Mol Pharmacol* **46**(3): 452–9.

15. Yokota H, Tamura S, Furuya H, Kimura S, Watanabe M, Kanazawa I *et al.* 1993. Evidence for a new variant CYP2D6 allele CYP2D6J in a Japanese population associated with lower in vivo rates of sparteine metabolism. *Pharmacogenetics* **3**(5): 256–63.

16. Nakamura K, Goto F, Ray WA, McAllister CB, Jacqz E, Wilkinson GR, Branch RA. 1985. Interethnic differences in genetic polymorphism of debrisoquin and mephenytoin hydroxylation between Japanese and Caucasian populations. *Clin Pharmacol Ther* **38**: 402–8.

17. Horai Y, Nakano M, Ishizaki T, Ishikawa K, Zhou HH, Zhou BJ *et al.* 1989. Metoprolol and mephenytoin oxidation polymorphisms in Far Eastern Oriental subjects: Japanese versus mainland Chinese. *Clin Pharmacol Ther* **46**: 198–207.

18. Wilkinson GR, Guengerich JP, Branch RA. 1989. Genetic polymorphism of S-mephenytoin hydroxylation. *Pharmacol Ther* **43**: 53–76.

19. Alván G, Bechtel P, Iselius L, Gundert-Remy U. 1990. Hydroxylation polymorphisms of debrisoquine and mephenytoin in European populations. *Eur J Clin Pharmacol* **39**: 533–7.

20. Skjelbo E, Brøsen K, Hallas J, Gram LF. 1991. The mephenytoin oxidation polymorphism is partially responsible for the *N*-demethylation of imipramine. *Clin Pharmacol Ther* **49**: 18–23.

21. Chiba K, Saitoh A, Koyama E, Tani M, Hayashi M, Ishizaki T. 1994. The role of *S*-mephenytoin 4'-hydroxylation in imipramine metabolism by human liver microsomes: a two-enzyme kinetic analysis of *N*-demethylation and 2-hydroxylation. *Br J Clin Pharmacol* **37**: 237–42.

22. Koyama E, Tanaka T, Chiba K, Kawakatsu S, Morinobu S, Totsuka S, Ishizaki T. 1996. Steady-state plasma concentrations of imipramine and desipramine in relation to *S*-mephenytoin 4'-hydroxylation status in Japanese depressive patients. *J Clin Psychopharmacol* **16**(4): 286–93.

23. Yamamoto J, Fung D, Lo S, Reece S. 1979. Psychopharmacology for Asian Americans and Pacific Islanders. *Psychopharmacol Bull* **15**: 29–31.

24. Yamashita I, Asano Y. 1979. Tricyclic antidepressants: therapeutic plasma level. *Psychopharmacol Bull* **15**: 40–4.

25. Pi EH, Jain A, Simpson GM. 1986. Review and survey of different prescribing practice in Asia. In: Shagass C, Josiasen RC, Bridger W, Weiss KJ, eds. *Biological Psychiatry*. New York: Elsevier Science Inc., pp. 1536–8.

26. Allen JJ, Rack PH, Vaddadi KS. 1977. Differences in the effects of clomipramine on English and Asian volunteers: preliminary report on a pilot study. *Postgrad Med J* **53**(S4): 79–86.

27. Lewis P, Rack PH, Vaddadi KS, Allen JJ. 1980. Ethnic differences in drug response. *Postgrad Med J* **56**(S1): 46–9.

28. Rudorfer MV, Lane EA, Chang WH, Zhang M, Potter WZ. 1984. Desipramine pharmacokinetics in Chinese and Caucasian volunteers. *Br J Clin Pharmacol* **17**: 433–40.

29. Rudorfer MV, Lane EA, Potter WZ. 1985. Interethnic dissociation between debrisoquine and desipramine hydroxylation. *J Clin Psychopharmacol* **5**: 89–92.

30. Pi EH, Wang AL, Gray GE. 1993. Asian/non-Asian transcultural tricyclic antidepressant psychopharmacology: a review. *Prog Neuropsychopharmacol Biol Psychiatry* **17**: 691–702.

31. Kishimoto A, Hollister LE. 1984. Nortriptyline kinetics in Japanese and Americans. *J Clin Psychopharmacol* **4**: 171–2.

32. Pi EH, Simpson GM, Cooper TB. 1986. Pharmacokinetics of desipramine in Caucasian and Asian volunteers. *Am J Psychiatry* **143**: 1174–6.

33. Pi EH, Tran-Johnson TK, Walker NR *et al.* 1989. Pharmacokinetics of desipramine in Asian and Caucasian volunteers. *Psychopharmacol Bull* **25**: 483–7.

34. Shimoda K, Noguchi T, Ozeki Y *et al.* 1995. Metabolism of clomipramine in a Japanese psychiatric population: hydroxylation, desmethylation, and glucoronidation. *Neuropsychopharmacology* **12**: 323–33.

35. Kinzie JD, Leung P, Boehnlein JK, Fleck J. 1987. Antidepressant blood levels in Southeast Asians: clinical and cultural implications. *J Nerv Ment Dis* **175**(8): 480–5.

36. Ziegler VE, Briggs JT. 1977. Tricyclic plasma levels—effect of age, race, sex, and smoking. *JAMA* **238**: 2167–9.

37. Rifkin A, Kline DF, Quitkin F. 1978. Possible effect of race on tricyclic plasma level (letter). *JAMA* **239**: 1845–6.

38. Bertschy G, Vandel S. 1992. Clomipramine plasma levels among depressed outpatient in Benin, West Africa: drug compliance and comparison with Caucasian patients. *J Clin Psychopharmacol* **12**(5): 334–6.

39. Strickland T, Lin KM, Fu P *et al.* 1995. Comparison of lithium ratio between African-American and Caucasian bipolar patients. *Biol Psychiatry* **37**: 325–30.
40. Okpaku S, Fraxer A, Mendels J. 1980. A pilot study of racial differences in erythrocyte lithium transport. *Am J Psychiatry* **137**: 120–1.
41. Chang SS, Pandey GN, Zhang MY *et al.* 1984. Racial differences in plasma and RBC lithium levels. Presented at the Annual Meeting of the American Psychiatric Association, May 5–11, Los Angeles, CA. Continuing Medical Education Syllabus and Scientific Proceedings, pp. 239–40.
42. Gaviria M, Gil AA, Javaid JI. 1986. Nortriptyline kinetics in Hispanic and Anglo subjects. *J Clin Psychopharmacol* **6**: 227–31.
43. Glassman AH, Perel JM, Shostak M *et al.* 1977. Clinical implications of imipramine plasma levels for depressive illness. *Arch Gen Psychiatry* **34**: 197–204.
44. Yang YY. 1985. Prophylactic efficacy of lithium and its effective plasma levels in Chinese bipolar patients. *Acta Psychiatr Scand* **71**: 171–5.
45. Chang SS, Pandey GN, Yang YY et al. 1985. Lithium pharmacokinetics: interracial comparison. Presented at the 138th Annual meeting of the American Psychiatric Association, May 19–24, Dallas, Texas.
46. Jefferson JW, Greist JH, Ackerman DL, Carrol JA, eds. 1987. *Lithium Encyclopedia for Clinical Practice*, 2nd ed. Washington, DC: American Psychiatric Press.
47. Kilonzo GP, Kaaya SF, Rweikiza JK, Kassam M, Moshi G. 1994. Determination of appropriate clomipramine dosage among depressed African outpatients in Dar es Salaam, Tanzania. *Centr Afr J Med* **40**(7): 178–82.
48. Raskin A, Crook T. 1975. Antidepressants in black and white inpatients. *Arch Gen Psychiatry* **32**: 643–9.
49. Strickland TL, Ranganath V, Lin K *et al.* 1991. Psychopharmacologic considerations in the treatment of Black American populations. *Psychopharmacol Bull* **27**(4): 441–8.
50. Henry BW, Overall JE, Markette J. 1971. Comparison of major drug therapies for alleviation of anxiety and depression. *Dis Nerv Syst* **32**: 655–67.
51. Overall JE, Hollister LE, Kimball I Jr *et al.* 1969. Extrinsic factors influencing psychotherapeutic drugs. *Arch Gen Psychiatry* **21**: 89–94.
52. Livingston RL, Zucker DK, Isenberg K, Wetzel RD. 1983. Tricyclic antidepressants and delirium. *J Clin Psychiatry* **44**: 173–6.
53. Rudorfer MV, Robins E. 1982. Amitriptyline overdose: clinical effects of tricyclic antidepressant plasma levels. *J Clin Psychiatry* **42**: 457–60.
54. Marcos LR, Cancro R. 1982. Pharmacotherapy of Hispanic depressed patients: clinical observations. *Am J Psychotherapy* **36**: 505–13.
55. Escobar JI. 1985. Are results on the dexamethasone suppression test affected by ethnic background? (letter) *Am J Psychiatry* **142**: 268.
56. de la Fuente JR, Sepulveda Amor J. 1986. Does ethnicity affect DST results? [letter] *Am J Psychiatry* **143**: 265–76.

19

Meta-Analysis of Safety of Fluoxetine in Asian Patients

Kenneth Kwong[a], Man C. Fung[a], Hsiao-hui Wu[b], John Plewes[a] and Rajinder Judge[a]

[a]*Eli Lilly and Company, Indianapolis, IN, USA;* [b]*Eli Lilly and Company, Taipei, Taiwan*

INTRODUCTION

Prevalence of Major Depression in Asian Populations

Depression is one of the most common mental disorders, affecting an estimated 2–4% of men and 5–9% of women at any point in time [1]. Up to one in six individuals may require treatment for depression during their lifetime [2]. Rates can be higher for at-risk populations, including elderly people, socioeconomically disadvantaged people, and those with a family history of depression. For example, it is estimated that 1–5% of elderly persons in the community and 5–43% of patients in nursing homes have major depression [3]. Persons of low income and with a history of alcohol abuse or dependence are 2–7 times more likely to develop major depressive disorder (MDD) [4]. MDD is in part a genetic disorder and individuals with a family history are up to three times more likely to develop the disorder than their counterparts [5]. Depression is a clinical syndrome, often chronic and recurring, diagnosed by the occurrence of at least one of the following three abnormal moods for a period longer than 2 weeks: a depressed mood, loss of interest or pleasure in activities, and extreme irritability (for people of 18 years old and younger) [6]. Associated disabling physical symptoms of MDD include sleep disturbance, psychomotor retardation, and changes in appetite or weight. Psychological symptoms of fatigue, self-reproach, poor concentration and morbid thoughts of death can accompany the disorder. MDD causes marked functional impairment, has a disruptive effect on family and social life, increases use of healthcare resources and causes economic losses due to occupational impairment. Despite the high prevalence of depression, recognition and diagnosis of the disorder in primary care patients by physicians is varied and suboptimal. Perhaps the underdiagnosis of depression in patients is due in part to the cultural stigma attached to the diagnosis of a mental

Cross Cultural Psychiatry. Edited by John M. Herrera, William B. Lawson and John J. Sramek.
© 1999 John Wiley & Sons Ltd.

disorder. Only 30% of persons with depression seek or receive treatment despite the treatable nature of the condition [7]. Evidence suggests that correct diagnosis, psychotherapy, pharmacotherapy, or a combined therapeutic approach of adequate duration correlates with improvements in symptomology, restoration of functioning and work performance, and the prevention of relapse [8–11].

Asian populations represent the world's largest ethnic group, comprising approximately 54% of the world's population [12]. According to the US Bureau of the Census, Asians and Pacific Islanders accounted for 3% of America's population in 1995, but, more importantly, they are the fastest growing minority group, doubling in size each decade since 1970 [13]. Depression in Asian cultures has generally been reported at lower incidence than in North American or European populations. For example, Lee *et al.* estimates the lifetime prevalence of major depression in Korea at 0.3% for men and 2.4% for women [14], using the epidemiological survey procedures of Robin and colleagues. For comparison, Robins *et al.* reported depression prevalence to be 2–4% for Asian men, and 5–9% for women, living in the USA [1]. In China, the frequency of depression was reported by the Hunan Medical College at only 1%, while the disorder of neurasthenia (all forms) was reported at 30% [15]. Similarly, Shen reported low rates of depressive disease in Chinese patients (0.03–0.09%) [16]. However, by employing a standardized procedure of symptom evaluation with a group of Japanese, Chinese, and Korean psychiatrists, Nakane and colleagues suggest that the actual prevalence in Asians may actually be no lower than those in the West [17]. Rather, the difference in incidence between countries may result from the differences in diagnostic criteria for this condition, cultural differences in the acceptance of depression as a treatable mental disorder, and the accessibility of psychiatric or medical care. A patient diagnosed with major depression in one culture may receive a diagnosis of neurasthenia (a general condition of weakness or exhaustion) in another. A follow-up study using diagnostic criteria from the Diagnostic Statistical Manual of Mental Disorders [6] established a prevalence of major depression for Japan, China and Korea to be between 5 and 16%, although differences in patient symptoms were noted [18].

In Japan, the lifetime prevalence of MDD is 5.8% in adults and is markedly similar to the rates in the USA [19]. Depressed patients in Japan were more likely to be women, aged 45 or older, or married. No seasonal dependence of depressive onset was noted, in stark contrast with patients in the USA, many of whom have recurrent fall–winter and spring–summer depression [20]. Of all the Japanese patients who met the criteria of clinical depression in this study, few had been previously diagnosed or treated. The authors suggest that the underdiagnosis of depression in Japanese patients may be due in part to cultural factors and an overburdened primary care system that is not conducive to the diagnosis of psychological distress/disorders. The major precipitating factor of depression in Japanese men was occupational change, responsible for 30% of the depressive onsets for men compared with only 1% for the women studied [21].

Mental health studies suggest that recently arrived and first-generation immigrants in the USA are at higher risk of depression than either Asians counterparts overseas or

Caucasian counterparts in the USA. Higher depression rates in such groups may be caused by stress related to immigration, cultural and language barriers, and educational and occupational difficulties. Seven per cent of newly arrived Vietnamese refugees were diagnosed with major depression [22]. Community-based studies of Chinese Americans (predominantly foreign-born) in San Francisco suggest that one-quarter of the population is clinically depressed as indicated by a score of 16 or higher on the Center for Epidemiological Studies-Depression Scale (CES-D) [23]. These results are in agreement with a community-based study of Chinese Americans in Seattle, which reported that 19% of the population was clinically depressed [24]. Ying [23] found a significant correlation between depression symptomology and socio-economic level, suggesting that higher educational/occupational levels can buffer against the stresses of daily life. However, the author also mentions that there is a lack of differentiation between psychological and bodily complaints in the Chinese-American sample. This may suggest that depression cannot be easily diagnosed or fully understood beyond the borders of the culture under study.

Statistical models suggest that the lifetime rate of depression is increasing, albeit gradually, in younger birth cohorts compared with older generations for all countries examined [25]. Studies involving college students in the USA suggest that Asian Americans suffer a higher rate of depression than Caucasians, a fact which may have an affect-specific explanation: ethnicity variables are linked to social anxiety and covariant with depression in Asian Americans [26]. A study of adolescents living in Los Angeles examined how interracial differences between Asian and Caucasian patients affected their psychiatric diagnoses [27]. Highest rates of depression were noted among Korean and Japanese men (20.9% and 6.4%, respectively), and Filipino, Japanese, and Chinese women (13.6%, 12.8%, and 12.5%, respectively). Lowest rates were found among Filipino and Vietnamese men (2.6% and 2.7%, respectively), and Southeast Asian, Cambodian, Laotian, and Hmong women (4.9%). Gender differences also proved significant, with 9.7% of Asian and 5.7% of Caucasian women diagnosed with MDD, while only 5.3% of Asian and 3.8% of Caucasian men were similarly diagnosed.

Owing to dramatic improvements in medical care, the world's elderly population is growing at a rapid pace. Although symptoms of depression in elderly people are remarkably similar to those seen in younger patients, elderly patients represent a particular challenge for pharmacotherapy because they are less tolerant of adverse effects, take one or more concomitant medications and have altered pharmacokinetics. In addition, concomitant medical illness obscures the diagnosis of depression in elderly patients, and as a result many go untreated. Depression continues to be the major cause of morbidity and mortality in elderly people [3].

Transcultural Differences in Antidepressant Metabolism

Presently there is a limited number of transcultural studies of pharmacokinetic responses to antidepressants, with those few primarily focusing on tricyclic antidepressants. However, differences in patient response will influence prescribed dosage, safety of use and patient compliance. There is debate as to whether Asian and Caucasian groups have different pharmacokinetic responses and side-effect sensitivities to antidepressants. Survey data suggest that the tricyclic antidepressants (TCAs) imipramine and amitriptyline are generally prescribed to Asians at a lower dosage with equivalent efficacy than for Caucasian patients in the USA [28]. Kleinman, in clinical practice with Chinese patients in the People's Republic of China, further found that therapeutic doses of TCA were generally half those required by Caucasians [15].

Single-dose kinetic studies with desipramine in healthy Chinese and Caucasian volunteers showed that oxidative metabolism was slower in gender- and age-matched Chinese than their Caucasian counterparts, thus supporting a pharmacokinetic mechanism for lower dosage requirements in Chinese patients [29]. A trimodal distribution of drug clearance was found, with only Chinese subjects in the slow clearance/poor metabolizer group, only Caucasians in fast clearance/rapid metabolizer group and the majority of patients (both Chinese and Caucasian) in the intermediate group. Body weight corrections did not remove the statistical significance of the findings. In a similar pattern, Pi *et al.* found differences in the mean time to peak plasma concentration for desipramine between Asian and Caucasian subjects, supporting the existence of a trimodal distribution of drug clearance [30, 31]. Single-dose kinetic studies involving British and Asian volunteers measured higher plasma drug concentrations in Asian volunteers 24 h after taking clomipramine, a TCA [32]. Other studies suggest that there is no difference between Asians and Caucasians in plasma concentration after the administration of TCAs: Japanese and Caucasian men had similar plasma concentrations following administration of the TCA nortriptyline [33]; Asian and Caucasian subjects also had similar plasma concentrations of imipramine and amitriptyline after administration [28]. The authors of these studies suggest that low-dose therapeutic effects in the Asian patients must therefore be pharmacodynamic or psychosocial in nature.

The cytochrome P-450 isoenzyme CYP2D6 is responsible for the metabolism of lipophilic bases, whereas CYP2C19 is involved in the metabolism of acids and bases (for example, imipramine). More than 25 drugs, including various tricyclic and selective serotonin reuptake inhibitor (SSRI) antidepressants are known to be metabolized by cytochrome CYP2D6, an enzyme with genetic polymorphism [34]. Fluoxetine and desipramine are metabolized predominantly by CYP2D6. A partially deficient CYP2D6 allele with a $Pro^{34} \rightarrow Ser$ amino acid exchange is found in as many as 50% Oriental alleles [34]. Consequently, the mean activity of CYP2D6 in Oriental extensive metabolizers (EMs) is lower than in Caucasian EMs, and this is thought to account for the slower metabolism of antidepressants and neuroleptics observed in Oriental patients. Koyama and colleagues reported that the metabolism of the TCA imipramine is pharmacogenetically controlled by CYP2C19 rather than CYP2D635, which might be more of a clinical concern for Japanese patients who have a prevalence for the recessive trait of 18–23%, compared with only 3–6% in Caucasian populations [35]. Currently, the major problem in the clinical use of imipramine is the intersubject differences in plasma concentrations; these may cause differences in clinical response and toxicity, particularly cardio-toxicity [37]. In contrast, the larger margin of safety of SSRIs minimizes the safety concerns arising from intersubject variability.

TREATMENT OF DEPRESSION USING FLUOXETINE

Clinical studies with depressed patients have shown lower than normal levels of 5-hydroxyindoleacetate (5-HIAA), a metabolite of the neurotransmitter serotonin, in their cerebrospinal fluid establishing a relationship between diminished serotoni-nergic function and depression [38]. Fluoxetine is a potent antidepressant because it selectively interferes with serotonin reuptake in the synaptic cleft, the junction of nerve terminals of the central nervous system, thereby enhancing steady-state concentrations of serotonin in the brain [39]. Fluoxetine and other SSRIs have greater pharmacological specificity than first and second-generation antidepressants such as the monoamine oxidase inhibitors (MAOIs) and TCAs in that they do not affect other important neurotransmitters such as dopamine, norepinephrine, histamine, acetylcholine, and r-aminobutyric acid. The MAOIs and TCAs inhibit the breakdown of amine neurotransmitters including norepinephrine, serotonin and dopamine. Clinical experience has shown that the efficacy of fluoxetine is com-parable to that of the tricyclic antidepressants in treating major depressive disorder, elderly depression, and depression in general practice. Fluoxetine has minimal anticholinergic, antihistaminergic and cardiac activity compared with TCAs, which translates into fewer adverse effects, and therefore better patient compliance [40]. Fluoxetine has no interaction with antacids, analgesics, anesthetics, antihistamines, diuretics, oral contraceptives, or thyroid hormones [41]. Fluoxetine is safe for patients with comorbid physical illnesses, with minimal impact on phospholipid levels, hepatic and renal function [42]. It can be administered safely at usual dosages to elderly patients and to patients with impaired renal function [43, 44]. Patients with comorbid anxiety and depression symptoms, who suffer intensified functional impairment, are found to benefit from treatment with fluoxetine and other SSRIs. Since its introduction 10 years ago as the first SSRI approved for patient use, fluoxetine has been prescribed to approximately 31 million patients world-wide (as of the end of 1997), and is one of the most frequently prescribed antidepressants.

Fluoxetine is efficacious at a dose of 20 mg once daily. Peak serum concen-trations are often achieved 6–8 h after oral administration [39]. The drug binds to plasma proteins with an efficiency of 95%, resulting in a plasma half-life of 2–3 days for the drug itself, and 7–9 days for its major active metabolite, desmethyl fluoxetine. Steady-state concentrations are achieved after 2–4 weeks of continuous treatment. The slower half-life of fluoxetine compared with that of other SSRI and TCA antidepressants renders discontinuation reactions (dizziness, paresthesia, headache, anxiety, and nausea) less likely in patients who discontinue it abruptly. Although fluoxetine has been available world-wide for some time there is no large-scale study to ascertain its safety profile and patient compliance in Asians. This chapter provides a meta-analysis on the clinical trial safety data from 460 patients in seven Asian countries who were exposed to 20 mg fluoxetine once daily. The safety of fluoxetine was compared with various tricyclic antidepressants in four of the 12 trials included in this analysis. To date, this meta-analysis represents the most complete evaluation in the literature of the safety of fluoxetine in Asians.

Methods

The safety profile of fluoxetine in the treatment of depression or dysthymia in Asian patients was examined using a descriptive statistical approach. Twelve clinical trials, sponsored by Eli Lilly and consisting entirely of Asian patients were included in the meta-analysis. Represented in those trials (Table 19.1) are 539 patients from seven Asian countries (China, Indonesia, Philippines, Singapore, South Korea, Taiwan, and Thailand).

In each of these trials, patients were diagnosed with major depression or dysthymia by a certified psychiatrist using the DSM criteria [6]. A minimum score of 18 was required on the Hamilton Rating Scale for Depression (HAM-D), or the HDRS, for patient inclusion in most cases [45]. Elevated Hamilton scores indicate the severity of depressive symptoms relative to that of normal patients. Patients in complete depressive remission will typically score an 8 or less.

Patients gave written informed consent and were permitted to discontinue treatment at any time. Routine measurements were made of the patient's vital signs including body weight, pulse, blood pressure, oral temperature, and electro-cardiogram. In addition to complete blood counts, laboratory tests for evaluating hepatic and renal function and urine content were performed. Patients received physical examinations and laboratory tests routinely as part of their follow-up. Noticeable changes in a patient's laboratory results or vital statistics were recorded. For safety reasons, patients were excluded from the clinical trials in many cases if they were:

- physically ill, or had a history of major physical illness;
- pregnant or nursing;
- already taking antidepressants, antiepileptics or antipsychotics;
- at risk of suicide, or had a history of suicide attempts; or
- had abnormal laboratory results.

A more detailed description of the selection criteria employed in each clinical trial can be obtained from the references [46–51].

For all the trials discussed here, a once-daily dose of 20 mg fluoxetine was self-administered in the morning. In some trials, adjustments were made to the delivery time for those patients who reported adverse effects of nausea (administering after meals) and daytime sleepiness (administering at bedtime). This alteration relieved

TABLE 19.1   Clinical trials used to evaluate safety of fluoxetine in Asian patients

Clinical trial	Duration of treatment (weeks)	Diagnosis	Positive control	Number of patients	
				Fluoxetine	TCA
Double-blinded, positive control					
1: Korea [46]	6	Depression	Amitriptyline	18	14
2: China	6		TCA[a]	30	30
Open-label, positive control					
3: Taiwan [47]	6	Depression	Imipramine	18	18
4: Taiwan	6	Depression	Imipramine	24	17
Open-label					
5: Taiwan	12	Depression	None	23	—
6: Taiwan	6	Depression	None	31	—
7: Korea [48]	4	Depression	None	186	—
8: Philippines	6	Depression	None	32	—
9: Singapore [49]	12	Depression	None	19	—
10: Indonesia	8	Depression	None	14	—
11: Korea [50]	8	Depression/dysthymia	None	46	—
12: Thailand [51]	8	Depression/dysthymia	None	19	—

[a] TCA: amitriptyline, maprotiline or clomipramine

symptoms for some patients. The duration of therapy in the various clinical trials ranged from 4 to 12 weeks.

In the comparator trials (two double-blind [46] and two open-label [47]), 169 psychiatric outpatients were randomly assigned to receive fluoxetine or TCA. The 90 patients in the fluoxetine group received a once-daily dose of 20 mg, while 79 patients received 25–150 mg/day, in 2–3 divided doses, of various tricyclic antidepressants (amitriptyline, imipramine, maprotiline, or clomipramine). TCA dose was adjusted during the trial depending on patient response and efficacy of the medication. All comparator trials lasted for 6 weeks. Patients were matched in terms of gender and age. One of these trials was composed exclusively of elderly patients (60 years of age and older) who were diagnosed with depression (Zhang; unpublished report). This particular trial had a higher than average age (69 years for the fluoxetine group and 70 years for the TCA group), and 30% of the patients within the trial were inpatients. Otherwise, patient demographics in the 12 clinical trials are quite similar.

Each individual study was examined in terms of patient demographics, dose response, patient compliance, and the frequency of self-reported adverse events. With the exception of the trials in Indonesia and Singapore, only treatment emergent adverse events were collected. Differences in adverse experiences between fluoxetine and TCAs were determined based on data from the comparator trials. Each patient responder from the 12 clinical trials was given equal weighting in the meta-analysis. To explore the differences in the safety profile of fluoxetine between

Asian and non-Asian populations, the frequency of reported adverse events in 460 Asian patients was compared with results from 2444 American patients (Eli Lilly clinical trial database with predominantly Caucasian patients) who participated in fluoxetine trials. In this meta-analysis, factors most responsible for patient attrition, and the fraction of patients who discontinued their treatment due to adverse side-effects of antidepressants, were determined.

Results

Patient Demographics

Patients who were lost to follow-up or dropped out for personal reasons were labeled as non-evaluable patients and were excluded from the analysis. In 12 separate clinical trials involving 539 Asian patients between the ages of 18 and 85, 443 (82%) completed the full treatment period of 4, 6, 8, or 12 weeks and were labeled evaluable patients. The average age of the combined population was 46 (±11) years. On average, 64% of the evaluable patients were female, reflecting the higher prevalence of depression in women. With the exception of the trial comparing the safety and efficacy of fluoxetine and TCAs (amitriptyline, maprotiline, or clomipramine) in elderly Chinese patients (all of whom were 60 years or older) (Zhang; unpublished report), there were no significant differences in patient age or gender profile for the separate clinical trials. Excluding the elderly patients from that one trial, which comprises 11% of the total number of evaluable patients, the mean age of the remaining patients was 43 years.

Patients in the four comparator trials taking various TCAs as controls were well matched in gender and age distribution to patients taking fluoxetine. In addition to the trial with elderly Chinese patients, there was a comparator trial involving psychiatric outpatients from Seoul taking either fluoxetine or the amitriptyline control [46]. The remaining two comparator trials involved psychiatric outpatients from Tri-Service General Hospital and psychiatric inpatients from NTUH hospital, Taiwan, comparing fluoxetine and imipramine [47, and Chen, unpublished report].

Four of the 12 trials reported the average body weight of the evaluable patients: the three Korean trials [46, 48, 50] and the trial in Singapore [49]. The average body weight of patients ranged from 54 to 60 kg. Asian patients are typically lighter in weight than their Western counterparts. In a study comparing the metabolism of desipramine in Chinese and Caucasian patients, Rudorfer et al. noticed a 14 kg (31 lb) weight difference between the two groups, with the Caucasian group weighing on average 72 kg (160 lb) [29].

Reports of Adverse Effects

The efficacy of fluoxetine in the four comparator trials was comparable to that of the TCAs in the treatment of depression and anxiety. Both drugs are already established as efficacious and reasonably fast-acting antidepressants [39, 52, 53]. The optimal choice between these two classes of antidepressants for Asian patients depends to a large part on their safety profiles. Asian patients taking TCAs in the comparator trials discussed here had considerably higher incidences of anti-cholinergic and central nervous system complaints than those taking fluoxetine (1.5% vs. 39% for dry mouth; 1.7% vs. 24% for constipation; 2.2% vs. 20% for drowsiness), and had frequent complaints of daytime sedation or drowsiness, constipation, dry mouth and visual disturbance or blurry vision (Table 19.2). On the other hand, nausea was reported more frequently among patients treated with fluoxetine (9.2% vs. 2.5%): this effect, however, was significantly reduced when the drug was taken after meals. For many patients taking fluoxetine, most of the adverse effects disappeared or lessened as the treatment continued. In one clinical study, 11 of 18 patients reported mild to severe side-effects after the first week of treatment, but 10 of these 11 reported no side-effects after 6 weeks of treatment [47]. In comparison, patients in the same trial taking imipramine ($n = 18$) reported mild to extreme effects after the first week of treatment and most (92%) still had mild to moderate symptoms at the sixth week of treatment. These results suggest that fluoxetine was better tolerated than any of the TCAs used in the comparator arm trials and had fewer treatment-emergent side-effects. This conclusion parallels a report by Tollefson *et al.*, which shows that fluoxetine is superior to TCAs in terms of its overall risk:benefit ratio in non-Asian patients [53].

In two of the Asian trials included in the present meta-analysis (the open-label trial with fluoxetine in Singapore [49] and the trial in Indonesia (Wibawa Roan; personal communication)), some of the adverse drug experiences collected from patients were present at baseline. These trials made no distinction between the depressive symptoms experienced by patients at baseline and those after the initiation of fluoxetine treatment. The incidence of treatment-emergent adverse events among fluoxetine recipients in these trials is expected to be lower than the total incidence of adverse events reported as some of these events might be part of the depressive symptoms rather than drug related. These two trials represent only 7% of all the evaluable patients.

Table 19.3 shows the number of patients who dropped out of each clinical trial. For the comparator trials, 16% of all patients receiving fluoxetine did not complete the trials and only one of 90 enrolled patients (1%) dropped out due to adverse effects (see Table 19.4 for symptoms responsible for patient discontinuation). In the TCA group (control), 22% of the patients did not complete the trials and 15% dropped out due to the adverse effects of the TCA medications—effects such as dry mouth, visual disturbance, constipation, and drowsiness. In the open-label clinical trials, 17% of the enrolled patients taking fluoxetine dropped out for various reasons (Table 19.3): 5% of drop-outs were due to insomnia, nausea, palpitations, or headache (Table 19.4). The other fluoxetine recipients who did not complete the full trial period were either lost to follow up or dropped out for personal issues. Of the 460 enrolled patients taking fluoxetine in the 12 clinical trials only 22 (5%) cited adverse effects, none of which were serious, as their reason for dropping out.

TABLE 19.2   Incidence of adverse effects in patients taking antidepressants

Adverse event	Percentage of Asian patients[a]		Percentage of American patients[b]
	Fluoxetine (n = 460)	TCA (n = 79)	Fluoxetine (n = 2444)
Anticholinergic			
Dry mouth	1.5	39.2	10.0
Constipation	1.7	24.1	5.1
Visual disturbance	0.5	14.0	2.8
Central nervous system			
Drowsiness	2.2	20.0	13.1
Dizziness	2.7	19.0	9.7
Insomnia	5.1	2.5	20.4
Anxiety	1.2	2.5	12.8
Agitation	1.7		1.0
Headache	2.2	3.0	21.0
Asthenia	1.2		11.7
Nervousness	0.7		13.5
Tremor	0.5		10.4
Vertigo	0.5		0.2
Persecutory idea	0.5		
Gastrointestinal			
Nausea	9.2	2.5	23.0
Appetite loss	5.6		11.0
Diarrhea	0.7		12.0
Dyspepsia	0.7		8.0
Cardiac			
Tachycardia	0.5	0.0	0.7
Palpitation	1.0	6.3	2.2
Postural hypotension	0.0	2.5	0.1
Skin			
Sweating	0.2		8.2
Urticaria	0.2		0.9
Body as a whole			
Weight loss	1.5		2.3
Flu syndrome	0.0		5.0

[a] Asian patients (460, 79): extracted from meta-analysis, see Table 19.1;
[b] US patients in placebo-controlled trials (2,444): US package insert and data on file at Lilly Research Labs

With respect to medication compliance, Asian patients appear to tolerate fluoxetine better than TCAs: although fluoxetine recipients did report adverse effects, few discontinued treatment, possibly because of the mildness of the symptoms and the reduction in severity after the first week.

TABLE 19.3   Patient attrition

	Number of patients		Total patient drop-out		Drop-outs due to adverse events	
Study	Fluoxetine	TCA	Fluoxetine	TCA	Fluoxetine	TCA
1	18	14	3	3	0	0
2	30	30	2	8	0	6
3	18	18	1	6	1	6
4	24	17	7	NA	0	NA
5	23	—	3	—	2	—
6	31	—	11	—	8	—
7	186	—	20	—	2	—
8	32	—	2	—	0	—
9	19	—	0	—	0	—
10	14	—	7	—	4	—
11	46	—	16	—	2	—
12	19	—	7	—	3	—

NA, Not appropriate for evaluating patient attrition because all patients were psychiatric inpatients

TABLE 19.4   Adverse events that caused patients to drop out from the trial

Trial	Reason for discontinuation
2	Dry mouth, visual disturbance, constipation, dizziness, and drowsiness
3	One patient in fluoxetine group dropped out due to nausea; six in imipramine group due to anticholinergic effects (drowsiness, dizziness, and dry mouth)
5	One patient dropped out due to nausea and insomnia; one due to loss of appetite and palpitations
6	Four patients dropped out in one day, citing general malaise and asthenia; four after 1–2 weeks citing the same reasons
7	Specific adverse effects not reported
10	Palpitations, sweating, or insomnia
11	One patient dropped out due to urticaria; one due to severe weight loss
12	Headache and insomnia

For the most part no significant physiological or laboratory changes were observed in patients treated with either fluoxetine or TCAs. However, the following changes were observed. A significant increase in body weight of 2.2 (±0.6) kg was noted for Korean patients taking amitriptyline ($t = 2.44$, df $= 23$, $p = 0.022$) [46]. No change was noted for the group taking imipramine, although a slight increase in heart rate (6.3 (±4.2) beats/min) was observed [47]. In comparison, no significant change in body weight was noted in patients taking fluoxetine. Two of the 45 patients enrolled in this Korean study had acute viral hepatitis, and with close monitoring and their informed consent, were administered fluoxetine. Each patient's hepatic functions returned to normal after taking fluoxetine for 3 months, suggesting that it is possible to administer fluoxetine, with caution, to depressed patients with acute hepatitis.

Seven of the 12 clinical trials reported no significant physiological or bio-chemical changes with fluoxetine. The following abnormal observations were noted in the remaining trials with fluoxetine. Mild elevation of transaminases were noted in two trials. Chen *et al.* noticed two patients out of 24 with slight elevation in SGOT and SGPT levels after the initiation of fluoxetine (unpublished report). One patient returned to normal by the end of the trial while the other still had slight abnormality (2–3 times the upper limit of normal) 2 months after discontinuation of fluoxetine. In one trial, the SGPT in two of 21 patients increased to 2–3 times normal after 12 weeks of fluoxetine therapy [49]. In the other trial, one patient out of 166 had an elevated SGOT value, from 36 IU/l at baseline to 56 IU/l after 6 weeks [48]. Min *et al.* reported an average increase in diastolic pressure of 5% and three of 46 patients lost approximately 3 kg, due to the loss of appetite [50]. None of the observed events were serious.

Comparison of Fluoxetine Safety in Asians and Caucasians

The frequency with which Asian patients reported common side-effects was 9.2–2.2% (ranked in descending order) for nausea, appetite loss, insomnia, dizziness, and drowsiness (Table 19.2). Similar to results of the US trials (Table 19.2), the most commonly reported adverse effects were complaints of the gastrointestinal and central nervous systems. The safety data from the US trial represent the integrated results from placebo-controlled trials of fluoxetine in treating depression, bulimia, and obsessive-compulsive disorders before its FDA approval. The most commonly reported side-effect among Asian patients was nausea, with an incidence of 9.2%; headache, nausea and insomnia were most common in US patients, with incidences of 21%, 23%, and 20.4%, respectively. In general, Asian patients reported fewer adverse effects than their Caucasian counterparts. These differences were not due to the treatment duration, as the mean duration of fluoxetine therapy was similar in both trials (Asian trial 43 days; US trial 50 days).

Discussion

Fluoxetine and other SSRIs are efficacious in the treatment of dysthymia, major depression and depression with symptoms of comorbid anxiety or panic disorder. These drugs have also been found useful in the treatment of obsessive-compulsive neurosis, bulimia, and cataplexy [43, 44]. Fluoxetine is as effective as TCAs in treating depression but is devoid of cardiotoxicity and the frequent anticholinergic side-effects (most commonly dry mouth, constipation or blurry vision) that were responsible for patient non-compliance with TCAs. A small percentage of patients who took fluoxetine did experience mild to moderate nausea, headache, insomnia, drowsiness, or anxiety but these effects generally disappeared or diminished after a few weeks of treatment. The safety of fluoxetine in Caucasians at daily doses of up to 80 mg has been established in numerous clinical trials in the USA, in elderly patients and in patients with impaired renal function. Until now, however, the safety of fluoxetine in Asian patients has not been fully evaluated. The 12 clinical trials in this report involved 539 patients from seven Asian countries and revealed the following.

1. No serious drug reactions were noted in 460 Asian patients treated with fluoxetine for up to 12 weeks.
2. The safety profile of fluoxetine among Asians is similar to that in non-Asian patients. The most commonly reported side-effects were mild gastrointestinal problems (nausea, appetite loss) and complaints of the central nervous system (insomnia, dizziness, drowsiness). In general, Asian patients reported fewer adverse effects than their Caucasian counterparts.
3. Compared with patients who were treated with various TCAs (amitriptyline, imipramine, maprotiline, and clomipramine), those receiving fluoxetine reported fewer adverse effects and were more compliant.

These findings support the finding that fluoxetine is safe for treating Asian patients with depression at a daily dose of 20 mg for up to 12 weeks. The recommended dose for the treatment of depression for Caucasian patients is 20 mg per day as higher doses do not offer a significantly higher antidepressant effect [54]. Fluoxetine, at a daily dose of up to 80 mg, is currently approved in numerous countries for various indications (depression, obsessive compulsive disorder, and bulimia nervosa). The established safety of fluoxetine at this dosage provides a large margin of safety for the treatment of depression in Asian patients at a daily dose of 20 mg, even for those patients who might be poor metabolizers of this antidepressant.

Fluoxetine was well tolerated among Asian patients—as evident by low incidence of adverse drug experiences and a low rate of attrition. This observation was also applicable to geriatric patients. In a trial comparing the safety and efficacy of fluoxetine and TCAs in Chinese patients with a mean age of 69 years (Zhang; unpublished report), none dropped out due to adverse drug experience, although 20% of the TCA-treated patients in the same trial did so. This study is particularly relevant for the evaluation of drug safety as geriatric patients are more likely to develop drug interactions because they tend to take more concomitant medications than younger patients.

Currently healthcare costs associated with depressive illness are comparable to those of major illnesses such as cancer, AIDS and coronary heart disease, although the indirect costs associated with depression are often hidden in lost productivity and suboptimal job performance [55]. It is estimated that 80% of patients suffering from a first depressive episode will experience recurrent episodes in their lifetime [56]. It is suspected that insufficient antidepressant therapy duration, suboptimal dosing during treatment, or prescription non-renewal issues may be partly responsible. In five of the clinical trials discussed here, patients were interviewed about their depressive history; more specifically, they were asked to report the number of depressive events they had experienced in their life and the age of onset of their first depressive event. Jung and colleagues reported 1.5 (±0.3) previous depressive episodes in depressed patients living in South Korea (mean age 48 years) [46]. Tsoi *et al.* found that 53% of Chinese patients from Singapore, currently being treated for depression, had one or two previous depressive episodes, with the remaining patients depression-free before this particular event (mean age 47 years) [49]. Jurilla and colleagues found that 57% of clinical outpatients in the Philippines, currently diagnosed with major depression, self-reported 1–3 previous events (mean age 41 years) (unpublished final report). Wen and Ko reported only that 13% of Taiwanese patients treated for depression in their study were recurrent sufferers (mean age 45 years) (unpublished report). Zhang found that 60% of elderly Chinese patients diagnosed with depression had a history of prior depressive events (mean age 69) (unpublished report). Depression causes significant financial loss, to both the affected person and their employer, as it often occurs during an employee's most productive years. For instance, clinical patients from Korea and the Philippines most often reported that their first depressive event occurred between the ages of 41 and 60, whereas Chinese patients in Singapore reported a mean age of onset of 36 years [49].

Depression can be treated with a variety of therapeutic approaches. Concerns about the high economic costs associated with treatment prompted studies examining more cost-effective treatment approaches. These pharmacoeconomic studies with Caucasian patients show that whereas SSRI and TCA antidepressants have comparable efficacy for short-term therapy [7, 57] SSRIs have better patient compliance and more stable usage patterns. Patients on SSRI therapy are more likely to receive adequate therapeutic doses, benefit from longer duration of therapy and require fewer changes in medication over the course of their illness [58–60]. The higher acquisition costs of the newer SSRI medications are thus offset by lower inpatient and outpatient costs (hospitalization, physician/psychiatrist visits and laboratory tests) [61, 62]. Studies suggest that direct healthcare costs for patients starting fluoxetine are similar to, or lower than, the costs associated with TCA treatment and that there is a reduced risk of work loss/absenteeism. There is considerable debate as to whether individual SSRIs can be distinguished from one another, either with regard to efficacy or from an economic perspective. The longer half-life of fluoxetine provides built-in protection against discontinuation syndromes and the recurrence of depressive symptoms during brief treatment interruptions. The favorable pharmacoeconomic outcome of fluoxetine relative to TCAs in Caucasian patients should also be applicable to Asian patients in view of the findings discussed above.

CONCLUSIONS

Meta-analysis of the 12 clinical trials involving Asian patients treated with fluoxetine or various TCAs for major depressive disorder or dysthymia suggest that fluoxetine is better tolerated, with greater patient compliance and fewer and less sustaining adverse effects than the TCAs. No serious adverse events were reported in the clinical trials. Only mild and infrequent gastrointestinal and central nervous system complaints of nausea, appetite loss, insomnia, dizziness and drowsiness (in order of reported frequency) were noted. Attrition due to adverse side-effects was considerably lower among patients treated with fluoxetine than those treated with TCAs.

Thus, for the treatment of depression, the large therapeutic index of fluoxetine provides a comfortable margin of safety for any discernible interracial differences between the Asians and the non-Asians in the clearance of this compound.

ACKNOWLEDGEMENTS

This study was supported by the Eli Lilly Company. The authors would like to acknowledge the editorial support from L. McInnes, PhD, and support from various Lilly affiliates in Asia in providing the clinical trial information.

REFERENCES

1. Robins LN, Helzer JE, Weissman MM *et al.* 1984. Lifetime prevalence of specific psychiatric disorders in three sites. *Arch Gen Psychiatry* **41**: 949–58.
2. Wittchen HY, Knäuper B, Kessler RD. 1994. Lifetime risk of depression. *Br J Psychiatry* **165**(Suppl 26): 16–22.
3. Stewart RB. 1993. Advances in pharmacotherapy: Depression in the elderly—Issues and advances in treatment. *J Clin Pharm Ther* **18**(4): 243–53.
4. Golding JM, Burnam MA, Benjamin B, Wells KB. 1993. Risk factors for secondary depression among Mexican Americans and Non-Hispanic Whites. Alcohol use, alcohol dependence, and reasons for drinking. *J Nerv Ment Dis* **181**(3): 166–75.
5. Kendler KS, Neale MC, Kessler RC *et al.* 1992. A population-based twin study of major depression in women. The impact of varying definition of illness. *Arch Gen Psychiatry* **49**(4): 257–66.
6. American Psychiatric Association. 1987. *Diagnostic and Statistical Manual of Mental Disorders*, 3rd ed. (revised). Washington DC: APA.
7. Wilde MI, Benfield P. 1998. Fluoxetine. A pharmacoeconomic review of its use in depression. *Pharmacoeconomics* **13**(1): 543–61.
8. Tollefson GD. 1991. Antidepressant treatment and side effect consideration. *J Clin Psychiatry* **52**: 4–13.
9. Kasper S, Fuger J, Moller HJ. 1992. Comparative efficacy of antidepressants. *Drugs* **43**: 11–22.
10. Mintz J, Mintz LI, Arruda MJ, Hwang SS. 1992. Treatments of depression and the functional capacity to work. *Arch Gen Psychiatry* **49**: 761–8.
11. Altamura A, Percudani M. 1993. The use of antidepressant for long-term treatment of recurrent depression: Rationale, current methodologies, and future direction. *J Clin Psychiatry* **54**(Suppl 8): 29–38.
12. Devitt TM. 1996. US Bureau of the Census, Report WP/96, *World Population Profile: 1996*. Washington DC: US Government Printing Office.
13. US Bureau of the Census. 1995. Current Population Reports, *Population Profile of the*

United States: 1995 (Series P. 23–189). Washington DC: US Government Printing Office.

14. Lee HY, Namkoong K, Lee MH *et al.* 1989. Psychiatric epidemiologic survey (III). Lifetime prevalence of psychiatric disorders. *J Korean Neuropsych Assoc* **28**(6): 984–99.

15. Kleinman A. 1982. Neurasthenia and depression: a study of somatization and culture in China. *Cult Med Psychiatry* **6**(2): 117–90.

16. Shen Y. 1981. The psychiatric services in the urban and rural areas of People's Republic of China. *Bull Neuroinform Lab Nagasaki Univ* **8**: 131–7.

17. Nakane Y, Ohta Y, Uchino J *et al.* 1988. Comparative study of affective disorders in three Asian countries. I. Differences in diagnostic classification. *Acta Psychiatr Scand* **78**(6): 698–705.

18. Nakane Y, Ohta Y, Radford M *et al.* 1991. Comparative study of affective disorders in three Asian countries. II. Differences in prevalence rates and symptom presentation. *Acta Psychiatr Scand* **84**(4): 313–19.

19. Mino Y, Aoyama H, Froom J. 1994. Depressive disorders in Japanese primary care patients. *Fam Pract* **11**(4): 363–7.

20. Kasper S, Wehr TA, Bartko JJ *et al.* 1989. Epidemiology findings of seasonal changes in mood and behavior. A telephone survey of Montgomery County Maryland. *Arch Gen Psychiatry* **46**: 823–33.

21. Kunugi H. 1993. Depressive disorder following personnel change—its clinical features, situational factors antecedent to recovery and treatment. *Seishin Shinkeigaku Zasshi* **95**(4): 325–42.

22. Hinton WL, Du N, Chen YC *et al.* 1994. Screening for major depression in Vietnamese refugees: A validation and comparison of two instruments in a health screening population. *J Gen Intern Med* **9**(4): 202–6.

23. Ying YW. 1988. Depressive symptomatology among Chinese-Americans as measured by the CES-D. *J Clin Psychiatry* **44**(5): 739–46.

24. Kuo WH. 1984. Prevalence of depression among Asian-Americans. *J Nerv Ment Dis* **172**(8): 449–57.

25. Anonymous. 1992. The changing rate of major depression. Cross-national comparisons. Cross-National Collaborative Group. *JAMA* **268**(21): 3098–105.

26. Okazaki S. 1997. Sources of ethnic differences between Asian American and white American college students on measures of depression and social anxiety. *J Abnorm Psychol* **106**(1): 52–60.

27. Kim LS, Chun CA. 1993. Ethnic differences in psychiatric diagnosis among Asian American adolescents. *J Nerv Ment Dis* **181**(10): 612–17.

28. Yamashita I, Asano Y. 1979. Tricyclic antidepressants: Therapeutic plasma level. *Psychopharmacol Bull* **15**: 40–1.

29. Rudorfer MV, Lane EA, Chang WH *et al.* 1984. Desipramine pharmacokinetics in Chinese and Caucasian volunteers. *Br J Clin Pharmacol* **17**(4): 433–40.

30. Pi EH, Simpson GH, Cooper TB. 1986. Pharmacokinetics of desipramine in Caucasian and Asian volunteers. *Am J Psychiatry* **143**: 1174–6.

31. Pi EH, Tran-Johnson TK, Walker NR *et al.* 1989. Pharmacokinetics of desipramine in Asian and Caucasian volunteers. *Psychopharmacol Bull* **25**: 483–7.

32. Lewis P, Vaddadi KS, Rack PH, Allen JJ. 1980. Ethnic differences in drug response. *Postgrad Med J* **56**(Suppl 1): 46–9.

33. Kishimoto A, Hollister LE. 1984. Nortriptyline kinetics in Japanese and Americans. *J Clin Psychopharmacol* **4**: 171–2.

34. Bertilsson L. 1995. Geographical/interracial differences in polymorphic drug oxidation: Current state of knowledge of cyctochromes P450 (CYP) 2D6 and 2C19. *Clin Pharmacokinet* **29**(3): 192–209.

35. Koyama E, Tanaka T, Chiba K *et al.* 1996. Steady-state plasma concentrations of

imipramine and desipramine in relation to *S*-mephenytoin 4'-hydroxylation status in Japanese depressive patients. *J Clin Psychopharmacol* **16**(4): 286–93.

36. Nakamura K, Goto F, Ray WA *et al.* 1985. Interethnic differences in genetic polymorphism of debrisoquin and mephenytoin hydroxylation between Japanese and Caucasian populations. *Clin Pharmacol Ther* **38**: 402–8.

37. Sallee FR, Pollack BG. 1990. Clinical pharmacokinetics of imipramine and desipramine. *Clin Pharmacokinet* **18**: 346–64.

38. Schatzberg AF, Rothschild AJ. 1992. Serotonin activity in psychotic (delusional) major depression. *J Clin Psychiatry* **53**(Suppl): 52–5.

39. Bergstrom RF, Lemberger L, Farid NA *et al.* 1988. Clinical pharmacology and pharmacokinetics of fluoxetine: a review. *Br J Psychiatry* **153**(Suppl 3): 47–50.

40. Stark P, Fuller RW, Wong DT. 1985. The pharmacologic profile of fluoxetine. *J Clin Psychiatry* **46**: 7–13.

41. Cooper GL. 1988. The safety of fluoxetine—an update. *Br J Psychiatry* **153**(Suppl 3): 77–86.

42. Wernicke JF. 1985. The side effect profile and safety of fluoxetine. *J Clin Psychiatry* **46**: 59–67.

43. Hale AS. 1993. New antidepressants: use in high risk patients. *J Clin Psychiatry* **64**(Suppl. 8): 61–70.

44. Leonard BE. 1993. The comparative pharmacology of new antidepressants. *J Clin Psychiatry* **54**(Suppl 8): 3–15.

45. Hamilton M. 1960. A rating scale for depression. *J Neurol Neurosurg Psychiatry* **23**: 56–62.

46. Jung HY, Bae JN, Kwon JS, Cho DY. 1995. Double-blind comparative trial of fluoxetine and amitriptyline in major depression. *Korean J Psychosomatic Med* **3**(1): 11–18.

47. Lu RB, Ko HC, Huang CC, Lin YT. 1991. Comparison of the clinical efficacy and safety of fluoxetine and imipramine in major depressive disorder. *JAMA SEA* (Suppl 7): 41–45.

48. Namkoong K, Yoo KJ. 1994. Effects of fluoxetine in major depressive disorders. *Korean J Psychopharmacol* **5**(1): 11–17.

49. Tsoi W.F, Tan CT, Kok LP. 1995. Fluoxetine in the treatment of depression in Asian (Chinese and Indian) patients in Singapore. *Singapore Med J* **36**: 397–9.

50. Min SK, Lee HY, Kim JJ, Shin JH. 1989. A clinical trial of fluoxetine. *New Med J* **32**(1): 116–22.

51. Aroon S, Nipatt K, Thani S. 1991. A clinical study of fluoxetine hydrochloride. *JAMA SEA* (Suppl 5): 39–40.

52. Richelson E. 1988. Synaptic pharmacology of antidepressants: an update. *McLean Hosp J* **13**: 26–47.

53. Tollefson GD, Holman SL, Sayler ME *et al.* 1994. Fluoxetine, placebo and tricyclic antidepressants in major depression with and without anxious features. *J Clin Psychiatry* **55**: 50–9.

54. Altamura AC, Montgomery SA, Wernicke JF. 1988. The evidence for 20 mg a day of fluoxetine as the optimal dose in treatment of depression. *Br J Psychiatry* **153**(Suppl 3): 109–12.

55. Greenberg P, Stiglin LE, Finkelstein SN, Berndt E. 1993. The economic burden of depression in 1990. *J Clin Psychiatry* **54**: 405–18.

56. Hale AS. 1994. Juggling cost and benefit in the long-term treatment of depression. *Postgrad Med J* **70**(Suppl 2): S2–8.

57. Hylan TR, Buesching DP, Tollefson GD. 1998. Health economic evaluations of antidepressants: A Review. *Depression and Anxiety* **7**: 53–64.

58. Lin EH, Van Korff M, Katon W *et al.* 1995. The role of the primary care physician in patients' adherence to antidepressant therapy. *Med Care* **33**: 67–74.

59. Katon W, Van Korff M, Lin E *et al.* 1992. Adequacy and duration of antidepressant treatment in primary care. *Med Care* **30**: 67–76.
60. McCombs JS, Nichol MB, Stimmel GL *et al.* 1990. The cost of antidepressant drug therapy failure: A study of antidepressant use patterns in a Medicaid population. *J Clin Psychiatry* **51**: 60–9.
61. Sclar DA, Robison LM, Skaer TL *et al.* 1995. Antidepressant pharmacotherapy: Economic evaluation of fluoxetine, paroxetine, and sertraline in a health maintenance organization. *J Int Med Res* **23**: 395–412.
62. Hylan TR, Crown WH, Meneades I *et al.* 1998. Tricyclic antidepressants and selective serotonin reuptake inhibitors antidepressant selection and health care costs in a naturalistic setting: A multivariate analyses. *J Affect Disord* **47**: 71–9.

20

Ethnicity and Mood Disorders

Emile Risby and Scott Van Sant
DeCamp Crisis Center, Decater, GA, USA

INTRODUCTION

There have been many debates as to the role or influence of ethnicity in psychiatric disorders. Studies that have attempted to address the association between ethnicity and mood disorders have had such significant methodological problems that generalization of the data to broader settings is difficult. Clearly the association between ethnicity and mood disorders involves multiple complex factors and interactions that are difficult to measure. Two major methodological issues include defining ethnic groups rather than racial groups, and sorting out the influence of culture rather than ethnicity *per se*. Unfortunately, the terms race and ethnicity are often used interchangeably and the influence of culture is seldom considered.

Race refers to the genetically determined characteristics that the individual is born with, including all biologically determined processes as well as physical characteristics. *Culture* refers to those attributes that are learned as a part of one's upbringing. Culture includes traits that are shaped by traditions and customs, such as language and religion. *Ethnicity* is the 'group' of which one identifies oneself as being a part. It is usually based on a combination of shared ancestry and cultural experience. Although ethnicity often combines race and culture, one's ethnicity may be independent of one's race or culture. Therefore, within a particular ethnic group, there may be individuals of different races and different cultures (e.g. Hispanic). Cultural differences—such as differences in socioeconomic status, regional influences, educational status, language, religion, and acculturation status—exist within racial or ethnic groups. All too often, racial and ethnic groups are treated as homogenous, leading to inappropriate generalizations, unmet needs, and unsuitable treatment [1].

Obviously, racial groups possess certain similarities because of their 'genetic' relatedness. Thus, one would think if there are going to be differences in the incidence, presentation or prognosis of biological conditions, such as mood disorders, then they would more probably be seen between racial groups than between ethnic or cultural groups. However, culture exerts powerful influences on diagnosis and treatment outcome. Culture shapes the general tone of emotional life within a

Cross Cultural Psychiatry. Edited by John M. Herrera, William B. Lawson and John J. Sramek.
© 1999 John Wiley & Sons Ltd.

society. Therefore the diagnostic 'cut-off points' for distinguishing common unremarkable mood symptoms from those that are unusual and noteworthy are modified by culture. Furthermore, most Western industrialized populations view people as 'egocentric'; unique, separate, and autonomous individuals. Many non-Western cultural traditions depict people in relational terms, as part of a collective interdependent kinship. One culture focuses on the individual, the other focuses on the interpersonal relationships. Hence, diagnostic criteria that depend exclusively on eliciting ego-oriented symptoms may be intrinsically constrained from identifying the same psychiatric symptoms that are 'sociocentric'. For example, persons from some cultural or ethnic groups may focus on the effects their illness has on others as opposed to its personal impact [2]. Clearly, culture affects the epidemiology of psychiatric disorders, especially the subjectively dependent mood disorders.

PHENOMENOLOGY

There is data to suggest that there may be racial and ethnic differences in the way psychiatric disorders present [3, 4]. It has been reported that in African Americans affective disorders are more likely to present with psychotic symptoms, mania with more irritable symptoms, and depression with more suspiciousness [5–7]. There is little ethnic variation in rates of bipolar disorder. Numerous epidemiological studies have compared symptoms of depression between Blacks and Whites in the USA. The Epidemiologic Catchment Area Study reported that, in regards to depressive symptoms, Blacks are more likely to report changes in appetite and retardation or agitation; Whites are most likely to report dysphoria, fatigue, guilt, and thoughts of death [8]. Other studies suggest that Blacks report more symptoms of depression than Whites in gross comparisons, but after adjusting for sociodemographic differences, Blacks report equal or even lower levels of depressive symptoms [9, 10]. This is a classic example of the influence of culture in the presentation and epidemiology of depression. In general, depressed patients from Western European backgrounds are more likely to report feelings of guilt than non-Western Europeans. Presumably guilt is a more Western European concept because it assumes a more individualistic view of the world and focuses on individual responsibility. People from tribal and many non-industrialized cultures assume a more communal responsibility and are more likely to experience shame than guilt. Consequently, when they do seek help for 'depression', they tend to present with more acceptable somatic symptoms than with psychological symptoms of depression [11, 12].

In general, Asian patients also report more somatic than psychological symptoms of depression. In many traditional Asian cultures, the pathogenesis of negative emotions is felt to be secondary to disturbances of internal organs and their functions, resulting in a tradition of expressing emotions in somatic metaphors [13]. The Confucian tradition of correct social behavior and the emphasis on inhibition of emotions may also influence the manner in which Asians express psychological distress. The tendency for Asian Americans to express depressive symptomatology in somatic terms is generally supported in the literature. In a study of four Asian-American groups (Chinese, Japanese, Korean, and Filipino), Kuo [14] reported that all four tended to combine depressive symptomatology with somatic complaints. However, within Asian subgroups in the Asian population there are differences in the 'symptom profile' of depression. In a study comparing depressive symptoms in China, Japan and Korea, Nakane and colleagues [15] found higher rates of neurasthenia, suicidal tendencies, gastrointestinal complaints and weight loss in the Chinese patients.

There are other reports of differences in the rates of somatic symptoms in depressed patients between ethnic and cultural groups. A greater percentage of depressed Turkish patients reported somatic symptoms than depressed German patients [16, 17]; island Puerto Ricans reported more somatization disorder than US born Mexican Americans or non-Hispanic whites living in the Los Angeles area [18]. Interestingly, some studies have found no significant differences in major depression or in the mood symptoms between Mexican Americans and non-Hispanic Whites [19]. These observations (as noted above for African Americans) suggest that 'culture' may have a more significant role in the presentation of depressive symptoms than 'ethnicity' *per se*.

The differences in the rates of depressive somatic symptoms varies with cultural background. In some cultures, to have a mental illness is considered unacceptable or shameful. If the symptoms can be attributed to natural or supranatural causes, then blame on the individual and the negative cultural impact on the family are minimized. Conversely, Western psychology emphasizes individual responsibility in the causation and recovery from emotional problems and discourages somatic expression.

The role of personality styles and psychosocial issues are all important to consider when discussing the symptoms of depression within individuals and ethnic groups. African Americans report more suspiciousness than non-Hispanic White populations on the Minnesota Multiphasic Personality Inventory. This increase in paranoid-type symptoms among African Americans has been interpreted as a 'healthy paranoia' or 'healthy cultural suspiciousness', due to the effects of long-standing racism [20]. This may explain the increase in paranoia reported in depressed African-American patients. As reviewed by Tabora and colleagues [21], Chinese-American students have been found to exhibit lower levels of verbal and emotional expressiveness than their Anglo-American counterparts. Asian-American students tend to be more somatic, less autonomous, and show greater introversion, self-restraint, and passivity. While these characteristics may be considered positive attributes in Chinese culture, in Western society they may be negatively interpreted as self-abasement, passive-aggressiveness, dependency, lack of self-confidence [21], or as symptoms of depression or a depressive personality.

EPIDEMIOLOGY

Approximately 30% of patients in primary care clinics in the USA have diagnosable psychiatric disorders [22]. Between 5% and 10% of patients in primary care settings suffer from major depression [23]. Large-scale studies using structured interviews such as the Epidemiological Catchment Area study and the National Comorbidity Study have found few racial or ethnic differences [8]. Nakane *et al.* [15] reported that the rates of depressive disorders in China, Japan, and Korea were similar to the rates reported in Western countries. Thus, when structured interviews are used, racial and ethnic differences tend to disappear. Differences in presenting symptoms may lead to problems in diagnosing conditions among different ethnic groups. The issue may not be whether individual symptoms are present or absent, but the extent to which a given group emphasize these symptoms or identify them as symptoms of an emotional disorder. For example, the word 'depression' is absent from the languages in some American Indian, Alaskan Native and Southeast Asian (India, Pakistan and Bangladesh) cultures; however, the symptom of 'low mood' is frequently expressed [2, 24].

Although there is no consistent data to suggest that the epidemiology of mood disorders differs among ethnic groups, there are some clinical issues within ethnic groups that may increase the risk for depression. In African Americans, issues such as drug abuse, break-up of the traditional family, and poverty all have a negative impact on emotional well-being and mental health. African-American women are felt to be at increased risk for developing depression because of their dual status of racial minority and female. Yet epidemiological data does not support the assumption that the rates of depression are higher in African Americans of either sex. There have been scattered but inconsistent reports that Jews are at higher risk for affective disorders than other religious groups; the reasons why, if this is true, are unclear [25, 26].

The negative aspects of the acculturation process may result in an increased risk among immigrants for developing depression [21]. Newly arrived immigrants may suffer stress due to a change in culture, social isolation, and problems with language, unemployment, and discrimination. Furthermore, premigration stresses may produce chronic psychiatric disorders, including depression [27]. For example, a survey of Cambodian refugees living in the USA 10 years after they had left their homes in Cambodia found extremely high levels of post-traumatic stress disorder, dissociation, depression, and anxiety: 90% of these refugees exhibited marked symptomatology in one or more of these categories [28]. This study highlights the difficulty in generalizing results from an ethnic subgroup to an entire ethnic group: Cambodians who are not refugees and who are second-generation US citizens will have a very different psychopathology profile. Again, the influence of culture, which may change with generations, is an important factor in the epidemiology of mood disorders.

ETHNICITY AND PSYCHOPHARMACOLOGY

Most psychotropic drugs are metabolized by one of the hepatic cytochrome P-450 (CYP) isoenzymes. Two of the most important are CYP2D6 and CYP2C19 [29].

CYP2D6 is responsible for the metabolism of many tricyclic antidepressants (TCAs), paroxetine, venlafaxine, to some extent nefazodone, and most antipsychotics [30]. Most individuals have a normal level of this enzyme and are called CYP2D6 extensive metabolizers (EMs). Individuals with very low levels of activity of this enzyme are called poor metabolizers (PMs) [30]. The percentage of individuals who are PMs for CYP2D6 varies considerably, but studies have consistently demonstrated a substantial contrast between Asians (0.5–2.4%) and Caucasians (2.9–10%). The percentage of CYP2D6 PMs among Blacks of different ethnic groups varies from 0% to 18% [31]. However, approximately one-third of Asians and African Americans have a gene alteration that gives this enzyme an intermediate rate between PMs and EMs. The end result is an overall lower rate of CYP2D6 activity. These ethnic differences in pharmacogenetics may partly explain the findings of ethnic differences in the pharmacokinetics of TCAs and neuroleptic agents [32]. The CYP2C19 isoenzyme is involved in the demethylation of the tertiary tricyclics [33]. While only 3% of Caucasians are CYP2C19 PMs, approximately one-fifth of African Americans and Asians are [34]. This would suggest a slower clearance of these drugs in a significant number of African-American and Asian patients. Ethnic comparisons of the pharmacokinetics of the TCAs have been inconclusive. Whereas some studies indicate that Asians metabolize TCAs slower than Caucasians, not all studies have replicated these findings. A possible explanation for the inconsistencies reported in the literature is the finding that the CYP isoenzymes and various conjugation enzymes are extremely responsive to environmental factors such as pharmaceutical agents, toxins, herbal medicines, steroids, tobacco, alcohol, caffeine, and various dietary factors. Thus, cultural lifestyle changes may modify metabolic and other biological functions [32].

Significant differences in the transport of lithium across cellular membranes have been reported between African Americans and Caucasians: African Americans have a less active sodium–lithium countertransport system than Caucasians. Therefore, African Americans are more likely to have significantly higher intracellular concentrations of lithium than Caucasians and consequently are more likely to have higher rates of lithium-induced side-effects [35].

TREATMENT ISSUES

In the USA, various ethnic groups have been observed to underuse mental health services, to drop out of therapy prematurely, or to seek treatment only when their problems have become severe. A lack of culturally responsive treatment options lies at the root of this problem. Issues to consider when developing culturally responsive treatments include matching ethnic group of patients and therapists, using compatible languages, and paying attention to beliefs about mental illness and how it should be treated. It has been reported that when these issues are addressed, utilization of services increases, dropout rates decrease, and outcomes improve [36]. Although there is no consensus among professionals, there is a general sense

that treatment by a therapist of the same ethnicity as the client increases compliance and improves clinical outcomes. A more fundamental issue deserving
further empirical investigation is the matching of the 'problem conceptualization'
between the service provider and the client. The ability of the clinician to recognize
the patient's view of their illness, and to present interventions in a way that fits that
view, is pivotal in the client's willingness to accept the diagnosis, to adhere to the
prescribed intervention, and, finally, to recover [37].

The stigma of mental illness within a culture or ethnic group not only influences
its expression but also influences the willingness of the patient to accept the
diagnosis and to receive treatment. In a study conducted by Cooper-Patrick and
colleagues [38], stigma was perceived as a particularly important barrier to getting
treatment for African Americans, who felt that the idea of seeking professional
mental health help was not acceptable among their family members or peers.
Another study found that African Americans and Caucasians had the same
perception of the stigma of mental illness, but that African Americans had more
fear related to mental health treatment [39]. This may explain why African
Americans with emotional problems are more likely to use clergy or other non-
mental health professionals for help.

Chinese Americans underuse mental health services in spite of indications that
they are likely to be in great need of them due to stresses of immigration, minority
status and discrimination [37]. This is partly a result of differences in the concept of
psychiatric conditions. The Chinese cultural conception of the person is relational.
Harmony in one's relationships as well as within oneself is paramount to the
mental health of a Chinese person. Imbalances in positive and negative forces
within oneself or with others can result in emotional symptoms [40]. With this
orientation, the Chinese base treatment on returning the individual into 'balance'
using herbs, rest, or appropriate exercises. In contrast to the Western psychometric
view of depression, depression is primarily experienced as somatic or interpersonal
difficulties in Chinese culture. In the study by Ying, Chinese Americans felt the
best way to treat depression was by increasing social support, pleasant and social
activities and by eating nutritious food. Thus, an intervention that espouses the
mutual relationship between psychological and physical health seems appropriate
for Chinese Americans. Cognitive behavioral techniques (thinking positive
thoughts, reducing negative thoughts, increasing pleasant and interpersonal activities, increasing and strengthening social supports) may be important and effective
strategies for treating depression in other minorities and patients from non-Western
cultures.

Like other US minorities, Chinese Americans tend to seek Western psychiatric
help only after their symptoms have progressed and significant deterioration has
occurred [37]. While cognitive and more holistic approaches seem appropriate for
these patients, it has been noted that when treating Asian patients for psychiatric
disorders the use of medications had the most significant impact on participation in
treatment. This is thought to be due to the fact that Asian patients are more likely
to focus on somatic complaints, suggesting that a 'medical model' would be the

most appropriate approach to treatment [36]. The same could be said for other minority groups.

There is a small body of literature suggesting that various racial/ethnic groups respond differently to psychotropic drugs. Studies have shown that non-Westerners (Chinese, East Indians, Indonesians, Japanese, Malaysians, Pakistanis, Turks) show improvements on much lower doses of psychotropic medications than Europeans or Caucasian Americans. The need for lower doses of TCAs in Asians, Hispanics, and African Americans than in Caucasians has been reported [41]. As reviewed by Lin *et al.* [42], Asian Americans and African Americans suffer more adverse effects from psychotropic agents than Caucasians.

SUMMARY

Ethnicity and culture are elements that are often overlooked in studies of psychiatric disorders. Clinicians should acknowledge these elements and be sensitive to a client's ethnic and cultural background. Although clinical decisions should be based on the clinical facts of the particular case, an understanding of how ethnic and cultural issues may affect expression and or vulnerability to mood disorders should help clinicians develop culturally relevant treatment regimens. This may be particularly true of patients with depressive disorders, where the patient's beliefs and expectations will have powerful effects on treatment compliance and clinical outcome. Any treatment plan should consider the patient's ethnicity and culture and their influences on illness expression and psychiatric treatment. It is important to eliminate the potential shame and stigma that seeking mental health services may entail. Therefore, community-based education and an emphasis on the 'medical model' is likely to reduce underuse and improve acceptance of psychiatric treatment in ethnic minorities.

REFERENCES

1. Rait G, Burns A. 1997. Appreciating background and culture: the South Asian elderly and mental health. *Int J Geriatr Psychiatry* **12**: 973–7.
2. Manson SM. 1995. Culture and major depression. Current Challenges in the Diagnosis of Mood Disorders. *Psychiatr Clin North Am* **18**: 487–501.
3. Lawson WB. 1986. Racial and ethnic factors in psychiatric research. *Hosp Community Psychiatry* **37**(1): 50–4.
4. Lawson WB, Cuffel B, Holladay J, Helper N. 1994. Race as a factor in inpatient and outpatient admissions and diagnosis. *Hosp Community Psychiatry* **45**(1): 72–4.
5. Adebimpe VR, Cohen E. 1989. Schizophrenia and affective disorder in black and white patients: a methologic note. *J Natl Med Assoc* **81**(7): 761–5.
6. Adebimpe VR, Hedlund JI, Cho DW *et al.* 1982. Symptomatology of depression in black and white patients. *J Natl Med Assoc* **74**: 185–90.
7. Adebimpe VR, Klein HE, Fried J. 1981. Hallucinations and depression in black psychiatric patients. *J Natl Med Assoc* **73**: 517–20.

8. Weissman MM, Bruce ML, Leaf PJ, Florio LP, Holzer C. 1991. Affective Disorders. In: Robins LN, Regier DA, eds. *Psychiatric Disorders in North America. The Epidemiologic Catchment Area Study.* New York: Free Press, pp. 53–69.

9. Jones-Webb RJ, Snowden LR. 1993. Symptoms of depression among blacks and whites. *Am J Publ Health* **83**: 240–4.

10. Brown C, Schulberg HC, Madonia MJ. 1996. Clinical presentations of major depression by African Americans and whites in primary medical care practice. *J Affect Disord* **41**: 181–91.

11. German GA. 1972. Aspects of clinical psychiatry in Sub-Saharan Africa. *Br J Psychiatry* **121**: 461–79.

12. Farooq S, Oyebode F, Sheikh AJ, Okyere E, Gahir MS. 1995. Somatization: a transcultural study. *J Psychosom Res* **39**(7): 883–8.

13. Ots T. 1990. The angry liver, the anxious heart, and the melancholy spleen. *Cult Med Psychiatry* **14**: 21–58.

14. Kuo W. 1984. Prevalence of depression among Asian Americans. *J Nerv Ment Dis* **172**: 449–57.

15. Nakane Y, Ohta Y, Radford M, Yan H, Wang X, Lee HY *et al.* 1991. Comparative study of affective disorders in 3 Asian countries: Differences in prevalence rates and symptom presentation. *Acta Psychol Scand* **84**: 313–19.

16. Diefenbacher A, Heim G. 1994. Somatic symptoms in Turkish and German depressed patients. *Psychosom Med* **56**(6): 551–6.

17. Ebert D, Martus P. 1994. Somatization as a core symptom of melancholic type depression. Evidence from cross-cultural study. *J Affect Disord* **32**(4): 253–6.

18. Shrout PE, Burnam MA, Bravo M, Rubio-Stipec M, Bird HR, Canino GJ. 1992. Mental health status among Puerto Ricans, Mexican Americans, and non-Hispanic whites. *Am J Community Psychol* **20**(6): 729–52.

19. Golding JM, Lipton RI. 1990. Depressed mood and major depressive disorder in two ethnic groups. *J Psychiatr Res* **24**(1): 65–82.

20. Lawson WB. 1996. The art and science of psychopharmacotherapy of African Americans. *Mt Sinai J Med* **63**(5,6): 301–5.

21. Tabora B, Flaskerud JH. 1994. Depression among Chinese Americans: A review of the literature. *Issues Ment Health Nurs* **15**: 569–84.

22. Kessler LG, Cleary PD, Burke JD. 1985. Psychiatric disorders in primary care. *Arch Gen Psychiatry* **42**: 583–7.

23. Katon W, Schulberg H. 1992. Epidemiology of depression in primary care. *Gen Hosp Psychiatry* **14**: 237–47.

24. German GA. 1987. Mental health in Africa: II. The nature of Mental disorder in Africa today. Some clinical observations. *Br J Psychiatry* **151**: 440–6.

25. Kohn R, Skodol AE, Shrout PE, Dohrenmend BP, Levav I. 1997. Jews and their intraethnic vulnerability to affective disorders. *Isr J Psychiatry Relat Sci* **34**(2): 149–56.

26. Levav I, Weissman MM, Golding JM, Kohn R. 1997. Vulnerability of Jews to affective disorders. *Am J Psychiatry* **154**(7): 941–7.

27. McKelvey RS, Mao AR, Webb JA. 1993. Premigratory risk factors in Vietnamese Amerasians. *Am J Psychiatry* **150**(3): 470–3.

28. Carlson EB, Rosser-Hogan R. 1993. Mental health status of Cambodian refugees ten years after leaving their homes. *Am J Orthopsychiatry* **63**(2): 223–31.

29. Kalow W. 1992. *Pharmacogenetics of Drug Metabolism.* New York: Pergamon Press.

30. Risby ED. 1996. Ethnic considerations in the pharmacotherapy of mood disorders. *Psychopharmacol Bull* **32**(2): 231–4.

31. Strickland TL, Ranganath V, Lin K-M, Poland RE, Mendoza R, Smith MW. 1991. Psychopharmacologic considerations in the treatment of Black American populations. *Psychopharmacol Bull* **27**(4): 441–8.

32. Lin K-M, Anderson D, Poland RE. 1995. Ethnicity and Psychopharmacology. *Psychiatr Clin North Am* **18**(3): 635–47.
33. Goldstein JA, Faletto MB, Romkes-Sparks M, Sullivan T, Kitareewan S, Raucy JL, Lasker JM. 1994. Evidence that CYP2C19 is the major (*S*)-mephenytoin 4'-hydroxylase in humans. *Biochemistry* **33**: 1743–52.
34. DeVane CL. 1994. Pharmacokinetics of the newer antidepressants: Clinical relevance. *Am J Med* **97**(6A): 12S–23S.
35. Strickland TL, Lin K-M, Fu P *et al.* 1995. Comparison of lithium ratio between African American and Caucasian bipolar patients. *Biol Psychiatry* **37**: 325–30.
36. Flaskerud JH, Hu Li-tze. 1994. Participation in an outcome of treatment for major depression among low income Asian Americans. *Psychiatry Res* **53**: 289–300.
37. Ying Y-W. 1990. Explanatory models of major depression and implications for help-seeking among immigrant Chinese American Women. *Cult Med Psychiatry* **14**: 393–408.
38. Cooper-Patrick L, Powe NR, Jenckes MW *et al.* 1997. Identification of patient attitudes and preferences regarding treatment for depression. *J. Gen Intern Med* **12**: 431–8.
39. Neighbors HW, Jackson JS. 1984. The use of informal and formal help: four patterns of illness behavior in the black community. *Am J Community Psychol* **12**: 629–44.
40. Tseng W. 1973. The development of psychiatric concepts in traditional Chinese medicine. *Arch Gen Psychiatry* **29**: 569–75.
41. Turner SM, Cooley-Quille MR. 1996. Socioecological and sociocultural variables in psychopharmacological research: methodological considerations. *Psychopharmacol Bull* **32**(2): 183–92.
42. Lin KM, Pollard RE, Lesser IM. 1986. Ethnicity and psychopharmacology. *Cult Med Psychiatry* **10**: 151–65.

21

A Double-Blind Comparison of Fluoxetine and Amitriptyline in the Treatment of Major Depression with Associated Anxiety ('Anxious Depression')

Marcio Versiani[a], Alfonso Ontiveros[b], Guido Mazzotti[b], Jorge Ospina[c], Jorge Dávila[d], Salvador Mata[e], Antonio Pacheco[f], John Plewes[g], Roy Tamura[g] and Moramay Palacios[g]

[a]*Federal University Rio De Janeiro, Brazil;* [b]*National Institute of Mental Health, Lima, Peru;* [c]*San Vicente de Paul Hospital, Medellin, Colombia;* [d]*San Ignacio Hospital, Bogota, Colombia;* [e]*Jose Maria Vargas Hospital, Caracas, Venezuela;* [f]*Centro de Orientacion y Docncia las Palmas, Caracas, Venezuela;* [g]*Eli Lilly and Company, Indianapolis, IN, USA*

INTRODUCTION

Epidemiological studies in Latin America place lifetime prevalence for depressive disorders at 12% in Argentina, 15.3% in Chile, 9.8% in the Dominican Republic, and 11% in Peru [1]. Several therapies appear to be effective in the treatment of depressive disorders; however, there appears to be a consensus that the therapy of choice for depressive disorders of moderate severity is the use of antidepressant drugs [2]. The selection of treatment for this common disorder is guided by a number of factors including, but not limited to, the presence or absence of features of anxiety. The overlap between anxious and depressive symptoms has long been a problem for patients, clinicians, and researchers. The patients and clinicians are concerned primarily with resolving all the symptoms while the goals of researchers have varied. Roth and colleagues have tried to demonstrate that depressive disorders are independent of anxiety disorders, employing principal component analyses and multivariate discriminant analyses [3]. Methodological difficulties

Cross Cultural Psychiatry. Edited by John M. Herrera, William B. Lawson and John J. Sramek.
© 1999 John Wiley & Sons Ltd.

hamper nosological conclusions from studies based on selected clinical samples. However, investigations by Roth and colleagues did yield a multivariate diagnostic scale that can be used for research purposes to separate anxious from depressive patients [3]. Frances *et al.* [4] have reviewed four possibilities, all supported by data, for the relationship between anxiety and depression: (1) co-occurrence; (2) one cause may underlie both; (3) one predisposes to the other; and (3) the association may be due to artifactual definitional overlap. It has been shown that, besides co-occurring frequently, comorbid anxiety and depression may depend on a particular structure of psychopathology, with possible etiological and neurophysiopathological implications [5–8]. Depression frequently appears after years of a previous anxiety disorder. The reverse is not true; anxiety disorders rarely supervene on the course of depressive disorders [8].

Another way to look at the co-occurrence of anxiety and depressive symptoms is the clinical picture often seen in primary care or in general medical settings, called 'mixed anxiety and depression'. In this condition patients suffer from both anxious and depressive symptoms but do not meet all the criteria for an anxiety disorder or for a depressive disorder. The DSM-IV field trial concluded that this condition does exist, is fairly common, can be differentiated from DSM-IV anxiety or depressive disorders and is associated with significant distress and impairment [9]. A criteria set derived from this trial has been included in the appendix of DSM-IV for further study [10]. Liebowitz has discussed the advantages and disadvantages of the diagnosis of 'mixed anxiety and depression', pointing out that primary-care physicians do encounter these patients frequently [11]. A similarly defined category, Mixed Anxiety and Depressive Disorder (F41.2), has been included in ICD-10 [12].

Anxiety symptoms may worsen the prognosis of depressive disorders [13, 14]. Naturalistic follow-up studies suggest that the prognosis for mixed panic disorder and major depression is poorer than for major depression alone [15–17]. Klein has discussed the various implications of the comorbidity between anxiety and depressive disorders, including family data showing increased genetic predisposition and worse prognosis [18].

The possibility that anxiety may predispose to early-onset depression or to a greater number of depressive episodes has important clinical implications [19]. Clinical assessment and treatment of anxiety symptoms in patients thus identified may be a more efficient and useful strategy than focusing primarily on the depressive disorder.

Treatment selection may be influenced by the comorbidity of anxious and depressive features. Anxious patients are often thought of as more likely to respond to more sedating tricyclic antidepressants [2]. It has also been suggested that monoamine oxidase inhibitors (MAOIs) may be more effective than tricyclic antidepressants (TCAs) in patients with major depression and prominent anxiety features [20, 21]. This relationship of anxious (psychomotor-agitated) patients responding to sedating agents and non-anxious (psychomotor-retarded) patients responding to more activating agents has not been demonstrated in the literature

[22, 23]. In fact, some investigators have suggested that a high score on the anxiety/agitation factor may be predictive of good response to selective serotonin reuptake inhibitors (SSRIs), which are typically thought of as being more activating than other antidepressants [24–28].

In a meta-analysis of double-blind studies comparing fluoxetine to a TCA, placebo, or both, Tollefson *et al.* demonstrated that fluoxetine was comparable to the TCAs in the treatment of both 'anxious depression' and 'non-anxious depression' [29]. In addition, fluoxetine was better tolerated than the TCAs in both patient subgroups, as demonstrated by discontinuation rates. A number of comparative trials have shown both amitriptyline and fluoxetine to be effective in the treatment of depression [30–34]. However, no studies have examined the comparative efficacy of amitriptyline and fluoxetine in depressed Latin American patients with anxious features.

The study reported in this chapter was designed to compare the efficacy, safety and tolerance of fluoxetine with amitriptyline in the treatment of major depression and associated anxiety.

METHOD

This was a parallel, double-blind, multicenter, randomized study comparing fluoxetine with amitriptyline in the treatment of major depression with associated anxiety. Studies were conducted in seven centers in five Latin American countries (Brazil, Colombia, Mexico, Peru and Venezuela). The protocol was approved by the institutional review board of each study site, and all patients signed the informed consent document before participating in the trial. The study consisted of two periods: a 2-week, single-blind placebo lead-in phase to eliminate placebo responders followed by an 8-week double-blind active therapy phase. Patients not eliminated in the single-blind phase were randomly assigned to one of two treatment groups: fluoxetine 20 mg/day or amitriptyline 50–250 mg/day.

Inclusion criteria were as follows: patients of either sex, aged 18 years or older, meeting DSM-IV criteria for major depression (except duration of illness of at least one month in the present study) with a minimum score of 18 on the Hamilton Rating Scale for Depression (HAMD) (the first 17 items of the 21-items version) and a minimum score of 18 on the Hamilton Rating Scale for Anxiety (HAMA). A structured clinical interview was employed to assure the reliability of the diagnosis at entry.

Exclusion criteria were: a woman who was pregnant or lactating, a woman with childbearing potential not using an approved contraceptive method, serious suicidal risk, significant medical disease, history of allergy to the study drugs, regular use of other psychopharmacological drugs within the preceding 2 weeks, previous participation in an antidepressant trial, or history of unresponsiveness to fluoxetine or amitriptyline. The following significant psychiatric disorders were excluded: organic mental disorder, substance-abuse disorders, psychotic disorders, bipolar disorder, melancholic disorder, panic disorder, obsessive-compulsive disorder. Patients taking concomitant medications with psychotropic effects were also excluded: vitamins, benzodiazepines, antihistamines, agents recognized as having anticholinergic activity, as well as other antidepressant treatments (including electroconvulsive therapy, phototherapy, or psychotherapy). Use of aspirin or acetaminophen was allowed.

Study drugs were administered on a twice-daily treatment regimen, morning and evening. For the fluoxetine group capsules labeled 'morning doses' contained 20 mg of the active drug and capsules labeled 'evening doses' contained placebo. For the amitriptyline group capsules labeled 'morning doses' contained placebo and capsules labeled 'evening doses' contained 50 mg of amitriptyline. Each patient was administered doses in a double-blind fashion during the active treatment period as follows: one capsule in the morning and evening for the first 7 days, one capsule in the morning and two in the evening for the next 7 days and one capsule in the morning and 1–5 capsules in the evening for the remainder of the study. As a result, fluoxetine was administered in a fixed dosage of 20 mg/morning (plus a varied number of placebo capsules in the evening) and amitriptyline in a range of 50–250 mg/evening (plus one capsule of placebo in the morning). Study visits occurred every week until week 4, then every 2 weeks until week 10 (study period: 2 weeks of placebo run-in plus 8 weeks of study drugs).

Efficacy assessments were analyzed for all randomized patients who had at least one post-baseline visit (intent-to treat basis). Assessment measures applied at each visit were: the $HAMD_{21}$, the HAMA, the Raskin–Covi Depression and Anxiety Scale, the Clinical Global Impression–Improvement (CGI) and Patient Global Impression (PGI). Adverse events were assessed at every visit and classified according to the Coding Symbol and Thesaurus for Adverse Reaction Terms (COSTART) dictionary. A laboratory test battery and electrocardiogram were performed at admission and at the final visit. Vital signs were assessed and recorded at each visit.

Efficacy scale data were analyzed as change from baseline (visit 3) to endpoint (last of visits 4–10) by an analysis of variance (ANOVA) with change as the dependent variable and treatment, investigator, and treatment-by-investigator interaction as the independent variables in the model. The F-test for treatment in this model was the basis for statistical comparisons of treatment groups. In addition to the total scores for the $HAMD_{21}$, HAMA, and Raskin–Covi scales, statistical analysis was conducted on the factors of the $HAMD_{21}$. These factors were: anxiety/somatization factor (sum of items 10, 11, 12, 13, 15, 17), cognition factor (sum of items 2, 3, 9, 19, 20, 21), retardation factor (sum of items 1, 7, 8, 14), sleep factor (sum of items 4, 5, 6) and core depression factor (sum of items 1, 2, 3, 7, 9, 10, 11, 14) [35–37].

Response was defined as a reduction of at least two points in the CGI improvement scale, a decrease greater than or equal to 50% in the HAMD (first 17 items), and a decrease greater than or equal to 25% in the HAMA. A partial response was defined as a reduction of at least two points in the CGI improvement scale, a decrease greater than or equal to 50% in the HAMD (first 17 items), and a decrease less than 25% in the HAMA. Patients not meeting one of these sets of criteria at endpoint were considered non-responders. Response rates were statistically analyzed across treatment groups using the χ^2 test.

Adverse events which either first appeared during the treatment phase or worsened in severity from the baseline period (visits 1–3) were considered treatment-emergent adverse events. Treatment-emergent adverse event rates were analyzed across treatment groups using the χ^2 test.

RESULTS

A total of 157 patients were randomized to one of the two treatment groups: fluoxetine 20 mg/day ($n = 77$) or amitriptyline 50–250 mg/day ($n = 80$). Seven centers from five countries contributed patients: Brazil (52), Mexico (36), Peru (28), Columbia (23) and Venezuela (18). Of the 157 randomized patients, 75.8% were women. Mean age was 41.3 years. Origins were Mestizo (44.6%), Caucasian (36.3%), Mulatto (5.7%), and 'other' (13.3%). There were no statistically significant differences across treatments at baseline in gender, age, origin, or number of years of completed education. The two treatment groups were also comparable at baseline relative to the mean scores in the assessment parameters (HAMD, HAMA, Raskin–Covi scales, CGI).

Of the 157 patients who were randomized, 82.8% completed the study (65 patients in each treatment group). The percentage of patients completing the study was not significantly different between treatment groups. Seven patients (8.8%) dropped out from the amitriptyline group compared with 3 (3.9%) from the fluoxetine group due to adverse events. Eight patients (5.1%) from the total sample were lost to follow-up. One patient in the amitriptyline group discontinued without recording any post-baseline efficacy information. Four patients discontinued due to lack of efficacy (one fluoxetine-treated, three amitriptyline-treated). Four patients (three receiving fluoxetine, one amitriptyline) discontinued for personal reasons and one amitriptyline patient was retired due to protocol requirement. Results relative to the outcome assessed with the HAMD, HAMA, CGI improvement, PGI improvement, Raskin Depression Scale and Covi Anxiety Scale are summarized in Table 21.1.

There were no statistically significant differences across treatments for the HAMD 21-item, HAMD 17-item, or HAMA total scores. There was a statistically significant difference in one single factor, the HAMD sleep factor ($p<0.001$), with a greater change from baseline to endpoint in the group receiving amitriptyline. The treatment difference in the sleep factor (approx. 1.4 points) accounts for most of the numerical differences in the change from baseline across treatments in $HAMD_{21}$ and $HAMD_{17}$ total scores. Within-group differences in all the parameters shown in Table 21.1 (i.e. differences between baseline and endpoint in each of the two treatment groups) were statistically significant at the $p<0.001$ level. Among fluoxetine-treated

TABLE 21.1 Measures of efficacy of fluoxetine and amitriptyline

Efficacy scale	Fluoxetine ($n = 77$)			Amitriptyline ($n = 79$)			
	Baseline mean (SD)	Endpoint mean (SD)	Change mean (SD)	Baseline mean (SD)	Endpoint mean (SD)	Change mean (SD)	p-value
HAMD$_{21}$ Total score	28.9 (4.7)	10.7 (9.2)	−18.2 (8.3)	28.6 (5.0)	9.0 (8.0)	−19.6 (8.4)	0.138
HAMD$_{17}$ Total score	26.5 (4.6)	9.9 (8.4)	−16.6 (7.3)	26.2 (4.4)	8.1 (7.0)	−18.1 (7.5)	0.095
HAMD Anxiety factor	9.6 (2.2)	3.9 (2.9)	−5.8 (2.7)	9.7 (2.1)	3.7 (3.0)	−6.0 (3.3)	0.275
HAMD Cognition factor	5.7 (2.4)	1.7 (2.3)	−4.0 (2.8)	5.2 (2.1)	1.4 (1.9)	−3.8 (2.6)	0.835
HAMD Retardation factor	8.6 (1.4)	3.1 (2.8)	−5.5 (2.8)	8.4 (1.7)	3.1 (2.9)	−5.4 (3.0)	0.512
HAMD Sleep factor	3.5 (1.9)	1.6 (1.8)	−1.9 (2.1)	3.7 (1.6)	0.4 (0.8)	−3.3 (1.8)	<0.001
HAMD Core depression factor	16.8 (3.0)	5.9 (5.1)	−11.0 (4.9)	16.4 (2.5)	5.6 (4.9)	−10.7 (4.9)	0.639
HAMA Total score	28.5 (6.4)	11.0 (9.0)	−17.5 (7.7)	27.7 (6.5)	9.9 (8.4)	−17.8 (8.7)	0.483
CGI Improvement	4.1 (0.5)	1.8 (1.2)	−2.3 (1.3)	4.0 (0.5)	1.8 (1.1)	−2.2 (1.1)	0.813
PGI Improvement	3.9 (0.7)	1.9 (1.3)	−2.0 (1.3)	3.8 (0.6)	1.9 (1.3)	−1.9 (1.2)	0.887
Raskin Depression scale	11.4 (2.0)	5.4 (2.8)	−6.0 (3.0)	11.3 (2.1)	5.3 (2.9)	−6.0 (2.9)	0.400
Covi Anxiety scale	10.8 (1.9)	5.8 (2.5)	−5.0 (2.4)	10.5 (1.8)	5.7 (2.6)	−4.8 (2.6)	0.730

patients, 57 (74.0%) responded to treatment and among amitriptyline-treated patients, 58 (74.4%) responded. This difference was not statistically significant ($p = 0.995$). There were no partial responders in either treatment group.

The average mean dose for amitriptyline was 114.1($\pm$29.9) mg/day and the average last dose was 138.1($\pm$49.8) mg/day (range: 50–250 mg/day). The fluoxetine dose was fixed at 20 mg/day, according to the protocol.

Adverse events that were reported by 3% or more of the patients, or that were statistically significant between treatments, are shown in Table 21.2. Events such as dry mouth, somnolence, constipation, tremor, amblyopia, and anxiety were reported by the amitriptyline-treated patients significantly more often than by the fluoxetine-treated patients. No events were reported significantly more often by fluoxetine-treated patients. No treatment-emergent anxiety was reported in the fluoxetine-treated patients.

There was a significant increase in orthostatic blood pressure (defined as the difference between supine and standing systolic blood pressure) in amitriptyline-treated patients (average increase of 2.4 mm at endpoint over baseline) compared with fluoxetine-treated patients. In other vital signs measures, there were no significant differences between the two groups. Patients treated with amitriptyline had a statistically significant increase in weight (average increase of 0.6 kg) but those treated with fluoxetine had a statistically significant decrease in weight (average decrease of 0.6 kg); weight gain was statistically significant between treatment groups. Clinical laboratory tests outside of the local laboratory reference range were classified as either clinically significant or not clinically significant by the investigator. Inspection of clinically significant abnormal laboratory results established that there were no significant treatment differences in any laboratory test.

DISCUSSION

The main objective of this study was to compare the efficacy of fluoxetine with that of amitriptyline in the treatment of major depression with associated anxious symptoms ('anxious depression'). The minimum score of 18 on the HAMA as an entry criterion was employed for the selection of a subsample of patients with major depression with high levels of anxious symptomatology.

Another way to study the levels of anxious symptomatology is to explore the scores on the HAMD Anxiety Factor. Tollefson *et al.* had classified patients as 'anxious' and 'non-anxious' based on a cut-off point of 7 on the HAMD anxiety/somatization factor [29]. In the present study, 143 of 157 patients (91.1%) had baseline HAMD anxiety/somatization factor scores higher than 7. The mean anxiety/somatization factor score for these 143 patients was 10.0 ($\pm$1.8). This mean is substantially higher than the mean score for anxious patients in the Tollefson meta-analysis, suggesting that patients in this study were more anxious than patients in typical clinical trials of major depression.

TABLE 21.2   Most commonly reported adverse events

Adverse event	Fluoxetine ($n = 77$) no. (%)	Amitriptyline ($n = 80$) no. (%)	p
Dry mouth*	16 (20.8)	57 (71.3)	<0.001
Somnolence*	11 (14.3)	32 (40.0)	<0.001
Constipation*	8 (10.4)	32 (40.0)	<0.001
Tremor*	5 (6.5)	22 (27.5)	<0.001
Headache	14 (18.2)	10 (12.5)	0.323
Dizziness	8 (10.4)	11 (13.8)	0.519
Libido decreased	8 (10.4)	9 (11.3)	0.862
Nausea	7 (9.1)	10 (12.5)	0.492
Amblyopia*	1 (1.3)	8 (10.0)	0.019
Gastritis	6 (7.8)	2 (2.5)	0.132
Asthenia	3 (3.9)	4 (5.0)	0.738
Sweating	4 (5.2)	2 (2.5)	0.379
Anxiety*	0 (0.0)	5 (6.3)	0.026
Insomnia	3 (3.9)	2 (2.5)	0.618
Diarrhea	1 (1.3)	4 (5.0)	0.187
Dyspepsia	1 (1.3)	4 (5.0)	0.187
Tachycardia	1 (1.3)	4 (5.0)	0.187
Abdominal pain	2 (2.6)	3 (3.8)	0.681
Weight gain*	0 (0.0)	4 (5.0)	0.047

* significant differences ($p<0.05$)

Fluoxetine was comparable to amitriptyline in the present study in almost all outcome measures except the factor 'Sleep' from the HAMD. The well known sedative properties of amitriptyline may explain why it was superior to fluoxetine in improving insomnia. In 'anxiety' outcome measures, including the 'Anxiety' factor from the HAMD, the HAMA total score and the Covi Anxiety Scale total score, fluoxetine and amitriptyline were comparable.

Adverse events, especially dry mouth, somnolence, constipation, tremor, amblyopia, anxiety, and weight gain, were statistically more common in the amitriptyline-treated patients. There were no reports of treatment-emergent anxiety in the fluoxetine-treated patients.

The results of this study support the conclusion that fluoxetine is as efficacious as amitriptyline in the treatment of major depression with associated anxiety. As fluoxetine was better tolerated than amitriptyline it may be an important alternative for the treatment of the frequent and disabling condition known as 'anxious depression.'

REFERENCES

1. Garcia AR. 1986. Epidemiology of depression in Latin America. *Psychopathology* **19**(Suppl 2z): 22–5.
2. Joyce PR, Paykel ES. 1989. Predictors of drug response in depression. *Arch Gen Psychiatry* **46**: 89–99.

3. Roth M, Gurney C, Garside R, Kerr T. 1972. Studies in the classification of affective disorders: the relationship between anxiety states and depressive illness. *Br J Psychiatry* **12**: 147–61.

4. Frances A, Manning D, Marin D, Kocsis J, McKinney K, Hall W, Kline M. 1992. Relationship of anxiety and depression. *Psychopharmacology (Berl)* **106**(Suppl): S82–S86.

5. Akiskal HS. 1990. Toward a clinical understanding of the relationship of anxiety and depressive disorders. In: Maser, JD, Cloninger CR, eds. *Comorbidity of Mood and Anxiety Disorders.* Washington, DC: American Psychiatric Press, pp. 597–607.

6. Akiskal HS. 1992. Le deprime avant la depression. *Encephale* **18**: 485–9.

7. Akiskal HS, Lemmi H, Dickson H, King D, Yerevanian B, Valkenburg CV. 1984. Chronic depressions. Part 2. Sleep EEG differentiation of primary dysthymic disorders from anxious depressions. *J Affect Disord* **6**: 287–95.

8. Cloninger CR, Martin RL, Guze SB, Clayton PL. 1990. The empirical structure of psychiatric comorbidity and its theoretical significance. In: Maser, JD, Cloninger CR, eds. *Comorbidity of Mood and Anxiety Disorders.* Washington, DC: American Psychiatric Press, pp. 439–62.

9. Zinbarg RE, Barlow DH, Liebowitz M, Street L, Broadhead E, Katon W *et al.* 1994. The DSM-IV field trial for mixed anxiety-depression. *Am J Psychiatry* **151**: 1153–62.

10. American Psychiatric Association. 1994. *Diagnostic and Statistical Manual of Mental Disorders,* 4th ed. Washington, DC: American Psychiatric Association, Inc.

11. Liebowitz MR, Keller MB. 1993. Depression with anxiety and atypical depression. *J Clin Psychiatry* **54**: 10–15.

12. World Health Organization. 1992. *The ICD-10 Classification of Mental and Behavioural Disorders. Clinical Descriptions and Diagnostic Guidelines.* Geneva: World Health Organization.

13. Schapira KM, Rogh M, Kerr T. 1972. The prognosis of affective disorders: the differentiation of anxiety states from depressive illness. *Br J Psychiatry* **121**: 175–81.

14. Van Valkenburg C, Akiskal HS, Puzantian V, Rosenthal T. 1984. Anxious depressions: clinical, family history, and naturalistic outcomes. Comparisons with panic and major depressive disorders. *J Affect Disord* **6**: 67–82.

15. Angst J, Vollrath M, Merikangas KR, Ernst C. 1990. Comorbidity of anxiety and depression in the Zurich cohort study of young adults. In: Maser JD, Cloninger CR, eds. *Comorbidity of mood and anxiety disorders.* Washington DC: American Psychiatric Press, pp. 123–37.

16. Clayton PJ, Grove WM, Coryell W, Keller M, Hirschfeld R, Fawcett J. 1991. Follow-up and family study of anxious depression. *Am J Psychiatry* **148**: 1512–17.

17. Coryell W, Endicott J, Andreasen NC, Keller MB, Clayton PJ, Hirschfeld RMA, Schfnerr WA, Winokur J. 1988. Depression and panic attacks: the significance of overlap as reflected in follow-up and family study data. *Am J Psychiatry* **145**: 293–300.

18. Klein DF. 1993. Mixed anxiety and depression, for and against. *Encephale* **19**: 493–5.

19. Parker G, Wilhelm K, Asghari A. 1997. Early onset depression: the relevance of anxiety. *Soc Psychiatry Psychiatr Epidemiol* **32**: 30–7.

20. Liebowitz MR, Quitkin FM, Stewart JH, McGrath PJ, Harrison W, Rabkin J *et al.* 1988. Antidepressant specificity in atypical depression. *Arch Gen Psychiatry* **45**: 129–37.

21. Robinson DS, Nies A, Ravaris CL, Lamborn KR. 1973. The monoamine oxidase inhibitor, phenelzine, in the treatment of depressive anxiety states. *Arch Gen Psychiatry* **29**: 407–13.

22. Davidson JR, Miller RD, Turnball CD. 1982. Atypical depression. *Arch Gen Psychiatry* **35**: 527–34.

23. Zisook S, Schuchter SR, Gallagher T. 1993. Atypical depression in an outpatient psychiatric population. *Depression* **1**: 268–74.

24. Dalery J, Bouhassira M, Kress J-P, Lancrenon S, Tafani A, Hantouche EG. 1995.

Agitated-anxious versus blunted-retarded major depressions: Different clinical effects of fluoxetine. *Encephale* **21**: 217–25.

25. Filteau MJ, Baruch P, Lapierre YD, Bakish D, Blanchard A. 1995. SSRIs in anxious-agitated depression: A post-hoc analysis of 279 patients. *Int Clin Psychopharmacol* **10**: 51–4.

26. Otto MW, Pollack MH, Fava M, Uccello R, Rosenbaum JF. 1995. Elevated anxiety sensitivity index scores in patients with major depression: Correlates and changes with antidepressant treatment. *J Anxiety Disord* **9**: 117–23.

27. Partiot A, Jouvent R, Pierson A, Brauch P, Beuzen JN, Ammar S, Widlocher D. 1997. Are there differential effects of fluoxetine in retarded/blunted affect versus agitated/anxious depressives? A clinical study. *Eur Psychiatry* **12**: 21–7.

28. Schatzberg AF. 1995. Fluoxetine in the treatment of comorbid anxiety and depression. *J Clin Psychiatry Monogr Ser* **13**: 2–12.

29. Tollefson GD, Holman SL, Sayler ME, Potvin JH. 1994. Fluoxetine, placebo, and tricyclic antidepressants in major depression with and without anxious features. *J Clin Psychiatry* **55**: 50–9.

30. Bressa GM, Grugnoli R, Pancheri P. 1989. A controlled comparison of fluoxetine and amitriptyline in major depression. *Clin Psychopharmacol* **4**: 69–73.

31. Chouinard G. 1985. A double-blind controlled clinical trial of fluoxetine and amitriptyline in patients with major depressive disorder. *J Clin Psychiatry* **46**: 32–7.

32. Potvin JH. 1993. Fluoxetine versus amitriptyline in the treatment of major depression: a multicenter trial. *Int Clin Psychopharmacol* **8**(3): 143–9.

33. Feighner JP, Cohn JB. 1985. A comparative trial of fluoxetine and amitriptyline in patients with major depressive disorder. *J Clin Psychiatry* **45**: 369–72.

34. Young JPR, Coleman A, Lader MH. 1987. A controlled comparison of fluoxetine and amitriptyline in depressed outpatients. *Br J Psychiatry* **150**: 340–77.

35. Cleary MA, Guy W. 1975. Factor analysis of the Hamilton depression scale. *Drugs Exp Clin Res* **1**: 115–20.

36. Gibbons RD, Clark DC, Kupfer DJ. 1993. Exactly what does the Hamilton depression rating scale measure? *J Psychiatr Res* **27**: 259–73.

37. Guy W. 1976. ECDEU Assessments Manual for Psychopharmacology. Rockville: National Institute of Mental Health.

Inpatient Treatment

22

Psychiatric Inpatient Care and Ethnic Minority Populations

Lonnie R. Snowden

University of California, Berkeley, CA, USA

INTRODUCTION

The need for hospital-based psychiatric care has long been subject to the winds of political and economic fortune. Critics have argued that, from the very founding of mental institutions to the era of deinstitutionalization and continuing to the present day, sociopolitical and economic factors have played a significant role in dictating how mental hospitals have been used. For example, by enlarging the definition of mental illness a century ago, local authorities shifted responsibility and cost for a variety of indigent populations to state government [1]; state government, with the advent of federal entitlement programs in the 1960s, later shifted responsibility and cost for these populations to the federal government [2].

The vulnerability of hospitalization to forces other than clinical necessity has aroused particular interest among scholars and activists concerned with ethnic minority populations [3]. They fear that cultural misunderstanding and societal efforts at marginalization and control of minorities may have guided hospital confinement—that the ambiguity surrounding when and for whom hospital-based care is appropriate has been used to serve a pernicious political agenda. Such fears have contributed to a cloud of skepticism around the issue of inpatient psychiatric care.

Lately, the practice of psychiatric hospitalization has been further challenged in the revolution that is managed care. Hospital-based care is costly and therefore has become a particular target of care managers seeking to curtail expenditures. As a result, psychiatric hospitalization is becoming a scarce resource. The resulting pressures on access to this type of care and lengths of hospital stays might interact with sociocultural factors and further complicate the question of how to make appropriate use of the psychiatric hospital in treating ethnic minorities.

Cross Cultural Psychiatry. Edited by John M. Herrera, William B. Lawson and John J. Sramek.
© 1999 John Wiley & Sons Ltd.

RATES OF PSYCHIATRIC HOSPITALIZATION IN MINORITIES

Concern over psychiatric hospitalization of minorities has a foundation in racial and ethnic disparities in rates of hospital admissions. Building on a body of previous research, Snowden and Cheung [3] documented the problem by demonstrating substantial racial and ethnic variation. Data from the National Institute of Mental Health Survey of Mental Health Organizations indicated that African Americans were admitted to psychiatric hospitals at a rate of 931.8 per 100 000 civilian population, and Native Americans at a rate of 818.7 per 100 000 [3]. Both rates were considerably higher than the rate for Whites (550.0 per 100 000) [3]. Rates for Latinos and Asian Americans/Pacific Islanders, on the other hand, were below the rate for Whites: 451.4 per 100 000 for Latinos, and 268.1 per 100 000 for Asian/Pacific Americans [3]. The pattern was most pronounced at state and county mental hospitals, but continued to appear at non-Federal general hospitals and VA medical centers [3]. At private psychiatric hospitals, admission rates for groups other than African Americans were lower than those for Whites; for Blacks and Whites they were roughly equal [3].

Additional evidence bearing on the extent and meaning of racial and ethnic disparities in rates of hospitalization has become available since Snowden and Cheung's report. Investigators have published data from community surveys, from mental health claims submitted to insurance companies (insurance plan studies), and from studies of health and mental health services systems that permit racial and ethnic comparison of psychiatric hospitalization rates (studies of recidivism). Researchers also have investigated a number of collateral questions—such as whether bias in clinician decision-making might influence rates of hospitalization—permitting further assessment of alternative explanations of racial and ethnic disparities.

Community Surveys

Evidence is now available from a number of community surveys that asked respondents about psychiatric hospitalization and included large numbers of minority participants. Community surveys represent a valuable source of information on psychiatric hospitalization but omit a group which is—as will be shown later—of particular importance: the homeless. Two surveys are of special note: the National Medical Expenditure Survey (NMES) and the Epidemiologic Catchment Area Surveys (ECA). Data from a third major study, the National Comorbidity Survey (NCS), are not available at present.

Sponsored by the Agency for Health Care Policy and Research, the NMES was conducted in 1987 as a successor to the 1977 NMES. Its purpose was to gather information on the health status of Americans, on healthcare financing, and on the utilization of healthcare services. The NMES included a community survey of

36 400 adults and children, forming a probability sample of American households, and was supplemented with companion surveys: the Medical Providers Survey (MPES) and the Health Insurance Plan Survey (HIPS). The MPES gathered supplementary data about respondents from their healthcare providers and the HIPS gathered data from insurance plans. African Americans and Latinos were oversampled (represented in disproportionately great numbers) as part of the community survey's sampling plan and, in turn, were overrepresented in the other surveys. A parallel survey was conducted on the American Indian and Alaska Native populations, The Survey of American Indian and Alaska Natives (SAIAN).

NMES respondents were asked about their use of mental health services during 1987, including psychiatric hospitalization. About 0.6% of African Americans received psychiatric inpatient care and about 0.1% of Latinos, compared to about 0.4% of Whites [4]. The disparities are gross, having not yet been adjusted for socioeconomic and other differences between groups.

Examination of other findings from this analysis suggests the probable outcome from controlled analysis. Persons with incomes below the poverty line were twice as likely to be hospitalized as those with high income; those with less than 12 years of education were 2.3 times more likely than those who had finished college; and persons on MEDICAID were almost three times as likely to be hospitalized as those with private insurance. These findings strongly imply that economic disadvantage plays a significant role in explaining racial and ethnic differences in hospitalization. They might largely account for Black–White differences in rates of inpatient care, and would reduce the Latino–White difference, although perhaps not to the point of eliminating it.

The ECA was the first comprehensive attempt to assess levels of mental illness using DSM criteria, and to determine patterns of mental health services use. Data were collected from community and institutional samples at five sites representing a cross-section of the USA: New Haven, Baltimore, St Louis, urban and rural areas of North Carolina, and Los Angeles. Special provision was made to obtain large samples of African and Mexican Americans.

Along with other types of services used, ECA respondents were asked about admission for an overnight stay at a 'hospital or other treatment program' for a mental health or substance abuse problem. Across the five sites, lifetime rates of admission were about 3.71% among African Americans and 4.02% among Whites [5]. One controlled analysis was performed: after adjusting for demographic and socioeconomic factors, diagnosis, and usual source of care, Whites proved significantly more likely to be hospitalized than African Americans [5]. Mexican Americans, who were concentrated at the Los Angeles site and made up about half of the sample, were hospitalized at a rate of 2.1%, and Whites in Los Angeles were hospitalized at a rate of 4.3% [5]. Asian Americans were not a focus of the study and were not sampled to include adequate representation for making rigorous estimates. Analysis of the naturally occurring Asian American portion of the sample—including about 161 persons of Asian heritage at Los Angeles—revealed no instances of psychiatric hospitalization [5].

Results from the NMES and ECA were in substantial agreement about relative hospitalization rates for Latinos but diverged somewhat regarding African Americans. The two surveys differ in numerous ways, which might help to explain the discrepancy in findings. Hospitalization reported on the ECA occurred because of substance abuse as well as mental illness; the wording of the question to respondents precludes determination of hospitalization for psychiatric reasons alone. African Americans might have underreported psychiatric hospitalization on the ECA; among persons surveyed in psychiatric facilities as part of the institutional sample about 95% of Whites but only 80% of African Americans indicated a history of inpatient psychiatric care [5]. The NMES respondents indicated 1-year hospitalization; ECA-reported hospitalization took place over a lifetime. In a given year, repeat users were more likely to appear than one-time users and, as a result, NMES-assessed hospitalization tended to overrepresent repeat users. (As will be discussed, African Americans are especially likely to be hospital recidivists.) Finally, hospitalization remains a relatively rare event and estimates are subject to much fluctuation.

Insurance Plan Studies

Padgett *et al.* [6] examined use of mental health services among members of the Blue Cross/Blue Shield Federal Employees Plan (FEP). The FEP was studied previously by Scheffler and Miller [7] in a sample drawn 2 years earlier and restricted to adult employees enrolled in that part of the plan providing the most generous mental health benefit. The findings of Scheffler and Miller indicated that African Americans and Latinos were more likely than Whites to experience psychiatric hospitalization. Among both minority groups, they discovered a greater likelihood of hospitalization than was found among Whites, and a lesser likelihood of receiving outpatient care. Padgett *et al.* failed to replicate the earlier finding. They found that African Americans were hospitalized at a rate of 0.97%, Latinos at 1.09%, and Whites at 0.78%; the difference, although in the expected direction, was not statistically significant [6]. In interpreting their finding, it is important to recall that Padgett *et al.* had included in their sample not only adult benefit holders (as had Scheffler and Miller) but also 'surviving annuitants, retirees, and dependent children and adolescents' [6]. Inclusion of children and adolescents, in particular, might have weakened any difference among adults: among children and youths aged 17 and under with private insurance, Whites are more likely than minorities to be hospitalized [8].

The RAND Health Insurance Experiment (HIE) [9] followed a large sample of subjects at six sites in order to understand the impact of financing on health care and health status. The investigators studied mental as well as physical healthcare, and discovered that African Americans were more likely than Whites to experience psychiatric hospitalization: 'Blacks are over four times as likely to have a hospitalization during a month of care . . . Yet the distribution of diagnoses are similar' [9]. However, the investigators were unable in their analysis to disentangle effects associated with race from those associated with other factors, including study location and socioeconomic standing.

Estimates For Native Americans

As noted previously, psychiatric hospitalization was, according to Snowden and Cheung [3], 1.6 times greater among American Indian/Alaska Natives than among Whites The disparity was greatest at state and county mental hospitals but remained notable at non-Federal general hospitals and VA medical centers. These data almost certainly provide an underestimate for they omit hospital care provided by a major source of mental health treatment, the Indian Health Service.

At present there is little basis to update Snowden and Cheung's estimate. Community-based surveys of services use, like those discussed above, included too few American Indian and Alaska Native peoples to permit meaningful analysis, and failed to carry out oversampling (drawing more such people than would be drawn naturally) to rectify the problem. Other sources of data, including the SAIAN, remain to be exploited. The problem arises because too few researchers concern themselves with American Indian/Alaska Native populations.

Another obstacle to better understanding psychiatric hospitalization of these groups is the complex structure of the populations and of the specialized programs serving them. Not only the Indian Health Service but also Tribal Health and Urban Indian Health Programs provide mental health treatment, reflecting complex and varying legal, geographic and sociocultural circumstances. Psychiatric hospitalization appears to occur at quite a high rate among American Indian/ Alaska Native populations, but little can be said at present to better define the magnitude of utilization or to better understand its origins.

Studies of Recidivists

Having a history of psychiatric hospitalization predicts future hospitalization. Because they count admissions into inpatient care rather than individuals who *might* have been admitted, studies such as the Survey of Mental Health Organizations are influenced by recidivists, who are counted repeatedly at each admission. Surveys that focus on a 1-year reporting period, like the NMES, are more likely than lifetime surveys to detect an episode of hospital-based care for recidivists; thus they tend to overrepresent repeat users. If African Americans are overrepresented among recidivists, then racial disparities in rates of psychiatric hospital admissions will be attributable, in part, to the racial difference among recidivists.

There are strong indications that mental hospital recidivists include a disproportionate number of African Americans. From a study of more than 40 000 patients discharged from state mental hospitals, Liginsky *et al.* [10] found that African Americans were substantially more likely than others, during the ensuing year, to experience one or more readmissions.

Studies of psychiatric emergency services have also documented a high incidence of repeat use, and an overrepresentation of African Americans among repeat users. African American recidivism appears to account for a paradoxical finding: in one study of psychiatric emergency services, emergency room clinicians proved less likely than warranted by circumstances to regard African Americans as dangerous [11]. The clinicians may have been unwilling to declare the patients dangerous and to involuntarily commit them if they felt that African Americans, in general, were caught in a 'revolving door' of crisis, emergency room visit, and commitment.

DIFFERENTIAL ACCESS TO RESOURCES: ASSETS, INSURANCE, HEALTH CARE AND COMMUNITY

As demonstrated earlier using the NMES [4], psychiatric hospitalization occurs most often among the poor; middle- and high-income persons are only half as likely to be hospitalized during a year as those who are poor. Hospitalization is expensive and, at first glance, would appear to require wealth. But severe mental illness, which precipitates hospitalization, is strongly associated with poverty and public insurance is a major payer for hospital care. The definition of poverty currently in use is: families with incomes below the federal poverty line. An estimated 29% of African Americans live below the federal poverty line; for this minority group, the relationship between economic disadvantage and rate of psychiatric hospital admissions is especially significant.

Neglected in measures of income is another important economic factor: total wealth [12]. Total wealth reflects a repertoire of available financial resources and provides a more comprehensive view of assets than does family income alone. Total wealth includes assets accumulated over a lifetime as well as wealth inherited from previous generations. It is sensitive to both income and expenses, to assets and liabilities, and reflects—better than income alone—the pool of resources available to cope with problems created by mental illness. There are marked racial differences in total wealth. The median net worth of African-American families was only about one-tenth that of White families in 1988, a differential that outstrips the roughly three times greater African American than White poverty rate [12]. The difference in total wealth reflects lower rates of home ownership and the lesser market value of homes owned; parents and grandparents who lived in the rural south in deep poverty and were unable to accumulate assets; high rates of current poverty and lower incomes among the poor. From this limited economic base, African-American families and individuals must cope with many crises and problems stemming from disability among family members and friends.

The wealth gap between blacks and whites provides a stark reflection of the tenuous economic circumstances facing blacks. Without an accumulation of assets to fall back on, sudden unemployment or a health care crisis that could be weathered by a family with more resources could push many black families past the breaking point.

O'Hare *et al.* [12]

In addition to economic disadvantage, African Americans are, more frequently than Whites, confronted by illness, incarceration, and other social stressors, and these stressors are more likely to make pressing demands. Juggling competing commitments and with fewer bonds of marriage as a source of support, caretakers of mentally ill persons may find themselves overwhelmed for reasons both financial and social.

Other sources of stress arise from the larger communities in which African Americans are likely to reside, and these stressors might aggravate a mental health problem or precipitate a mental health crisis. For example, African Americans are more likely than Whites to live in areas marked by high rates of poverty. In central metropolitan cities in 1989, more than 70% of African Americans lived in areas characterized by high rates of poverty, whereas only 40% of poor Whites lived in such areas [12]. Living in high poverty areas has been shown to have adverse consequences going beyond those associated with individual and family-level poverty. In a study of negative consequences of alcohol use, Jones-Webb *et al.* [13] found that African American men living in impoverished neighborhoods lived in areas with lower family incomes and fewer people in the labor market than White men or Latinos living in impoverished neighborhoods, and they reported more legal, work, and social problems from drinking than White men or Latinos who also lived in poor neighborhoods and drank alcohol at similar levels. Areas marked by high levels of poverty are plagued by social and economic instability [14], by higher rates of violence and victimization, and by closer monitoring by the police. Any of these factors might push a mental health problem toward psychiatric crisis and precipitate an episode requiring hospital-based treatment.

Finally, health insurance and healthcare are related to poverty in ways that might contribute to greater African American psychiatric hospitalization. Persons on MEDICAID are, as noted previously, especially likely to be hospitalized. Resorting to MEDICAID can be a result of hospitalization which, in turn, may result in a loss of private insurance coverage due to downward social mobility. MEDICAID coverage may also encourage hospitalization, even if inadvertently, by reimbursing hospital-based care but not programs and services aimed at community support.

Perhaps the most telling indication of African American social fragility having demonstrable implications for rates of hospitalization is the heavy Black representation among the homeless. Using the best evidence available, Jencks [15] estimated that about 350 000 people were homeless at any moment in 1987. He estimated that about 44% of homeless people were African American. Under this calculation, the proportion of African Americans among the homeless is more than 3.5 times the proportion of African Americans in the population at large.

Moreover, many homeless people have at some point been residents of psychiatric hospitals. According to Jencks, about 24% of the homeless have been admitted for inpatient care at least once [15]. It follows that a disproportionately great number of African Americans who have been hospitalized have become homeless.

CULTURAL FACTORS IN HOSPITALIZATION

A socioeconomic interpretation of disparities in rates of psychiatric hospitalization is consistent with facts describing African American overrepresentation, but is unsatisfactory in accounting for Latino and Asian American underrepresentation. Latinos are poor like African Americans but are underrepresented. Asian Americans are somewhat wealthier, but this difference in resources cannot begin to explain their very low rates of inpatient care. Studying differences in services use among individual groups of Asian Americans, Hu *et al.* [16] discovered that the wealthiest of the groups, Japanese Americans, had the highest rate of psychiatric hospitalization. The relationship between resources and incidence of inpatient treatment in general was reversed among the Asian American groups that were included in the study.

Low rates of psychiatric hospitalization among Latinos and Asian Americans may be explained by looking at cultural factors. The pattern of underrepresentation displayed by these groups is consistent with their lack of involvement in outpatient mental health treatment. Takeuchi and Uehara [17] asserted confidently that 'it is well established that Asian Americans make less use of community mental health services than White Americans (see Leong, 1986, for a review)' [16]. A recent study by Zhang and co-workers [18] again documented this conclusion, finding little evidence of Asian American help-seeking even when directed toward family and friends or religious figures. Careful studies have also demonstrated that Latinos, especially Mexican Americans, make less use of community mental health services than Whites.

Data from the NMES demonstrate the extent of minority underrepresentation in outpatient care and suggest a rank ordering of underrepresentation among groups [5]. As indicated on the NMES, the highest rate of services use occurred among Caucasians, at 4.9%. Second highest were Latinos at 2.57%, and African Americans were slightly below at 2.29%. Asian American/Pacific Islander rates of use were lowest by far, at 1.33%. The analysis was not controlled but this rank ordering was repeated when studied under a variety of financing arrangements, strongly reflecting socioeconomic standing and which can usefully be thought of as proxies.

Huba [19] described a number of the cultural barriers to the use of mental health services by Asian Americans, including stigma, suspiciousness, and a lack of awareness as to the availability of services. It is reasonable to expect that levels of stigma and suspiciousness would be especially high in connection with a form of treatment as noticeable and disruptive of day-to-day routines as psychiatric hospitalization. Huba further noted the lack of treatment providers who were aware of cultural norms and attuned to the expectations and experiences of Asian cultural groups.

In light of what appear to be considerable cultural obstacles preventing timely and effective use of inpatient care by Asian Americans and Latinos, culturally specialized treatment units have appeal. Achieving linguistic proficiency and cultural awareness at levels promoting comfort and acceptance may justify the creation of specialized treatment units and forms of treatment. Minority-focused inpatient units report experiences that appear to warrant the adoption of these specialized care centers as a means to overcome culturally rooted rejection of inpatient treatment.

MINORITY PSYCHIATRIC HOSPITALIZATION IN AN ERA OF MANAGED CARE

Managed care originated in the general health sector over the past two decades and its growing practice is credited with helping to check a growth rate for healthcare spending that had been increasing well beyond the overall rate of inflation. The shift towards managed care has been driven in part by changes in public insurance programs including MEDICAID [20]. The previously discussed link between MEDICAID and inpatient treatment has contributed to escalating costs and has prompted a wave of attempts at reform. Many states have sought and been granted waivers in order to carry out demonstration projects designed to reduce the cost of MEDICAID-financed treatment, often emphasizing reductions on levels of inpatient care, especially Medicare.

Since the inception of managed care, psychiatric hospitalization has become an increasingly scarce resource and, as managed care continues to be adopted, is expected to decline further still. Inpatient psychiatric care is costly: in 1987 the average annual expenditure for persons admitted to a hospital was $9676. The average annual expenditure for outpatient care, by contrast, was only $517 [4].

The term 'managed care' refers not to a specific organizational form or administrative technique but to a family of structures and policies potentially deployed individually or in combination under a variety of arrangements. Familiar examples of organizations constructed on managed care principles are Health Maintenance Organizations and Preferred Provider Organizations. Gaining prominence in recent years have been firms specializing in 'carve out': using managed care principles to administer a mental health or other benefit of special concern and/or which is provided by an insurance company. Although managed care originated and remains most widely practiced in the private sector, public sector managers are turning increasingly to managed care. They sometimes purchase the services of managed care specialty firms operating on for-profit or not-for-profit bases to provide services ranging from technical assistance to complete operational control of services (e.g. management information system design). For this reason (and others), the boundary between public and private is less than hard and fast. The public–private distinction continues to be important, nevertheless: the public system remains an accountable agent of multiple and overlapping constituencies [21].

Despite the diversity of managed care, both in principle and practice, most observers would recognize a number of features as characteristic:

1. Persons enrolled in managed care plans are encouraged, and are often required, to seek care from a designated group of providers. The providers are either employed by a managed care organization or have entered into agreements requiring them to adhere to policies that limit their fees and otherwise constrain their styles of practice. The organization thereby retains control over client use of services and provider patterns of practice.

2. Access to care is limited to people enrolled in the managed care plan or otherwise meeting eligibility criteria. The organization is obligated for its part to offer or make available a package of services.

3. An active role is taken toward monitoring the status of clients and the provision of care. Mechanisms are established to screen clients for eligibility and evaluate their needs, and for monitoring their movement through a system.

4. The decision-making ability of providers is overtly constrained. Policies are established that include limits on certain forms of care, and review of treatment is performed by people employed directly by the managed care organization or engaged by the organization under contract.

5. Incentives may be introduced to reduce costs, including paying providers a salary rather than using a fee-for-service basis, creation of bonus plans, and requirements for cost sharing. All are designed to encourage conservative styles of practice.

6. Emphasis is placed on using interventions of proven effectiveness, particularly those that are cost-effective.

Capitated financing goes hand-in-hand with managed care [22]. Under capitation, providers are paid by the client rather than by the procedure. They receive a fixed amount per client and must, within limits, provide all necessary care. Providers stand to lose money if costs exceed the per-client rate at which they are being paid and, for this reason, they are vulnerable and operate at financial risk. Capitation is often seen as a financial incentive for providers to undertreat—to skimp on care—a controversy which has received widespread attention in the popular press.

Managed care is controversial in other ways. Incentives are felt within the organization to enroll only clients who are least needy and easiest to serve, in order to 'cream' the population. Consumers complain of restrictions on their freedom of choice; under some arrangements they are no longer able to select a provider they prefer, to seek help from specialists at will, or otherwise to dictate the terms of their care. All managed-care organizations must somehow strike a balance between provider and client autonomy on the one hand and centralized control and conformity to policy on the other.

PSYCHIATRIC HOSPITALIZATION AS A SCARCE RESOURCE

The remaining role of the psychiatric hospital and its appropriate use in the treatment of psychiatric disorders for any patient, minority or White, has yet to be fully worked out. Despite continuing uncertainty about the future of psychiatric hospitals, several considerations seem useful for thinking about race and ethnicity in the use of inpatient care.

Among African Americans, excess psychiatric hospitalization appears to occur. High levels of inpatient care may well be associated with the social fragility of African Americans—with regard not only to poverty but also to a constellation of interrelated factors including low levels of overall wealth, homelessness, and stressful neighborhood environments. Because of high levels of stress and low levels of support, such factors have given rise to repeat use of the psychiatric hospital, especially publicly supported hospitals by mentally ill African Americans. When confronted with African-American repeat users whose problems appear socially based and intractable, clinicians appear to have been at least sometimes less rather than more likely to hospitalize.

The decline in psychiatric hospitalization under managed care will have a disproportionately great effect on mentally ill African Americans, because this group is already overrepresented in mental hospitals. Special efforts may be necessary to insure substitution of high-quality clinical care, housing, employment, and other resources necessary for successful functioning in the community. Community support-based alternatives, such as the well established Program of Assertive Community Treatment, take precisely this approach and ought therefore to be especially beneficial to African Americans.

The challenge in realizing this promise is twofold. First, mentally ill African Americans must be successfully identified as needing treatment and thereafter successfully engaged in receiving it. Obstacles to overcome include mistrust of agents of authority (who often will be identified with a criminal justice system in which African Americans are greatly overrepresented), a paucity of existing resources on which to build, and community and cultural norms that might conflict with underlying program assumptions. The translation of community-support programs of care for implementation in African American and other ethnic minorities, and the evaluation of proposed modifications, remains an important, unfinished task.

In an era of managed care, different concerns arise in thinking about psychiatric hospitalization of Asian Americans and Latinos. As inpatient treatment is avoided by clinicians who are following policies designed to minimize treatment costs, there will be a tendency to overlook people who naturally shy away from this form of treatment despite legitimate need. The problem is one of recognizing and providing inpatient care when appropriate, in spite of pressure—based on cost considerations—from the mental health treatment system and pressure—based on fear and culture, hesitancy and incompatible belief—from the patient and community. Especially in the case of Asian Americans, it may be difficult to separate problems leading to unwarranted minimization of inpatient psychiatric care from larger problems of limited participation in mental health programs and use of health services of all kinds. Cultural beliefs and practices and patterns of institutional rejection, in whatever combination they occur, appear to exercise a pervasive impact for this group. There may be a particularly great stigma associated with psychiatric hospitalization but this stigma must share in a concentration of forces that inhibit use of other mental health interventions, and even general health care services.

The problem to overcome in insuring appropriate psychiatric hospitalization of minority populations historically underrepresented in such care is how to engage their members in any form of mental health treatment in the first instance. Groups disinclined by cultural orientation, and possibly also by adverse historical experience, must be actively sought out and engaged. Extra effort must be made to reach these groups, and the pressure to satisfy expectations of limited hospitalization by failing to consider the legitimate needs of those whose inclination might be to avoid participation must be resisted.

REFERENCES

1. Grob G. 1994. *The Mad Among Us: A History of the Care of America's Mentally Ill.* New York: Free Press.
2. Mechanic D. 1989. The evolution of mental health services and mental health services research. In: Taube CA, Mechanic D, Hohman A, eds. *The Future of Mental Health Services Research.* Washington, DC: US Government Printing Office, DHHS Pub. No. (ADM) 89–1600.
3. Snowden LR, Cheung FK. 1990. Use of inpatient mental health services by members of ethnic minority groups. *Am Psychol* **45**: 347–55.
4. Freiman M, Cunningham P, Cornelius L. 1994. *Use and Expenditures for the Treatment of Mental Health Problems.* Rockville, MD: Agency for Health Care Policy and Research, Pub. No. 94–0085.
5. Snowden LR. African American service use for mental health problems. *J Community Psychol* (submitted).
6. Padgett DK, Patrick C, Burns BJ, Schlesinger HJ. 1994. Ethnic differences in use of inpatient mental health services by blacks, whites, and Hispanics in a national insured population. *Health Serv Res* **29**: 135–53.
7. Scheffler RK, Miller AB. 1989. Demand analysis of mental health service use among ethnic subpopulations. *Inquiry* **26**: 202–15.
8. Mason MA, Gibbs JT. 1992. Patterns of adolescent psychiatric hospitalization: implications for social policy. *Am J Orthopsychiatry* **62**: 447–57.

9. Keeler EB, Wells KB, Manning WG, Rumpel JD, Hanley JM. 1986. The Demand for Episodes of Mental Health Services. Santa Monica, CA: RAND Pub. No. R-3432–NIMH.
10. Leginsky WA, Manderscheid RW, Henderson PR. 1990. Patients served in state mental hospitals: results from a longitudinal data base. In: Manderscheid RW, Sonnenschein MA, eds. *Mental Health United States*. Washington, DC: Superintendent of Documents, DHHS Pub. No. (ADM) 90–1708.
11. Snowden LR, Segal S, Watson M. African Americans in the psychiatric emergency service: bias, dangerousness, and involuntary civil commitment (submitted).
12. O'Hare WP, Pollard KM, Mann TL, Kent M. 1991. African Americans in the 1990's. *Pop Bull* 46: 1–40.
13. Jones-Webb R, Snowden LR, Herd D, Short B, Hannan P. 1997. Alcohol related problems among black, Hispanic and white men: the contribution of neighborhood poverty. *J Stud Alcohol* 58(5): 539–45.
14. Wilson WJ. 1987. *The Truly Disadvantaged*. Chicago: University of Chicago Press.
15. Jencks C. 1994. *The Homeless*. Cambridge, MA: Harvard University Press.
16. Hu TW, Snowden LR, Jerrell JJ. 1993. Public mental health services to Asian American ethnic groups in two California counties. *Asian American and Pacific Islander Journal of Health* 1: 78–89.
17. Takeuchi D, Uehara ES. 1996. Ethnic minority mental health services: current research and future conceptual directions. In: Levin BE, Petrila J, eds. *Mental Health Services: A Public Health Perspective*. New York: Oxford University Press.
18. Zhang AY, Snowden LR, Sue S. Differences between Asian and white Americans help seeking and utilization patterns in the Los Angeles Area. *J Commun Psychol* (submitted).
19. Huba L. 1994. *Asian Americans. Personality Patterns, Identity, and Mental Health*. New York: The Guilford Press.
20. Sturm R. 1997. How expensive is unlimited mental health care coverage under managed care? Working paper 107. Santa Monica, CA: Research Center on Managed Care for Psychiatric Disorders, RAND.
21. Cuffel B, Snowden LR, Masland M, Piccagli G. 1996. Managed care in the public mental health system. *Community Ment Health J* 31: 425–36.
22. Masland M, Piccagli G, Snowden LR, Cuffel B. 1996. Planning and implementation of capitated mental health services in the public sector. *Evaluation and Program Planning* 19: 253–62.

23

The Asian Focus Unit at UCSF: An 18-year Perspective

Kenneth K. Gee, Nang Du, Kathy Akiyama and Francis Lu

University of California at San Francisco, CA, USA

INTRODUCTION

San Francisco General Hospital (SFGH) is the only public hospital in San Francisco to serve urban poor, chronically ill, and numerous ethnic and minority groups. The psychiatric inpatient services comprised five locked inpatient units with 97 beds. Each unit has developed a focus which reflects the cultural diversity of both San Francisco and the patients served by SFGH. In 1987, the American Psychiatric Association awarded a Certificate of Significant Achievement to these ethnic and minority psychiatric inpatient programs 'in recognition of the innovative model program that provides specialized services for four previously under-served groups, including Asian/Asian-American, Latino, African-American, and AIDS/HIV patients as well as services geared to the special needs of women.' The Asian focus program was the first of these focus programs at SFGH and became the model for the Latino, African-American, AIDS/HIV, and women's programs that followed.

The 22-bed Asian Focus psychiatric inpatient program began in March 1980 and was the first inpatient psychiatric program in the United States designed especially for Asians/Asian Americans. The formation of the unit was driven, in large part, by the burgeoning number of Asian/Asian Americans in San Francisco at the time. According to the 1980 census, 21% of San Francisco's 685 000 residents were Asian or Asian American. Since then, this population has grown to nearly 30% of San Francisco's 725 000 residents (1990 census). This is the largest percentage within a total population of any major city in the USA. This explosive growth has resulted in an even greater need for our services.

Program activities are designed to address the following specific goals.

1. To provide culturally competent clinical services sensitive to the particular needs of the Asian and Asian-American residents of San Francisco.

Cross Cultural Psychiatry. Edited by John M. Herrera, William B. Lawson and John J. Sramek.
© 1999 John Wiley & Sons Ltd.

2. To provide cross cultural multidisciplinary training opportunities for students and clinicians interested in delivering such care to Asian and Asian-American patients.
3. To provide consultation services to other departments and agencies within SFGH and the larger Department of Mental Health services in San Francisco.
4. To promote and conduct research on the psychiatric treatment of Asian and Asian-American populations.

The elements that we feel are critical to culturally competent clinical services are outlined below.

CULTURALLY COMPETENT CLINICAL SERVICES

Bicultural Staffing

Studies have demonstrated that service utilization is greatly enhanced when bilingual, bicultural personnel are employed. Ethnic, linguistic, and cultural similarities between client and therapist decrease the dropout rate and improve the effectiveness of care [1–3]. Throughout the program's 15 years, a high priority was placed on hiring bilingual, bicultural Asian staff and faculty. Currently, over 28 staff members and trainees are Asian or Asian Americans. Administrative and clinical leadership as well as programming are provided by the unit chief attending psychiatrist. Other Asian staff consist of two team leader attending psychiatrists, two social workers, 30 nurses or psychiatric technicians, one occupational therapist, one psychologist, two unit clerks, and four Asian student interns. Most of our staff were born, raised, and educated in Hong Kong, Taiwan, the People's Republic of China, Malaysia, the Philippines, or Vietnam. They are very familiar with the cultural background of their patients, because many are immigrants or refugees themselves.

Asian Language Coverage

The ability to communicate with monolingual Asian patients in their own language is a vital part of our program. Currently, the program's on-site staff can communicate fluently in 11 Asian languages (Cantonese, Mandarin, Shanghainese, Chungsunese, Toisan, Hakka, Chiu Chow, Fukienese, Tagalog, Malay, and Vietnamese). The SFGH interpreter services also provide language backup for our patients. A training manual for interpreters working with psychiatric patients has been developed by our program to improve the quality of the interpreting service. A communication skills workshop is also available for clinicians who want to improve their interviewing skills with the help of interpreters. According to our experience, the staff's ability to speak with patients and their family members in their primary language is essential in establishing a therapeutic relationship, gathering accurate data, and formulating culturally relevant treatment plans.

Family Involvement

Family assessment, intervention, and education are strongly emphasized in our treatment program. Because of the traditional importance of the family in Asian culture, family members are encouraged to participate in the family intervention program. Family assessments based on a social systems approach are used frequently by clinicians to gain an understanding of family dynamics [2]. As most of our patients are acutely psychotic at admission, the history and information provided by family members is very important. Work by McGill *et al.* showing the importance of family education in reducing relapse in schizophrenic patients has encouraged us to increase our efforts to educate families in the management of our patients [4]. More culturally sensitive and meaningful care is provided, with success measured in the ability of the staff to keep the patient and family engaged in their treatment. The staff's sensitivity to the enormous importance of families to our Asian and Asian-American patients and the high availability of bilingual, bicultural staff who can communicate directly with family members helps to maximize the patient's ability to utilize his family as a source of support. Without adequate communication, the family may come to distrust the staff and serve as an obstacle to treatment. We have also developed family education materials in different Asian languages to enhance the family members' understanding of psychiatric disorders and have helped form the Chinese Family Alliance, a consumer-driven support group for families with mentally ill members.

Asian Focus Milieu Program

The milieu and group activities in our program are designed to provide multi-lingual, multicultural diagnostic and therapeutic services in a short-term inpatient unit. Program activities can be divided into two major groups:

- activities offered to all patients on the unit;
- activities designed especially for the monolingual patients whose primary language is not English.

All patients are encouraged to join the general group activities, which include community meetings, self-improvement meetings, small discussion groups, patio activities, recreational groups, medication groups, occupational therapy groups, and special issues groups. Asian patients have opportunities to interact with non-Asian patients and with staff. Their participation in such activities is made possible with the help of our bilingual staff members and volunteers. For example, at community meetings, which are held three times a week, staff members simultaneously translate the discussion into several Asian languages. When Asian patients are selected as patient community meeting leaders, they conduct the meetings in their native language, while the staff leader translates simultaneously into English. Occupational therapy activities are conducted by a Mandarin and Cantonese-speaking occupational therapist and various other Asian language speaking interns. Both provide Asian patients with much-needed daily support during hospitalization.

For many of the immigrant and less acculturated patients, special efforts are made to create a therapeutic living environment that is more compatible with their cultural backgrounds. For example, at the time of admission, whenever possible, bilingual staff members conduct the admission procedures and orientation to the unit. Patient brochures, descriptions of patients' rights, legal forms, community meeting agenda, and unit signs and schedules are translated into several Asian languages. Small discussion groups with members who share the same language offer refugee and new immigrant patients opportunities to provide emotional support to each other and to minimize their fear and sense of helplessness about being on a locked psychiatric unit. Discussion content usually includes past life experiences in home countries, separation and losses during migration, joys or disappointments of being new immigrants or refugees, family and community perception of mental illness, past hospitalization and treatment experiences, attitudes toward herbal medicine and Western medicine, questions about diagnosis, and discharge planning. The Asian/Asian American patients become much more verbal, open, and expressive in small groups that are conducted solely in their native language.

Patients participate actively in the activities with which they are familiar, such as table tennis, cooking, meditation, and physical exercise. They celebrate traditional Asian holidays and appreciate the availability of newspapers, books, and music from their ethnic communities or home countries. The unit has some aspects of an oriental decor, and rice and tea are routinely served to Asian patients with their regular meals. The staff frequently prepares oriental food during weekend brunches. Family members are allowed to bring in home-cooked meals during their visits.

Diagnosis and Treatment

In many acute, short-term inpatient psychiatric hospitals, the immediate history of present illness and the mental status examination are the major determinants of diagnosis, and rapid stabilization with medication is the major form of treatment. Based on our clinical experience with Asian and Asian-American patients, this solely biomedical approach is not sufficient and, at times, may lead to inappropriate diagnosis and ineffective treatment. In our program we attempt to incorporate a cultural formulation model, which assesses, among other things, the patient's cultural identity, cultural support systems, and expectations of treatment from Western clinicians. Specific approaches to diagnosis and treatment based on understanding of the cultural expression of mental illness are strongly emphasized. The DSM-IV Outline for Cultural Formulation in the *Annual Review of Psychiatry*, Volume 14, entitled 'Issues in the Assessment and Diagnosis of Culturally Diverse Individuals', details this assessment process.

The following illustrates two aspects of our cultural approach.

1. Asian immigrants and refugees often retain their traditional cultural beliefs and health practices regardless of the degree of assimilation into the host society. Although there is no one set of beliefs held universally by all Asian immigrants and refugees, in general their beliefs involve the concept that disease is caused by an excess or deficit of yin or yang principles. Supernatural intervention by demons, malevolent spirits, wind, etc., is still perceived by many patients as the major cause of mental illness. They frequently visit traditional herbal doctors, temple mediums, and folk healers who know little of Western medicine. In our clinical practice, it has been helpful to explore the patients' and the family members' conceptual orientation of mental illness, their health seeking behavior, and their expectations of treatment by Western clinicians.

2. Secondly, a crisis and symptom-oriented approach is used in our program. It is not aimed at uncovering personal, intrapsychic dynamics; rather, our goal is to understand the symptoms and difficulties as perceived by the patient and to focus on symptom reduction through medication, supportive individual and family therapy, and a structured milieu therapy program.

Medication

Many Asian health beliefs and practices center on balancing yin and yang or hot and cold. Asians often perceive Western medications as 'too hot' or 'too strong.' When common side-effects occur, patients interpret this as further imbalance in the body and thus discontinue the medication. Even more importantly, the need for long term medications may be a painful reminder of their mental illness, and the number of pills may be misequated with the severity of the mental illness. As one patient put it, 'you must think I'm really crazy to make me take so many pills!'

In short, the tremendous stigma of mental illness for Asians/Asian Americans and its pervasive impact on all aspects of treatment cannot be overstated. Several studies, and our own experience, have shown that medication non-compliance is high and, because Asians strongly value respect for authority and do not want to offend the doctor, they often will not inform him of their non-compliance. Our program uses a symptom-oriented and active educational approach when using medications. We recommend gently encouraging the patient to identify symptoms he can admit to having and then explaining the medication as a means to relieve his troubling symptoms. Discussion of dosage changes, potential adverse effects, and the need to continue the medication even if the patient feels fully recovered, is very important and should be done frequently.

Medications are usually initiated at one-half the usual starting dose and titrated slowly to minimize adverse effects and allow very gradual adjustment to each higher dose. Antiparkinsonian agents are used aggressively to counteract extrapyramidal symptoms. Minimizing the number of pills and active inquiry of side effects is critical. Routine blood levels of tricyclic antidepressants and mood stabilizers should be obtained, if possible, until there is some assurance that the patient is taking the medication.

As mentioned earlier, Asian families are generally close-knit and extended in nature. The family is often the single most important source of care for ill family members. The family's involvement and assistance in treatment and compliance must be actively sought and nurtured.

Lastly, a significant number of our Asian patients believe in herbal medicine. A detailed medication history can help to prevent untoward and unexpected side-effects that may further impair compliance.

Community Linkage

During the past 15 years, the program has developed extensive liaisons with post-hospital care agencies. Our discharged patients are usually referred to outpatient community mental health centers, partial hospitalization programs, day treatment programs, residential care facilities, and board and care homes. Many of these outpatient programs also provide bilingual and bicultural services to our patients. Those who need long-term hospitalization are often referred to Napa State Hospital and other locked facilities, all of which are currently located outside San Francisco. Whenever possible, we try to place our Asian and Asian-American patients in community settings, where bilingual, bicultural mental health staff are available. In our experience, several linkage activities have been very helpful in facilitating a smooth transition for both the patients and the agencies.

1. Weekly visits by our inpatient staff to an outpatient clinic and treatment program in Chinatown. This affords our staff the opportunity to give progress reports on our patients and receive input regarding treatment and discharge planning from an outpatient therapist.
2. Weekly inpatient hospital visits by outpatient staff. The liaison staff attends our team rounds and visits with patients who either will be returning to the clinic or will be referred there as new patients. Other case managers and outpatient therapists are encouraged to visit their hospitalized patients and attend case conferences.
3. Preplacement visits to treatment facilities before discharge. Bilingual staff are available to escort our patients to the post-hospital care agencies where they can participate in program activities before discharge. This allows them to

gradually acquaint themselves with the program and staff, making their transition that much easier.

4. Training of multidisciplinary mental health workers. Many of our trainees go on to work in community agencies, bringing with them a keen knowledge of the continuum of services available to patients. This results in more efficient and effective utilization of services by patients.

TRAINING AND RESEARCH ACTIVITIES

As one of the training sites of the Department of Psychiatry, University of California at San Francisco, our program offers unique learning opportunities for mental health professionals who are interested in working with Asian and Asian-American patients. Since 1980 over 450 students, 50% of whom were Asian, received their training on the unit.

Our Asian Focus Unit is an integral part of University of California, San Francisco psychiatric residency, medical student and psychology fellow training programs. In addition, training opportunities are available for students of social work, nursing, and occupational therapy. A large number of trainees of all ethnicities are attracted to SFGH because of our Asian and other specially focused inpatient programs.

All 14–16 PGY-I residents have two 3-month rotations on two of the SFGH inpatient units, learning interviewing, differential diagnosis, inpatient management, and treatment planning focused on ethnic minority patients of the specific program. They are assigned to a multidisciplinary team led by a UCSF faculty attending psychiatrist. Under an apprenticeship model of on-unit supervision, both minority and non-minority residents learn the knowledge, skills, and attitudes needed to work with minority patients in an inpatient setting. Team-based case reviews, led by the attending psychiatrist, provide opportunities for the treatment team to review the history, diagnosis, assessment and treatment plan. In addition, a weekly unit-based teaching conference alternates between a formal case conference and a journal club. Each resident has one off-unit supervisor who pays specific attention to issues of transference/countertransference with minority patients and a community mental health systems perspective in the treatment of minority patients.

This unique training environment allows trainees to observe and practice culturally sensitive approaches taught from a multidisciplinary staff. Critical role modeling is provided for Asian men and women seeking to enter the field, which is traditionally heavily stigmatized and devalued by Asian culture. As a result, staff retention and recruitment has been greatly facilitated with many staff being with the unit over 12 years and all three of our Asian psychiatrists being graduates of the psychiatry residency training program. These programs have greatly assisted our efforts to recruit minority residents; 33–50% of our 62 residents are of ethnic minorities.

Our staff has participated in collaborative research projects with other research centers, such as the National Asian-American Mental Health Research Center at the

University of California, Los Angeles, and the National Asian-American Psychology Training Program based at Richmond Adult Maxi Services in San Francisco. Current research activities with Asian/Asian-American populations include the development of program evaluation criteria and patient satisfaction questionnaires, and a research project studying somatization in Chinese with major depressive disorders.

CONSULTATION SERVICES

The program faculty and staff offer a wide range of consultation services to other clinicians who are interested in improving their services to Asian and refugee patients. Consultation services are provided in the form of individual consultation, group consultation, in-service training for staff members, workshops, program consultations, etc. Consultation services are frequently requested by other focus inpatient units, the jail psychiatric ward, medical inpatient units, other psychiatric hospitals, and post-hospital care agencies.

DIAGNOSIS

The primary diagnoses are summarized in Table 23.2. A few points bear mentioning. First, there is a lower than expected number of major depressive episodes. Again, because of the stigma of mental illness and the high frequency of somatization, these patients may be presenting to general practitioners or not at all. The number of diagnoses of post-traumatic stress is also low but reflects an ongoing trend in this direction. As we move away in time from the Vietnam War, there is both attenuation of the syndrome and also more bilingual community treatment centers are available to provide treatment and avert inpatient hospitalization. Lastly, there are very few diagnoses of substance abuse, possibly because this is usually the secondary diagnosis, and is thus not routinely coded.

CAVEATS

Some caveats are worth mentioning regarding bicultural units. First, clinicians and staff of the same ethnic and/or cultural background as their patients should keep in mind the potential for countertransference. One example involves rescue fantasies and over-involvement with the patient such that the patient's ability to help themselves is not recognized. This dilemma is further magnified when, due to unique language or cultural barriers, only a few staff (or perhaps only one member) can communicate with the patient in their own language, perpetuating the fantasy that only those people can rescue the patient.

Second, a bicultural unit may not be a therapeutic setting for Asian/Asian-American patients who do not identify with their Asian heritage and prefer not to

TABLE 23.1   Demographics, financial year
1994–1995

Group (n = 412)	No. (%)
Asian	207 (52)
White	149 (36)
African American	22 (5)
Hispanic	11 (3)
Other ethnicity	23 (5)
Female	177 (43)
Male	235 (57)
Elderly (over 65 years)	46 (11)
Preferred language	
English	293 (71)
Asian	98 (24)
Other	21 (5)

TABLE 23.2   DSM-IIIR primary diagnoses, financial
year 1994–1995 (n = 412)

Diagnosis	No.	(%)
Schizophrenia	56	14
Schizoaffective disorder	81	20
Psychosis NOS	82	20
Other psychotic disorders	5	1.2
Major depressive episode	38	9
Bipolar affective disorder	82	20
Other mood disorders	4	1
Organic mental disorders	16	3.9
Post-traumatic stress disorder	4	1.0
Substance abuse/dependence	5	1.2

see themselves as Asian. The relationships of such individuals with various Asian staff may symbolize an ambivalently held mother or father figure to such a strong and painful degree that their current task of coping with problems of psychosis, etc. becomes a less imminent concern. Their recovery is thus prolonged due to overwhelming interpersonal conflict and acting out.

Thirdly, bicultural units are sometimes difficult for non-Asians who have issues of mistrust or dislike for Asians. It is difficult for these patients to develop a working alliance with the staff; in such cases, interunit transfers are often helpful.

RECOMMENDATIONS

In summary, our 18-year experience in providing inpatient psychiatric services to Asians and Asian Americans at SFGH has yielded a number of important insights and recommendations that may be of value to the future design and implementation of inpatient psychiatric services.

1. We strongly recommend that specialized bilingual, bicultural programs be developed in major cities or areas with a large Asian/Asian-American population. If necessary, these specialized services should be made available on a city-wide or region-wide basis, unrestricted by catchment area boundaries.

2. Evaluation and therapy should be provided, using a multidisciplinary team approach, by staff members whose ethnic, linguistic, and cultural backgrounds are similar to those of their patient population. A sufficient number of bilingual, bicultural mental health personnel should be employed to permit their assignment to teams or units to maximize their visibility and impact upon service delivery systems. Special effort should be made in the employment of interpreters and in the hiring and retention of bilingual mental health professionals in major disciplines [5]. Language coverage on a 24-h basis is also essential in a psychiatric inpatient setting.

3. Services available in the program should be comprehensive, including emergency services, consultation and liaison services, partial hospitalization, day treatment programs, medical referrals, and case management.

4. Therapeutic milieu programs should include culturally relevant activities.

5. Family members should be actively involved in evaluation and treatment processes. Family intervention with a psychoeducational approach can be effective in reducing relapse in mentally ill patients.

6. Strong links and good collaboration with outpatient community mental health programs and other health and human services are very important for providing continuity of care. Every attempt should be made to maintain patients in their community after discharge.

7. Ongoing in-service training, supervision, and consultation, with special emphasis on Asians and Asian Americans, should be provided to clinicians to minimize transcultural misunderstanding.

8. Training opportunities for inpatient psychiatry should be available to psychiatric residents or interns who are interested in cross cultural psychiatry. Most important, special efforts should be made to recruit Asian/Asian-American trainees, especially in the fields of psychiatry, psychology, social work, and psychiatric nursing.

9. Research opportunities should be provided for community clinicians as well as for university researchers who are interested in inpatient populations.

10. Strong links should be established with the Asian/Asian-American community's organizations and leaders. Their understanding and support are key factors in destigmatizing mental illness and fostering the program.

Our special, focused program located in a general hospital has brought many new and exciting treatment possibilities to our community. This Asian-focused inpatient unit model has been successful in San Francisco for a number of reasons.

Foremost is the tremendous need arising from the large heterogeneous Asian/ Asian-American population in San Francisco. Additionally, support from the hospital administration and community mental health system has been critical to our success.

This, of course, is not intended to provide the only 'recipe' for the inpatient treatment of Asians and Asian Americans. Program design should be tailored to the needs of each community's unique characteristics. It is hoped, however, that the recommendations presented here can stimulate more discussion about the provision of inpatient service in Asian communities and lead to more culturally relevant services for psychiatric patients in these groups.

REFERENCES

1. Lee E. 1980. *Mental health services for the Asian Americans: Problems and alternatives. Civil Right Issues of Asian and Pacific Americans: Myths and Realities.* Washington, DC: US Government Printing Office, pp. 734–56.
2. Lee E. 1982. A social system approach to assessment and treatment for Chinese American families. In: McGoldrick M., ed. *Ethnicity and Family Therapy.* New York: Guilford Press.
3. Wong HZ. 1982. Mental health services to Asian and Pacific Americans. In: Snowden LR, ed. *Reaching the Underserved: Mental Health Needs of Neglected Populations.* Los Angeles: Sage.
4. McGill C, Falloon IR, Boyd JL, Wood-Siverio C. 1983. Family educational intervention in the treatment of schizophrenia. *Hosp Community Psychiatry* **34**: 934–8.
5. Lee E. 1982. *Survey on Community Mental Health Service Manpower for Asian/Pacific Americans.* Ann Arbor, MI: University Microfilm International.

24

Development of a Client-centered Inpatient Service For African Americans

Michelle Clark

University of California at San Francisco, CA, USA

INTRODUCTION

In 1980 the chief of Psychiatry at the San Francisco General Hospital, Dr Frank Johnson, determined from the census data that by the year 2000 the population served would be predominantly ethnicities other than the national majority. Until this time training and practice in psychiatry were based almost entirely upon majority norms. He sought to prepare the department for service to these special populations by creating several task forces, which were directed to advise the department on ways to prepare for service to these special populations. Five task forces were created for addressing Asian, African American, Latino, gay–lesbian and women's issues. The group ultimately coalesced to form the Ethnic and Other Minority Issues Committee (EMIC). The continuing work of that coalition led to the development of the Cultural Competence and Diversity Programs (CCDP). This chapter will describe the development of the Black Task Force (BTF), with emphasis on events associated with the development and implementation of the model for inpatient services to patients of African descent: the Black Focus Program (BFP).

DEVELOPMENT OF THE MODEL

The early participants in the BTF were clinical and administrative staff of African descent. In spite of affirmative action the UCSF Department of Psychiatry had no full-time compensated faculty of African descent and there were no other faculty members who had knowledge and skills unique to work with this group.

Cross Cultural Psychiatry. Edited by John M. Herrera, William B. Lawson and John J. Sramek.

Initially, the task force organized and presented educational conferences to improve the awareness of clinicians regarding African-American culture. It also presented and interpreted the literature available regarding psychiatric treatment and African Americans. Over several years the task force sponsored a total of five continuing medical education courses. The second task force conference expanded upon the academic component. Grant funding was obtained to hold a policy workshop. The workshop included administrators, educators, and clinicians, who worked together to produce a document directing the department toward several goals and objectives that were to be achieved while working with African Americans. Among these was the recommendation that an inpatient service be established with an African-American focus [1]. There have been no other situations, to our knowledge, where an inpatient program was developed with the explicit task of forwarding expertise in working with the African-American population. Approximately 1 year later the department expanded its inpatient service and built an additional unit on another floor in the hospital. The chief of the service at that time presented to the BTF the opportunity to begin a Black Focus Program. The department recruited a psychiatrist from the Charles R. Drew University of Medicine and Science to fill the position of the founding director of the BFP. This team, along with another team, began the inpatient service on Unit 6B in 1985.

Because there was no model for the development of this program, the BFP team leader recruited volunteers from mental health service providers of African descent in the San Francisco bay area. Ultimately, 12 or more members met on a semimonthly basis to review literature, share information, and draft the initial statement of goals and objectives and a bibliography for the program [2, 3]. The group called themselves the Community Clinicians' Advisory Group and met for approximately 1 year during the initiation of the program. This was a multidisciplinary group consisting of physicians, clinical psychologists, licensed psychiatric technicians, and various levels of nurses (including clinical nurse specialists, head nurses, and line staff nurses). Also included were social workers, an occupational therapist, and a medical anthropologist.

In addition to drafting a structure for the program the unit had to hire a completely new staff. Positions were open to all in the department and only those who were interested in beginning work in this program were hired. At its inception the program had the advantage of a rich administrative staff on the unit. The Unit Executive Committee consisted of a unit chief (a senior attending psychiatrist), a head nurse, two clinical nurse specialists, and a program director. Two members of this group were African Americans. The BFP team consisted of a team leader psychiatrist, a clinical nurse specialist, a licensed clinical social worker, an occupational therapist, a discharge coordinator (shared by both teams), and a senior resident on an elective rotation for the year. The attending psychiatrist, the clinical nurse specialist, the senior resident, and the discharge coordinator were African Americans. The BFP team members met with the Executive Committee and, using the information compiled by the Community Clinicians' Advisory Group, drafted some objectives and goals toward the selection of patients to be forwarded to the BTF.

Of note is the fact that concern was raised, even before the development of the program, regarding segregating populations of patients in the special focus program. The program is at SFGH, the only public hospital in the city and county of San Francisco. The hospital accepts all patients for treatment, denying service to none. Patients are admitted to beds as they come available and according to need. These policies and procedures prevent isolation of any one population on any unit. In addition to being multidisciplinary all of the staff on each of the units are multicultural. The BTF noted certain criteria that they felt would be useful in identifying patients who might benefit most from their expertise and thus could be admitted. Among these were those with stressors that were associated with psychiatric illness in the African-American community. The stressors were cited in works from the BTF conferences and by the Community Clinicians' Advisory Group.

EARLY IMPLEMENTATION

The opening of the new unit occurred with much enthusiasm and excitement. In addition to their clinical duties, the BFP team met to discuss continuing issues in implementing the program in their Black Focus Steering Committee meeting. They also met with the BTF on a monthly basis to coordinate other activities. Most of the staff lacked formal training and knowledge in working with African Americans, so one of the first tasks of the team leader was to begin in-service training for all of the staff. Much of the training was a continuation of the information and discussions that had occurred in BTF conferences. In addition to didactic sessions, discussions on issues specific to African-American patients were held in case conferences and during team meeting case presentations.

Another aspect of the program was to establish what would be known as a Black Inpatient Milieu. This concept came as a result of consultation from one member of the Community Clinicians' Advisory Group who was an occupational therapist. In most institutions the decor and resources provided for activities other than direct clinical service were usually Eurocentric: such things as the art on the walls, the table games that were available, the menus, and the music played tended to be those that were preferred by the majority culture. Many of the arts and leisure activities of African Americans differ greatly from those of the majority culture and thus additional work was needed to make these things available. The most challenging and significant effort was made on the part of the staff to obtain the appropriate products for their African-American patients to groom themselves. The necessary hair-combing instruments, haircare products, and products for shaving were not part of the standard hospital issue. It took several months to find a resource of these products and arrange to order them. Ultimately there was success, and now these things are standard issue at the hospital. Volunteers have supplied artwork which reflects African-American life and culture. Several videos have also been donated that relate to African as well as African-American art and culture.

Therapeutic groups on the unit were planned with an eye toward making the subject material culturally relevant. This is not limited to African-American issues: we often have people of other races and ethnicities and so attempt to address anything of cultural relevance. For example, staff assisted one of our Jewish clients with preparing a Seder celebration during Passover.

Another unique aspect of the program was the development of the Black Awareness Group. This group was co-led by two staff members and attended on a voluntary basis by all patients who could maintain themselves in a group setting. The goal of the group was to model respectful and successful communications among people and to provide accurate information about living and working in the African-American community. We started this group because we recognized that the creation of the unit represented a microcosm of the African-American community. For many clients as well as staff the experience of working or living with a critical mass of people of African descent was unique. This experience, we felt, would necessitate some support and explanation. The group was initially held on a weekly basis, began with the statement of respectful and accurate communication, and encouraged clients to raise topics or questions of concern to them. Other therapeutic group activities offered on the unit were relatively standard; however, explicit culturally relevant content was applied to each.

Initially the referrals to the unit did not reflect attention to the focus of the program. The great need for services in the community and the limited number of beds available meant that referrals flowed in at a constant pace. Over time staff throughout the department began to recognize the special services and benefits that were offered by the program. We initially suggested that referrals were patients of African descent, particularly those for whom race was identified as an issue in their concerns surrounding hospitalization. We also welcomed referrals who were subject to the common stressors that we had identified were associated with illness among African Americans—such as recent migration to the area, single parenting, unemployment, and trauma. Later, the initial focus of the program was met, with referrals being mostly people of African descent. Similar patients who were hospitalized on other units with different focuses were seen by the BFP team upon request. We also often participated in case conferences on other units.

CHALLENGES AND CONTROVERSIES

The BFP has been in existence for 13 years. On our tenth anniversary we began to reflect on our experiences. At the beginning of our endeavor many questions were raised regarding the clinical, administrative, educational and political issues that were to be faced. We have learned much and seek to confirm our findings through research analysis.

Educators in psychiatry have emphasized the 'bio-psycho-social' approach for some time. We have found that for African Americans this model should be expanded, and we now use an 'anthro-bio-psycho-socio-spiritual' method to address everything that impacts on the mental health, or lack thereof, of our patients. We have noted that we must consider the historical impact of environment upon this special population. Inclusion of an anthropologic perspective pays particular attention to the unique experience of forced migration (the miafa) and the resultant unnatural disruption of cultural evolution in the presence of extreme human–human conflict. This has proven valuable to both clients and staff for understanding the cultural differences as manifested in symptom presentation and help-seeking, and it must be considered in treatment planning. Spiritual issues are prominent in African-American lifestyles and underlie basic beliefs in cause and effect. They also form the basis for the hope that has sustained this group through centuries of oppression. We feel that this is critical for competent clinical services to African Americans, as well as other groups [4, 5].

Early in our program we began participating in various forums that presented our work. In one debate on the controversy regarding benefits of culturally focusing, rather than mainstreaming, services, we were challenged on our recruitment and retention of culturally competent staff. Recruitment and retention has been a unique administrative problem in our location but presents a special issue in general. The percentage of African Americans in the population of San Francisco numbers less than the national average. This not only limits numbers for selection but also causes the area to be less attractive for recruitment. The percentage of African Americans decreases even more as one looks at the academic community. Recent political attacks on affirmative action at the university and state level make the future look dim. These realities, coupled with the shrinking number of residents in training and the fading of emphasis on development programs at the national level, are disturbing. Our response is to focus on the importance of cultural competence in the absence of biculturality.

The two most important aspects of our curriculum have been the presentation of accurate historical and clinical research regarding the African-American subculture and training in cultural competence. Historically, clinical research about most so-called 'minority' groups has been limited due to focus on study samples limited to majority populations. This lack of accurate information is paralleled in our society's overall blindness to African and African-American history and culture. Some of our more rewarding experiences have come from the exchanges generated in sharing this information with students, trainees, staff and patients. We have been stunned, however, by some of the resistance we have met to this information and lack of acceptance of our curriculum as valid within the training program. First-year residents in training in psychiatry have had the most difficulty with this program and have required us to seek outside consultation. Analysis of the issues included the observation that our program violates society's taboo regarding discussions of personal prejudice and institutional racism. Challenging the myths and stereotypes associated with White supremacist racism threatens the core identity of this majority group. We are aware that identity struggles are common for the period between medical school graduation and licensure for physicians. This is particularly true for psychiatrists as they enter a specialty that is sometimes denigrated. For some, the additional challenge of facing the realities of racism seems to be too disorganizing.

Training in cultural competence has been important because it provides a paradigm for staff, students and trainees. It allows them to conceptualize their needs regarding these curricula. Cultural competence training for the entire department was recommended as a result of the consultant's analysis of issues occurring with residents. We have been most successful with the Pinderhughes model, which emphasizes the individual's need to identify with their own culture [6]. Members of the majority culture tended to have difficulty with this. Once one's culture is identified, an experience with cultural dissonance occurs when one who was discriminated against is now accepted. While quite emotional, these exercises help members to achieve the empathy necessary to appreciate the experience of racism. The closing of the training focuses on identifying occasions where the members have colluded with discrimination, personally or institutionally. Once they become aware of these mechanisms people can choose to consciously avoid racist actions. Through this training, the members of the staff have been able to appreciate the importance of their cultural competence with all groups, particularly non-African-American trainees. Training has also helped people to conceptualize cultural competence along a continuum which stresses progression from cultural destructiveness to cultural proficiency. The continuum model reinforces the developmental aspects of this particular set of skills.

Our program was the first in the department to sponsor a formal seminar series. This was initially designed as in-service training for the staff but it has evolved into a full curriculum encompassing forums of supervision, team treatment planning meetings, case conferences, didactic education and patient education. The core module lists objectives divided into three areas: attitudes, knowledge and skills. These objectives are the goal of our educational program and are used for recruitment of faculty and staff.

In summary, it is clear that the absence of a culturally proficient faculty and staff at upper levels of administration has historically impeded development of novel programs such as those described in this chapter. As we near yet another anniversary of our African-American program, we continue to provoke controversy and face challenges, we look behind us to our ancestors for strength and guidance, we look around us to our allies for developing competence, and we look forward in faith and hope.

REFERENCES

1. Fallileve MT. 1985. *The Black Family: Mental Health Perspectives. Proceedings of the Second Annual Black Task Force Mental Health Conference, October 13 and 14, 1984*. San Francisco, California.
2. Bradshaw WH. 1978. Training psychiatrists of working with blacks in basic residency programs. *Am J Psychiatry* **135**(12): 1520–4.

3. Chunn JC, Dunston PJ, Ron-Sheriff F, eds. 1985. *Mental Health and People of Color: Curriculum Development and Change.* Washington DC.: Harvard University Press, Inc.
4. Griffith EH, Baker M. 1993. *Psychiatry Care of African Americans: Culture, Ethnicity and Mental Illness.* Washington, DC: APA Press.
5. Thomas A, Sellen S. 1972. *Racism and Psychiatry.* New York: Bruner and Maze.
6. Pinderhughes E. 1989. *Understanding Race, Ethnicity and Power.* New York: Free Press.

25

The Effectiveness of a Culturally Sensitive Milieu on Hospitalized Hispanic Patients

John M. Herrera[a] and Yasmine Collazo[b]

[a]Eli Lilly and Company, Indianapolis, IN, USA; [b]Mount Sinai School of Medicine, Elmhurst, NY, USA

INTRODUCTION

In recent years, studies examining the appropriateness of inpatient psychiatric treatment for Hispanics have reported a disproportionate rate of error in the diagnosis of major psychiatric disorders [1, 2] and poor response to treatment. Related outpatient studies have found that Hispanics, as other minorities, often shun psychiatric treatment until late in the course of their disorder [3, 4] and then terminate prematurely. Dolgin *et al.* [5] randomly selected Hispanic and Anglo case records from a state psychiatric hospital and found that Hispanic inpatients were more likely to refuse medication and resist treatment and reported more inter-personal difficulties and lower self-concepts than Anglo controls. In a comprehensive series of cross cultural studies on community mental health services to ethnic minorities, Sue and his colleagues [6, 7] examined detailed information on approximately 14 000 clients seen in 17 community mental health centers over a 3-year period in the greater Seattle area. One index of therapeutic responsiveness examined was the 'failure to return rate', defined as those patients who dropped out after *one* contact with the mental health outpatient facility. Suffice it to say that the reported 'failure to return' rate for Hispanics was over 50%.

One significant response by the psychiatric community to this problem has been the development of ethnic-specific psychiatric programs, designed to be more responsive to minority patients by providing culturally sensitive treatment [8–10]. Two related studies are presented in this chapter, assessing the inpatient milieus of psychiatric programs which were designed for Hispanic patients. The Ward Atmosphere Scale (WAS) [11], an instrument widely utilized and designed to assess the environments of hospital clinical programs, was used in both studies. In the first study, the therapeutic milieu of a long-established Hispanic inpatient unit was

---

Cross Cultural Psychiatry. Edited by John M. Herrera, William B. Lawson and John J. Sramek.
© 1999 John Wiley & Sons Ltd.

TABLE 25.1 Biodemographic profile of subjects of Study One

	Patient population			Diagnosis		
	Unit	Male	Female	Schizophrenia	Affective	Other
Hispanic	37	18	19	18	7	12
Female	45	—	45	29	9	7
Male	46	46	—	32	6	8

compared with the standard treatment milieus of two conventional psychiatric hospital units [12]; in the second, the therapeutic milieu of a newly developed inpatient Hispanic unit [13] was compared with the pre-existing conventional unit. The results of both studies clearly indicate that tailoring the psychiatric milieu to become more culturally responsive can successfully improve the inpatient experience of ethnic minority patients.

STUDY ONE

Site and Subjects

Metropolitan State Hospital (MSH) is a licensed, acute psychiatric hospital with a 1372-bed capacity (at the time of the study) that serves Los Angeles and Orange Counties, California. The Hispanic unit at MSH had been developed to provide treatment for those psychiatric patients whose primary language is Spanish or whose cultural identification is Hispanic. As seen in Table 25.1, the population of the Hispanic unit was 37 patients (18 males and 19 females) with an age range of 18–62 years (mean age 37). Two conventional psychiatric hospital units (a female and a male unit) housed in the same facility were chosen for purposes of comparison. The female unit's population was 45 patients with an age range of 18–63 years (mean age 37); the male unit's population was 46 patients with an age range of 18–67 years (mean 35).

Instrument and Precedes

The WAS [11] is a 40-item (short-form) true and false questionnaire that assesses the psychosocial environment of hospital-based clinical programs. Moos [11] has derived 10 subscales of the WAS which assess four dimensions of the treatment milieu. As seen in Table 25.2, the first three subscales (involvement, support and spontaneity) measure a 'relationship' dimension in that they assess the extent to which patients are involved in the milieu. The next four subscales (autonomy, practical orientation, personal problem orientation, and anger and aggression) measure a 'treatment dimension'. The last three subscales (order and organization, program clarity, and staff control) measure a 'system maintenance' dimension

TABLE 25.2 WAS subscale definitions

1 **Involvement**: measures how active and energetic patients are in the day-to-day social functioning of the ward. Patient attitudes such as pride in the ward, feelings of group spirit are assessed.

2 **Support**: measures how helpful and supportive patients are towards other patients, how well the staff understand patient needs and are willing to help and encourage patients, and how encouraging and considerate doctors are towards patients.

3 **Spontaneity**: measures the extent to which the environment encourages patients to act openly and to freely express their feelings towards other patients and staff.

4 **Autonomy**: assesses how self-sufficient and independent patients are encouraged to be in their personal affairs and in their relationships with staff, and how much responsibility and self-direction patients are encouraged to exercise.

5 **Practical orientation**: assesses the extent to which the program orients patients towards preparing themselves for release from the hospital and for the future. Such things as training for new kinds of jobs, looking to the future and setting and working toward practical goals are considered.

6 **Personal problem orientation**: measures the extent to which patients are encouraged to be concerned with their feelings and problems, and to seek to understand them through openly talking to other patients and staff about themselves and their past.

7 **Anger and aggression**: measures the extent to which a patient is allowed and encouraged to argue with patients and staff, to become openly angry and to display other expressions of anger.

8 **Order and organization**: measures how important order and organization is on the unit—i.e. do patients follow regular schedules, is the ward well kept, do staff keep appointments, are activities carefully planned?

9 **Program clarity**: measures the extent to which the patient knows what to expect in the day-to-day routine of the ward and how explicit the ward rules and procedures are.

10 **Staff control**: measures the extent to which it is necessary for the staff to restrict patients—i.e. in the strictness of rules and schedules, in the relationships between patient and staff, and in measures taken to keep patients under effective control.

related to program functioning. The study rationale provided to the three units was that feedback about how patients perceived the therapeutic milieu would facilitate the staff's treatment approach. A taped version (including a Spanish translation) of the WAS was administered to minimize the effects of differential reading abilities and to increase compliance. Patients were seated comfortably in the unit's day hall and provided with consent forms, a questionnaire, and answer sheets. Instructions and WAS items were then presented on the taped version. Nursing staff were available to manage the more difficult and disorganized patients. In the Hispanic unit 17 patients (7 male and 10 females) were able to complete the WAS and on the female and male units 21 and 18 patients, respectively, completed the WAS.

Results

Results of the comparisons of the Hispanic unit to the two traditional hospital milieus are provided in Table 25.3. Significantly higher mean values were reported

TABLE 25.3 WAS subscale scores

	Hispanic	Female		Male	
WAS subscale	Mean	Mean	T	Mean	T
Involvement	2.35	2.05	0.035	2.16	0.494
Support	2.71	1.90	0.018*	1.70	0.008*
Spontaneity	1.82	2.67	0.018*	2.68	0.007
Autonomy	2.06	2.19	0.718	2.33	0.422
Practical orientation	2.24	2.00	0.457	2.56	0.368
Personal problem orientation	2.06	1.71	0.197	1.50	0.079
Anger and aggression	1.65	2.52	0.006	2.50	0.019*
Order and organization	3.12	2.43	0.044*	2.94	0.612
Program clarity	3.06	2.19	0.022*	2.56	0.016*
Staff control	2.65	2.33	0.319	2.38	0.336

*$p<0.05$

by Hispanic patients on the support subscale and on the program clarity subscale. A significantly higher mean value on the order and organization subscale was also found on the Hispanic unit than in the female conventional unit.

These results suggest that the Hispanic unit is perceived by patients as more supportive, better organized and more clear in terms of therapeutic expectations. Significantly lower mean values were also reported by Hispanic patients on the anger and aggression subscale, and on the spontaneity subscale. These findings suggest that patients on the two conventional units perceived their milieus as more unpredictable and violent than patients on the Hispanic unit.

STUDY TWO

Site and Staff

The newly developed Hispanic inpatient program [13] was implemented in the context of a Psychiatry Department reorganization at Elmhurst Hospital Center (EHC, Elmhurst, NY), an academic affiliate of the Mount Sinai School of Medicine (MSMS, New York). EHC is located in a large multiethnic community with approximately 40% Hispanic and 20% Asian population(s). In an effort to more adequately serve this diverse clientele, the Department of Psychiatry (EHC) developed specialized clinical programs reflective of this service community, including a Hispanic inpatient unit (see below) and outpatient clinic and an Asian inpatient unit and outpatient clinic, staffed by Hispanic and/or Asian psychiatrists, psychologists, social workers, nursing and support staff [9, 10].

Milieu

A major goal of the newly developed inpatient Hispanic program was to structure the treatment environment in order to provide an optimum therapeutic experience for Hispanic patients. An existing 15-bed ward was designated as the site and minor construction was scheduled in order to convert the unit into a 'coed' facility (a review of projected occupancy patterns had revealed that a 'coed' program would best serve this community). At the onset of the reorganization, a staff survey had been conducted in order to better accommodate worksite preferences. Bilingual and bicultural staff who had expressed an interest in the program were reassigned from existing positions within the department. The inpatient Hispanic unit included the traditional community meeting, which was now educational in format (i.e. clarification of cultural misconceptions of mental illness) and taking place in Spanish. The interdisciplinary conference continued to represent the standard utilization of a treatment team approach but also included discussions of appropriate interventions with extended and traditional Hispanic families and other community resources (i.e. local folk healers). Rehabilitation activities on the unit now included current events groups where special topics about specific Latin American countries were obtained from Hispanic newspapers. Group treatments were now conducted in Spanish by members of the inpatient psychiatry staff and included medication, supportive therapy, and discharge planning groups. The program also included other ethnic-specific programs, such as extended family evening sessions, weekly Hispanic meals, appreciation of Latin music sessions, and recognition of Latin American holidays.

Procedure

The WAS [11] (see Table 25.2) was administered to patients and staff on two occasions. The reference unit's reorganization had been preceded by administration of the WAS and the scale was readministered 9 months later. As in study one, the rationale given was that feedback about how patients perceived their psychiatric inpatient units would aid staff in development of better treatment approaches. Patients were seated comfortably in a day hall and provided questionnaires and answer sheets. Instructions and items were also provided in a video taped version, administered to minimize the effects of differential reading abilities and to increase compliance. On the Hispanic inpatient unit, a Spanish video was used.

Results

The Hispanic inpatient service provided care to 140 psychiatric patients in the first 9 months of operation. Table 25.4 provides a profile of patient demographics, including diagnosis (DSM-IV) length of stay, sex, and age.

In the Hispanic unit 10 patients (six men and four women) were able to complete the WAS and on the pre-existing conventional unit 12 patients (all men)

TABLE 25.4   Biodemographic 9-month review of Hispanic inpatient unit

Diagnosis	Female	Age	Male	Age	Length of stay Female	Length of stay Male
Dementia	2	83.3	2	78.0	18.5	32.0
Substance OMD*	2	27.5	3	31.3	37.5	14.3
Other OMD*	2	43.5	0	0	31.5	0
Substance use	2	28.0	1	32.0	9.5	20.0
Schizophrenia	23	37.0	16	32.5	40.4	36.6
Affective disorder	35	44.3	14	42.3	30.6	30.3
Other psychology	7	32.4	2	27.5	15.4	31.0
Adjustment	12	35.6	6	36.0	16.2	26.5
All others	4	28.7	0	0	22.2	0
Total	93	39.3	47	41.0	24.8	24.9

* Organic mental disorder

had completed the WAS. t-Test comparisons of the conventional and Hispanic units revealed a number of significant differences on the WAS subscales; these are illustrated in Figure 25.1.

In comparison with the conventional unit patient ratings, patients on the Hispanic unit perceived a more relationship-oriented therapeutic environment, as indicated by the direction of significant mean differences (Figure 25.1) on the involvement and support WAS subscales. Significant differences were also found on the autonomy and personal problem orientation WAS subscales, suggesting that the Hispanic milieu was more directed toward individual self-growth as a treatment approach. Significant differences on the order and organization, program clarity, and staff control WAS subscales between the conventional and Hispanic unit suggest that the latter was better organized and well managed. Mean differences on the anger and aggression subscale were in the direction of less expression of anger on the Hispanic inpatient unit; however, these differences did not reach significant levels.

DISCUSSION

In the first study, the therapeutic milieu of a Hispanic unit was compared with the standard treatment milieus of two conventional hospital units. The Hispanic unit was found to differ significantly from the conventional units in that staff were perceived by patients as being more understanding and supportive of their clinical concerns. Hispanic patients also reported more clarity in terms of treatment goals and organization of the unit. The two conventional units did not differ from each other, but patients on both units perceived more anger and aggressive episodes than did patients on the Hispanic unit. In the second study, the therapeutic milieu of a newly developed inpatient Hispanic unit was compared with a pre-existing

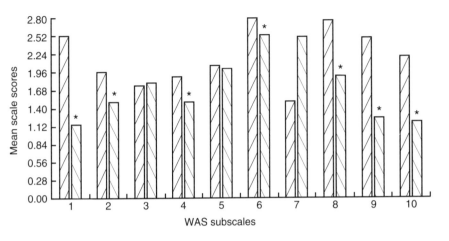

FIGURE 25.1 Ward atmosphere scale in Hispanic (▨) and conventional (▧) units. Subscale definitions: 1, involvement; 2, support; 3, spontaneity; 4, autonomy; 5, practical orientation; 6, personal problem orientation; 7, anger and aggression; 8, order and organization; 9, program clarity; 10, staff control. *$p<0.05$

conventional inpatient unit. The Hispanic unit differed significantly from the conventional unit in that it inspired more feelings of group spirit, and staff were perceived as more supportive and considerate. Hispanic patients also reported more sense of order and clarity in terms of the unit's routine, perhaps to the extent of strictness.

In a (now classic) review, Padilla *et al.* [14] reported that mental healthcare to Hispanics is generally 'of a different kind, of a lower quality, and in lesser proportions than that of any other ethnically identifiable population'. Hispanics have been found to enter inpatient psychiatric settings only reluctantly, where language and cultural barriers caused serious problems, including misdiagnosis and medication non-compliance. In a related study, Flaherty and Meagher [15] examined the inpatient experience of African-American and Anglo-American patients on a conventional unit using the WAS; they found that the former reported significantly less involvement, including less encouragement to act openly and express their feelings and less preparation for being released from the hospital. In the studies reported here, both Hispanic milieus had been specifically developed to meet unique language and cultural needs, and the findings suggest that the units were successful in providing sensitive healing environments in which patients were aware of therapeutic expectations and actively involved in their treatment. Generalization of these findings is limited by the variable of gender, which was only partially controlled in Study One, and by the small sample sizes. An additional criticism is the failure to examine outcome variables. The results of both studies do indicate, however, that making the treatment milieu more culturally responsive can greatly aid the inpatient treatment of ethnic minority patients.

REFERENCES

1. Lawson WB, Herrera JM, Costa J. 1992. The dexamethasone suppression test as an adjunct in diagnosing depression. *J Ass Acad Minor Phys* **3**(1): 17–19.
2. Mukherjee S, Shukla S, Woodle J, Rosen AM, Olaret S. 1983. Misdiagnosis of schizophrenia in bipolar patients: a multiethnic comparison. *Am J Psychiatry* **140**(12): 1571–4.
3. Karno M, Morales A. 1971. A community mental health service for Mexican-Americans in a metropolis. *Compr Psychiatry* **12**(2): 116–21.
4. Yamamoto J, James QC, Palley N. 1968. Cultural problems in psychiatric therapy. *Arch Gen Psychiatry* **19**(1): 45–9.
5. Dolgin D, Grosser R, Cruz-Martinez S, Garcia. 1982. Discriminant analysis of behavior symptomatology in hospitalized Hispanic and Anglo patients. *Hispanic J Behav Sci* **4**: 329–37.
6. Sue S, McKinney H, Allen D, Hall J. 1974. Delivery of community mental health services to black and white clients. *J Consult Clin Psychol* **42**(6): 794–801.
7. Sue S, Allen DB, Conaway L. 1978. The responsiveness and equality of mental health care to Chicanos and Native Americans. *Am J Community Psychol* **6**(2): 137–46.
8. Collazo J. 1996. Transcultural inpatient settings. Symposium presentation, American Psychiatric Association, May 1996.
9. Ruiz S, Chu P, Sramek J, Herrera J. 1996. Neuroleptic dosing with outpatient Hispanic and Asian schizophrenics. In: Herrera J, Lawson B, eds. Cross-Cultural Issues in Biological Psychiatry. *Mt Sinai J Med* **63**: 306–9.
10. Collazo J, Tam R, Sramek J, Herrera J. 1996. Neuroleptic dosing with inpatient Hispanic and Asian schizophrenics. In: Herrera J, Lawson B, eds. Cross-Cultural Issues in Biological Psychiatry. *Mt Sinai J Med* **63**: 310–13.
11. Moos RH. 1974. Determinants of physiological responses to symbolic stimuli: the role of the social environment. *Int J Psychiatr Med* **5**(4): 389–99.
12. Herrera JM. 1987. The effectiveness of a cultural milieu on hospitalized Hispanic patients. *Int J Psychosom* **34**(1): 6–8.
13. Herrera J, Collazo J. 1996. Cross-cultural therapeutic milieu. Symposium presentation, American Psychiatric Association, May 1996.
14. Padilla AM, Ruiz RA, Alvarez R. 1975. Community mental health services for Spanish-speaking/surnamed population. *Am Psychol* **30**(9): 892–905.
15. Flaherty JA, Meagher R. 1980. Measuring racial bias in inpatient treatment. *Am J Psychiatry* **137**(6): 679–82.

26

Anthropological Issues on Ethnic Units

Peter J. Guarnaccia

Rutgers University, New Brunswick, NJ, USA

TOWARDS A DEFINITION OF CULTURE

In order to develop culturally competent mental health services, program planners and mental health professionals need to come to terms with what they mean by 'culture' and how they will use culture in their services. By 'culturally competent mental health services', I mean services that respect cultural differences and have developed program adaptations which take cultural differences into account [1]. Cultural competence goes beyond attitudes and staffing patterns to include skills and program elements which enhance services to culturally diverse clients. It is my contention that previous work in the area of culturally competent mental health services, both in the literature and in practice, has given insufficient attention to an in-depth understanding of culture. This has inhibited the full development of programs and has often resulted in an impoverished understanding of the multiple and complex interactions of culture in the development of programs.

The purpose of this chapter is to review the different ways in which culture has been used in developing the notion of culturally competent mental health services and to provide an enhanced definition of culture through a critical review of these ideas. The issues raised here will inform the future development of inpatient ethnic units as these programs continue to develop. Because of my previous research experience, and because the data used in this paper comes from an evaluation study of three Hispanic bilingual/bicultural inpatient psychiatric programs, my examples will be primarily from the Hispanic mental health literature [2, 3]. However, many of the issues apply broadly to multicultural populations.

I felt it was critical to provide an extended discussion of the concept of culture as, both in my reviews of the literature and in my experience in the program evaluation, I found that not enough attention has been paid to conceptualizing culture within the development of culturally competent mental health services. The lack of this conception has led to several kinds of problems in designing and

Cross Cultural Psychiatry. Edited by John M. Herrera, William B. Lawson and John J. Sramek.
© 1999 John Wiley & Sons Ltd.

implementing culturally competent mental health programs. For example, it is not sufficient to bring together Hispanic staff with Hispanic clients and have everyone speak Spanish; nor is it sufficient to focus on a set of generalized values and illness concepts—this approach frequently becomes stereotypical rather than a base for program development. Careful assessment needs to be made of the multiple contexts which shape the program and the lives of both the clients and professionals who work in them. Given this approach, the definition of culture I provide is multifaceted and cannot be summarized in a neat paragraph.

In reviewing classic works on culturally competent mental health services, writers have often turned to earlier work by anthropologists to present a definition of culture [4–6]. In general, these definitions have reflected a static view of culture as a distinctive set of beliefs, values, morals, customs and institutions that people inherit through growing up in a culture. These definitions have also focused on a 'top-down' notion of culture as coming from a generalized 'society' and have not focused on the role of individual innovation and the dynamics of everyday lived experience on generating culture. Mental health professionals should not be unduly criticized for the problems within anthropology of defining a core concept.

More recent approaches to culture in anthropology provide a more dynamic perspective than earlier writing, and can more fully inform the development of culturally competent mental health programs. Recent views of culture, while not discarding the importance of a person's cultural inheritance of ideas, values, feelings, ways of relating and behaviors, have focused equally on the importance of viewing culture as a process in which views and practices are dynamically affected by social transformations, social conflicts, power relationships, and migrations [7, 8]. More recent approaches have also focused on the emergence of culture from the daily social practices and life experiences of individuals and small groups [9]. Culture is a product of both group values, norms and experiences and of individual innovations and life histories.

POLITICAL CONTEXT OF PROGRAM DEVELOPMENT

One of the hallmarks of an anthropological approach is to focus on a community context for examining any issue. One of the first anthropological issues in thinking about developing bicultural inpatient units is to understand the community dynamics surrounding the development and maintenance of such units [2]. The political context of developing a program is critical to its success, yet is often under-analyzed in thinking about bicultural inpatient units.

In the case of the bilingual/bicultural psychiatric programs (BBPP) in New York, key actors included the State Office of Mental Health, Association of Hispanic Mental Health Professionals (which included members in key decision-making positions in the City's mental health system), local administrations of the different hospitals, and advocacy groups for different ethnic communities. Support from these groups was critical to the establishment of the program, particularly advocacy

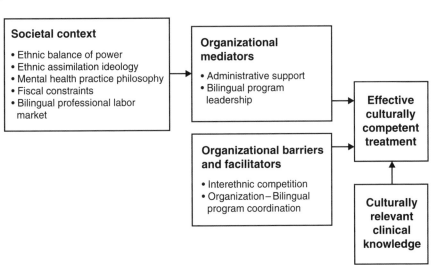

FIGURE 26.1 Societal and organization contexts of culturally sensitive mental health services. Adapted from [2] by permission of Sage Publications

by the Association of Hispanic Mental Health Professionals. At the same time, the programs were delayed because of opposition from other ethnic communities within the city and the hospitals. The National Association for the Advancement of Colored People (NAACP) blocked the implementation of the programs because of concerns that they would lead to a 'ghettoization' of minority patients within the hospital and to separate and potentially unequal services. Concerns were also raised about why the Office of Mental Health was supporting programs for Hispanics but not for other ethnic groups.

This conflict led the programs to argue for their need on the basis primarily of language and for programs directed to monolingual Spanish speakers. While the emphasis on language is clearly critical, an overemphasis on language, separate from culture, led to conceptual problems about how to integrate culture into assessment and treatment and who were appropriate clients for the program given the wide range of language abilities and acculturation statuses of Latinos in New York City.

Related to this issue is the question of whether the program implements a cultural sensitivity, cultural diversity, or cultural competence approach. *Cultural sensitivity* involves staff exploring their own ethnic/cultural backgrounds and their attitudes towards people from different backgrounds. While cultural sensitivity is an important first step in providing more effective services to culturally diverse clients, cultural sensitivity programs do not usually provide specific guidance and skills in how to deliver mental health services to multicultural clients. *Cultural diversity* issues focus more on the particular staffing patterns of service organizations and the fit between the cultural backgrounds of staff and clients. One aspect of cultural diversity involves 'affirmative action' policies and practices; another involves issues of 'ethnic matching' between staff and clients. As stated earlier, *cultural competence* addresses a range of organizational and system-level issues in serving a multicultural population. Cultural competence incorporates cultural sensitivity and cultural diversity issues. It goes beyond attitudes and staffing patterns, to include skills and program elements that enhance services to a diverse client population. The distinctions among these approaches lead to important differences in how culture is conceptualized and how it is implemented in developing treatment programs. A similar tension is reflected in the use of 'bilingual' or 'bicultural', or a combination of the terms. This discussion leads back to issues of how culture is conceptualized in developing bicultural inpatient programs and what program model(s) guide the development and implementation of such units.

APPROACHES TO CULTURE

'Culture' has been used in a variety of ways in the literature on culturally competent mental health services [10]. As a way of thinking about how varying definitions of culture affect mental health practice, I classify these varying definitions in terms of their actual implementation. The following list represents different aspects of implementing culture in mental health services: ethnic identity [2]; language [11]; material signs and symbols; events and celebrations; shared values [12, 13]; and views of mental illness [14, 15]. I will briefly discuss each of these aspects of culture.

In using the word culture to mean ethnic identity, it is often used as a synonym for nationality. Writers may refer to Hispanic or Asian culture, but the question immediately arises as to the level of cultural specificity that is appropriate for developing mental health services. While most researchers and clinicians quickly agree that thinking about developing services for Hispanics is an inappropriate level of generality, the question immediately arises as to whether talking about Puerto Ricans or Mexicans is specific enough for clinical purposes. Members of each of these groups vary significantly on the basis of social class, educational background and migration experience; all factors that might significantly affect the clinical encounter. Ethnic identity is a preliminary step to developing a culturally effective program.

Language issues are key aspects of developing bilingual/bicultural psychiatric inpatient programs. Language is a key encoder of culture and a major vehicle for its transformation. It is also a major tool used in psychiatric treatment for assessment, psychoeducation and therapy. A key question is: What does it mean to speak a client's language? While having a clinician and client who are both able to speak Spanish is a major advance for communication, subtle differences in language use and style—shaped by ethnicity, education, social class, and acculturation—may complicate communication during the therapeutic process. Attention to the subtleties of language is vital in developing an effective program.

Material signs and symbols of a cultural group are often used to mark out the space of a program as being special and welcoming to that group, particularly when the group is in the minority. Programs will decorate the walls with flags and crafts from the countries of origin of clients, play the music of those cultures, use books and magazines in the native language, and, when possible, serve foods familiar to and enjoyed by people from that culture. All of these efforts can make clients feel more at home in the program and emphasize that the staff appreciate the clients' cultures. At the same time, issues arise in selecting these material signs and symbols both, in terms of the countries to represent and whether the images and materials are from the popular or professional sectors of the countries represented.

Cultural events and celebrations often structure the lives of individuals and communities. These events are windows into the dynamic ways that people create meaning in their lives, reinforce old or establish new social ties, and manage social conflicts and tensions. Culture serves as a script for guiding people in dealing with important life changes. Engaging people in culturally driven events and celebrations can be a powerful way to create a sense of community on a unit and can provide scripts for therapeutic interventions. Attention to issues of cultural diversity is needed when selecting the events that are celebrated on the inpatient unit.

An understanding of important shared cultural values and styles of interaction is important in establishing a bicultural inpatient program. Awareness of ways to show respect for another person and of issues of cultural distance in social interactions can make an inpatient unit function much more smoothly. At the same time, practitioners need to be careful that they are not engaging in stereotypical thinking. Many of these value orientations undergo rapid change in the face of migration and acculturation. There is a danger in romanticizing traditional values and resisting change.

Views of mental illness are strongly shaped by culture. Different cultures use different idioms or forms of expressing psychological distress. Cultures differ in their understanding of the causes of mental illness and their attitudes towards those who suffer with psychiatric disorder. Some of these conceptions diverge strongly from professional views of mental illness and skill is needed by clinicians to move among these different understandings.

Two factors of social life further influence how ethnically derived culture shapes views and behavior: the role of different social status (age, gender, social class) in structuring subcultures within a broader cultural framework, and the processes of acculturation [16, 17]. A focus on only a single interpretation of culture is inadequate to understand what culturally competent mental health services are about, to respond adequately to the needs of multicultural clients—and, consequently, to integrate these definitions of culture into the provision of mental health services.

The issues raised above can be restated as a series of questions to guide program development:

1. Whose ethnicity is represented on a bilingual/bicultural inpatient unit and how is that ethnicity expressed?

2. How are issues of bilingualism addressed and what methods are used to assess language abilities *and* preferences?
3. Is some type of cultural assessment or formulation used by this program? How are cultural issues integrated into diagnosis, treatment and discharge planning?
4. How are tensions within ethnic group cultures and between ethnic and professional cultures resolved?

I conclude by restating my perspective on culture and describing an example to illustrate the complexity of cultural dynamics on an ethnic inpatient unit.

THE VALUE OF A MULTICULTURAL APPROACH

A key feature of my discussion of culture is that there is no such thing as culture as a static phenomenon. Most social settings involve multiple cultures in interaction—influencing, changing, and conflicting with each other. Culture is as much a process as a thing and thus attempts to freeze culture into a set of generalized value orientations or behaviors will constantly misrepresent what culture is. Culture is a dynamic and creative phenomenon, some aspects of which are shared by large groups of people and others are the creations of small groups and individuals resulting from particular circumstances. In developing culturally competent mental health services, providers and program planners need to develop a multicultural perspective, involving the multiple cultures of clients, the cultures of professionals, and the cultures of institutions. Another feature of this perspective is that the cultures of these interacting groups often conflict. The tensions across groups and institutions are frequently due to differential access to resources and power, where an institution may have considerable power to define clients' lives; clients' power may come through the support of a strong social network or through resistance to professional and institutional programs. At the same time, a goal of developing culturally competent mental health services is to bring these different cultures closer together so that people in need can be helped, professionals can experience efficacy and satisfaction, and institutions can provide the services they were designed for.

Even within a particular cultural group there is considerable diversity, and the use of a general label is both conceptually and practically inappropriate. The dimensions of difference among members of ethnic groups are grounded in national origin and history; in the particular social formations within each country of origin that shape age, gender and class relationships; in the pressures within each country that have led to migration and the differing waves of migration; and in the differing relationships with the USA that have affected how those migrants were received. At the same time, changes within US society and cultures have affected where migrants have gone, how they have been received, the opportunities they have had to develop themselves as individuals and groups, and the cultures with which they have interacted [18, 19]. Developing methods to fully assess and work with the diverse cultures is a core task of developing culturally competent mental health services.

Professional cultures are another significant part of this multicultural dynamic. Within the mental health professions there are different perspectives on what mental illness is, how to assess it, what interventions are appropriate, how to relate to clients, and how to work with other professionals. These cultures are reflected in, modified by, and passed on by training programs, internships and other practical experiences, clinical programs, and continuing education. Professional cultures are far from monolithic and are subject to multiple pressures for change from both within and without. Professional cultures reflect the dominant value system of the society and the historical period within which they develop. At the same time, in the person of practitioners, professional cultures interact with personal cultures. In developing culturally competent mental health services, professionals need to examine how they view the knowledge and insights they have received from their cultural and professional backgrounds, to analyze how they will employ the strengths from each to best help their clients, and to reconcile how they will manage situations when personal and professional cultures conflict.

Institutions play an important role in society as enforcers of social norms, as sources of social control, and as creators of culture. Major social institutions have always played a central role in acculturating new immigrants and in dealing with the problems of unsuccessful adaptation and adjustment. Social institutions have multiple goals: providing designated services, monitoring and carrying out programs, interacting with other institutions, extending government into the community, insuring their own survival, and maintaining and enforcing social control. Institutional cultures arise from the ways institutions are structured, the purposes the institution serves, the mix of professions involved, and the mix of individuals working there. Institutional cultures reflect the cultures of the dominant social classes; one of their roles is to maintain and impose the dominant culture on groups in society. Part of planning culturally competent mental health services is to assess where and how well the programs will fit into the overall institutional culture and structure.

Case Example

A case from the evaluation of the Bilingual/Bicultural Psychiatric Programs highlights many of the issues discussed in this chapter. The case identifies the multiple, and (at times) conflicting frames of reference among professionals from different backgrounds. The staff responses demonstrate how ethnic, class, and professional cultures shape conceptions of and responses to mental illness. This case illustrates how professional training acculturates members of ethnic groups to dominant professional cultures. It illustrates the need for a dynamic, multicultural understanding of the processes of assessment and treatment and the inclusion of ethnic and professional cultures into that analysis. The case is presented to illustrate the complexity of the issues involved, not to judge the particular participants.

A client had a seizure-like episode during a social event at one of the BBPP. For some of the staff, this event was referred to as an *ataque de nervios* (attack of nerves); others saw it as a hysterical episode; and the notes mentioned potential neurological disorder or seizures and referred frequently to the client as 'agitated'. This type of episode represents a challenge to mental health programs in integrating knowledge of culture into a psychiatric unit. It raises questions of how to understand and respond to such events from psychiatric, medical and cultural perspectives.

The front-line mental health staff who took care of the client responded, according to traditional cultural prescriptions, by holding the client's hand, rubbing the client's head and arms with medicinal alcohol (*alcoholado*), and talking in quiet, reassuring voices. These staff shared the client's Puerto Rican ethnicity and, as para-professionals, were only partly acculturated to the dominant professional cultural conceptions and norms. In a subsequent interview, a staff member reported knowing how to handle an *ataque de nervios* because of observing family members' responses to the ataques of a cousin. The staff member also attributed the client's improvement to medication administered after the 'seizure'. Staff members said they had not received specific training in dealing with such incidents, but had received training in dealing with epileptic seizures, which were similar. In the records of the episode written by the attending psychiatrist (who was a second-generation Puerto Rican and considerably more highly acculturated to professional conceptions and norms) the terms 'agitation', 'fainting', and 'hysterical reactions' were used to refer to the event and similar previous experiences. The word *ataque* was never mentioned in the written notes. The only treatment identified was intramuscular medication.

This case highlights the multiple perspectives on such episodes within a psychiatric and cultural context. There is a long psychiatric and anthropological literature about *ataques de nervios* [20–23]. The challenges to culturally competent services include integrating community and professional perspectives on mental illness and negotiating among different and sometimes conflicting popular and professional perspectives on forms of expressing distress. The ultimate goal is to effectively alleviate the client's suffering.

CONCLUSIONS

In this chapter I have presented a notion of culture which attempts to reflect the complexity of the concept, its multiple influences on people's lives, and the diversity of cultures that must be taken into account in developing culturally competent mental health services.

Culture serves as the web which structures human thought, emotion, and interaction. Culture provides a variety of resources for dealing with major changes and challenges, including serious illness and hospitalization. Culture is continuously being shaped by social processes such as migration and acculturation. Cultures vary not only by national, regional or ethnic background but also by age, gender and social class. Much of culture is embedded in and communicated by language; language cannot be understood or used outside of its cultural context.

It is my contention that a fuller understanding of culture can only enhance program planning, development, and implementation in the area of culturally competent mental health services. The developmental phases of programs should analyze and discuss what they mean by culture, how they will use culture in their programs, and how they will continue to assess the multiple impacts of culture on the program's development.

In the development of culturally competent mental health services, program planners need to move beyond a simplistic view of culture as creating a physical atmosphere and hiring people who speak the language to incorporate in a more detailed way the multiple dimensions of culture outlined in this chapter. For clinicians, some guidelines to interpreting culturally influenced expressions of mental illness are available within the diagnostic sections and Appendix I of DSM-IV [24]. The future program and research agenda involves continuing to document the impact of culture on mental health services and to evaluate programs and practices which effectively integrate a complex understanding of culture into mental health practice.

REFERENCES

1. Cross T. 1988. Services to minority populations: cultural competent curriculum. *Focal Point* **3**: 1–4.
2. Rodriguez O, Lessinger J, Guarnaccia P. 1992. The societal and organizational contexts of culturally sensitive mental health services: findings from an evaluation of bilingual/bicultural psychiatric programs. *J. Ment Health Admin* **19**: 213–23.
3. Guarnaccia PJ, Rodriguez O. 1996. Concepts of culture and their role in the development of culturally competent mental health services. *Hisp J Behav Sci* **18**: 419–43.
4. Favazza A, Oman M. 1977. *Anthropological and Cross-cultural Themes in Mental Health.* Colombia: University of Missouri Press.
5. Helman C. 1990. *Culture, Health and Illness.* Oxford: Butterworth-Heinemann.
6. Sue DW, Sue D. 1990. *Counseling the Culturally Different.* New York: Wiley.
7. Geertz C. 1973. *The Interpretation of Cultures.* New York: Basic Books.
8. Good BJ. 1994. *Medicine, Rationality and Experience: An Anthropological Perspective.* Cambridge: Cambridge University Press.
9. Ware N, Kleinman A. 1992. Culture and somatic experience: the social course of illness in neurasthenia and chronic fatigue syndrome. *Psychosom Med* **54**: 546–60.
10. Fabrega H. 1990. Hispanic mental health research: a case for cultural psychiatry. *Hisp J Behav Sci* **12**: 339–65.
11. Marcos L. 1994. The psychiatric examination of Hispanics: across the language barrier. In: Malgady RG, Rodriguez O, eds. *Theoretical and Conceptual Issues in Hispanic Mental Health.* Malabar, FL: Krieger, pp. 143–53.
12. Casas JM, Keefe SE. 1978. *Family and Mental Health in the Mexican American Community.* Los Angeles: Spanish-Speaking Mental Health Research Center.
13. Garcia-Preto N. 1982. Puerto Rican families. In: McGoldrick M, Pearce JK, Giordano J, eds. *Ethnicity and Family Therapy.* New York: Guilford Press, pp. 164–86.

14. Guarnaccia PJ, Parra P, Deschamps A, Milstein G, Argiles N. 1992. Si Dios quiere: Hispanic families' experiences of caring for a seriously mentally ill family member. *Cult Med Psychiatry* **16**: 187–215.

15. Jenkins J. 1988. Ethnopsychiatric interpretations of schizophrenic illness: the problem of nervios within Mexican-American families. *Cult Med Psychiatry* **12**: 303–31.

16. Rogler LH, Cortes DE, Malgady RG. 1991. Acculturation and mental health status among Hispanics: convergence and new directions for research. *Am Psychol* **46**: 585–97.

17. Harwood A. 1994. Acculturation in the post modern world: implications for mental health research. In: Malgady RG, Rodriguez O, eds. *Theoretical and Conceptual Issues in Hispanic Mental Health*. Malabar, FL: Krieger, pp. 3–17.

18. Guarnaccia PJ. 1997. Social stress and psychological distress among Latinos in the United States. In: Al-Issa I, Tousignant M, eds. *Ethnicity, Immigration and Psychopathology*. New York: Plenum, pp. 71–94.

19. Portes A, Rumbaut RG. 1990. *Immigrant America*. Los Angeles: University of California Press.

20. Goffman E. 1961. *Asylums*. New York: Doubleday.

21. Guarnaccia PJ, DeLaCancela V, Carrillo E. 1989. The multiple meanings of ataques de nervios in the Latino community. *Med Anthropol* **11**: 47–62.

22. Guarnaccia PJ, Canino G, Rubio-Stipec M, Bravo M. 1993. The prevalence of ataques de nervios in Puerto Rico: the role of culture in psychiatric epidemiology. *J Nerv Ment Dis* **181**: 157–65.

23. Guarnaccia PJ, Rivera M, Franco F, Neighbors C. 1996. The experiences of ataques de nervios: towards an anthropology of emotions in Puerto Rico. *Cult Med Psychiatry* **20**: 343–67.

24. American Psychiatric Association. 1994. *Diagnostic and Statistical Manual of Mental Disorders*, 4th ed. Washington, DC: American Psychiatric Association.

27

Gender Differences in Psychotropic Medications

Freda Lewis-Hall

Eli Lilly and Company, Indianapolis, IN, USA

INTRODUCTION

Despite significant gender differences in prevalence of psychiatric disease, symptom presentations, treatment-seeking behavior, and receipt of psychotropic medication, little research has been conducted into the potential gender differences in efficacy, dosage, and side-effects of psychotropic medications. This chapter will briefly review the literature on gender differences in psychotropic medications.

ANTIPSYCHOTIC AGENTS

The literature analyzing potential gender differences is more substantial for antipsychotic agents than for other psychotropic drugs. Four major areas have been investigated: overall efficacy, dose requirements, plasma levels, and side-effects. Chouinard and Annable [1] evaluated efficacy with antipsychotic medications in a small population and noted a greater improvement in women treated with pimozide and chlorpromazine than in men. The authors hypothesized that this differential response was caused by the presumed antidopaminergic effect of estrogen [2, 3], which is borne out by other research. Chouinard *et al.* [4] examined the dosage requirements of fluspirilene, a long-acting injectable neuroleptic agent. They noted that women required significantly lower doses (nearly half) than men despite similarities in weight and age. Using a survey-type design, Seeman [5] examined dosage requirements for neuroleptic agents (reported in chlorpromazine equivalents) for women. Women in their 20s and 30s were reported as requiring lower doses of antipsychotropic medications. Similar results were reported in a retrospective review of uncontrolled treatments by DiMello and MacNeil [6]: younger men and older women were reported as having received higher doses.

Cross Cultural Psychiatry. Edited by John M. Herrera, William B. Lawson and John J. Sramek.
© 1999 John Wiley & Sons Ltd.

Several significant questions arose in these studies. The assumption that the prescribed dose represented the therapeutic dose is significant, but questionable, because no consistent outcome variables were described. Further, the diagnoses varied within and between studies. Effective doses were recognized as varying across diagnoses, further obscuring the accuracy of the therapeutic dose. Unfortunately, plasma levels were not available to correlate differences with therapeutic responses, but some studies have examined plasma levels of antipsychotics agents. Simpson *et al.* [7] examined levels of fluphenazine in women and found higher plasma levels even though no significant differences in dose were noted. Ereshefsky *et al.* [8] also noted higher levels of thiothixene in women. In addition to higher plasma levels, women were noted to have significantly lower clearance of thiothixene than men.

Haring [9] reported that female patients being treated for schizophrenia with clozapine have higher plasma levels than men; according to Dawkins and Potter [10], clozapine plasma concentrations were 45% higher in women even when corrected for body weight and dose.

Differences in adverse effects induced by antipsychotics have also supported the possibility of gender differences in these medications. Four side-effects have been noted to be variably expressed by gender: tardive dyskinesia (TD), Parkinson's disorder, hematologic events, and sexual and neuroendocrine events. The incidence of TD has been reported as greater in women than in men in several studies [11–13], and women have also been reported to suffer more severe TD. Smith *et al.* [13] reported that the severity of TD increased significantly in women older than 67 years, and a gender–age relationship was further described by Chouinard *et al.* [14], who noted that young men reported a higher prevalence of severe dyskinesias than women. One potential explanation was that postmenopausal status increases exposure to the development of TD [13]. This would be consistent with hypotheses that estrogen acts at the dopamine receptor, protecting premenopausal women from TD. Yassar and Jeste [15] combined data from independent studies on prevalence, age, and sex differences in TD. Results indicate that TD is more prevalent in women and in old age. The authors raised several points, which suggested that these findings are complicated by differences in diagnosis and length of exposure to medications.

The impact on gender in the development of parkinsonism has been evaluated only infrequently. Jeste [16], in a close examination of rates and severity of movement disorders, reported that with lower doses of neuroleptic medications the risks of parkinsonism in women remain similar to or lower than those in men.

Hematologic events associated with treatment with newer neuroleptic therapies have been important in the clinical management of patients. Careful monitoring has provided some significant gender relationship differences. Banov *et al.* [17] reported that the incidence of eosinophilia in women treated with clozapine was significantly higher than in men. He also noted that eosinophilia occurred early in therapy, resolved spontaneously, and was not associated with known clinical complications. Clozapine-induced agranulocytosis also appears to occur at higher rates in women.

Studies have demonstrated that the incidence of adverse sexual effects is high during antipsychotic treatment. Variability in rate estimates across compounds and studies range from 25% to 100%. An overall lower incidence has been reported for women. Recently, increased attention has been given to the neuroendocrine impact of antipsychotic medication. For example, antipsychotics have been noted to have differential effects on prolactin, with the typical antipsychotics and the atypical risperidone predictably affecting prolactin level and the atypical agents clozapine and olanzapine producing little or no increase in prolactin levels. Antipsychotic-induced hyperprolactinemia may result in orgasmic dysfunction, reduced libido, galactorrhea, and ammenorrhea. Although galactorrhea may affect both men and women, premenopausal women appear to be disproportionately affected [18]. Ammenorrhea and a range of menstrual disorders affect 15–50% [18] of women treated with antipsychotics. This is believed to be mediated by hypoestrogenism caused by elevations in prolactin. Long-term effects of elevated prolactin levels may include osteoporosis.

Although sparse, the available literature in this area supports gender-related findings and suggest a need for a further, more aggressive research agenda to examine the critical interaction between age and gender more closely. Menstrual status, menstrual cycle effects, and exogenous hormone administration also need careful definition in studies.

ANTIDEPRESSANTS

Although the overall prevalence of depressive disorders is higher in women, there is little clarifying information on potential gender differences. Most studies in this area have focused on efficacy, dosage, and plasma levels as issues affected by gender. Overall efficacy of antidepressant medications in women has been evaluated in several studies. Davidson and Pelton [19] reported that women with depression who have panic attacks have a greater response to monoamine oxidase inhibitors than to tricyclic antidepressants. Men with depression and panic attacks, however, had a more favorable response to tricyclic antidepressant agents. Raskin [20] noted that women older than 40 and men had a better response to imipramine than younger women. Young men also responded better to chlorpromazine. Younger women in the study responded better to phenelzine than younger men. This study highlighted the importance of the gender–age relationship that is also seen in antipsychotic medications. Of note in this retrospective analysis is the fact that the subjects did not necessarily have a diagnosis of depression, that there is evidence for significant interdiagnosis differences in dose requirements, and that failure to standardize diagnoses and further specify diagnostic criteria are issues for future study.

Dose requirements and plasma levels have been examined in several studies, and the findings have been inconsistent. Burrows et al. [21] found no significant gender differences with nortriptyline. Zeigler and Biggs [22] noted similar findings with nortriptyline; they also examined plasma levels in a small sample of subjects given amitriptyline and noted no gender differences. Preskorn and Mac [23] examined 110 patients in a naturalistic study of inpatients and noted that women had higher plasma levels per milligram of drug than men. Moody *et al.* [24] noted non-significantly higher plasma levels of imipramine in women patients. In the area of newer antidepressant medications, Geenblatt *et al.* [25] investigated gender differences in trazodone, reporting that the volume of distribution was greater in women and that clearance was reduced in older men. A number of factors contributed to the variability of these findings:

- some of the studies had retrospective and 'naturalistic' study designs, which failed to account for diagnosis or standardized therapeutic dose by a specific metric (pz equivalents);
- small sample size and failure to control for variables such as coadministration of medication, smoking, hormone replacement therapy, or hormone status may have had an impact on outcomes; and
- several studies supported a relationship between plasma level and coadministration of oral contraceptives. Abernathy *et al.* [26] noted that oral contraceptives inhibited the hepatic metabolism of intravenous imipramine. This demonstrated that oral contraceptives and other hormonal products can produce a significant effect on the metabolism of antidepressant medications [27].

Lithium is one of the few psychotropic medications that has been the subject of reports related to menstrual cycle effect. In two case reports [28, 29] lithium levels were higher in women in the post-menstrual phase of the menstrual cycle than in the premenstrual phase. Volunteers without bipolar disorder (studied by Chamberlain *et al.* [29]) showed no difference between mean lithium levels regardless of whether lithium was given during the follicular or luteal phases of their cycle. Of note, several individuals evidenced phasic differences. Individual reports by women with bipolar disorder of phasic changes in symptoms may suggest those 'at risk' for cycle-dependent differences; further study is warranted.

ANTIANXIETY AGENTS

Much of the research on antipsychotic and antidepressant agents has been in efficacy, dosage, and side-effects; little has been done regarding pharmacokinetic and pharmacodynamic differences. Conversely, in the antianxiety agents little research has been conducted in the area of therapeutic affects and closer attention has been paid to kinetics. This series of studies has given greater consideration to the metabolic pathway as a factor to consider in evaluating gender differences. Greenblatt *et al.* [30] found that diazepam, a benzodiazepine metabolized through oxidation, had a higher clearance in younger women than in men. This study also noted that the statistical significance of this finding disappeared in women of 62–84 years. The study used a single intravenous dose, but did not assess metabolites. In a similar study, MacLeod et al. [31] noted no significant impact of age, finding that women metabolized diazepam slower than men regardless of age. Triazolam, also oxidatively metabolized, was found to evidence no gender differences in metabolism [32]. Nitrazepam, metabolized by reduction, was not found to have any gender-related differences in clearance [33]. Divoll et al. [34] found that the elimination half-life of temazepam, metabolized by glucuronidation, is longer in women than in men after single dose administration. Oxazepam, also metabolized by glucuronidation, was noted by Greenblatt et al. [35] to have a longer elimination half-life in women than in men. Half-life increased with age in women, but did not seem to be associated with age in men.

Several studies of benzodiazepines have examined the impact of the menstrual cycle and exogenous hormone administration on metabolism. Giles et al. [36] reported that the clearance of diazepam was lower in oral contraceptive users than in control subjects. Ellinwood et al. [37] found that the greatest psychomotor and cognitive impairment occurred on Day 28 of the menstrual cycle in women taking oral contraceptives. They postulated the oral contraceptives decrease the rate absorption of diazepam and during the week off hormones the plasma levels quickly rose to become more intoxicating. Jochemsen et al. [33] noted that women taking contraceptives and nitrazepam had higher steady-state levels than either men or women not taking oral contraceptives. Future studies in this area will require control gender-related effects on enzymatic function as some differences may depend on metabolic pathways. There also seems to be a great degree of interindividual variability, which implies a need to reduce reliance on reporting group findings in which individual differences may provide important information on how differences are mediated.

CONCLUSION

Several studies suggest that gender-related differences have an impact on clinically relevant parameters in psychotropic medication action. Recently, Dawkins and Potter [36] reviewed the substantial existing animal literature which supports the significant gender differences in animal models in both metabolism and response. Together, these two sources of information provide both provocation and caution to this field of research. The studies to date have generally been in small, poorly characterized populations. Future studies will require larger populations and those characterized by age, psychosocial factors, body weight, hormonal status, presence of exogenous hormones, concomitant illnesses and medications, and nutritional status (including alcohol and tobacco use). Further, stabilization of parameters used in diagnosis, therapeutic affect, and adverse events are required. The diversity and complexity of psychotropic medications have made it important to recognize that information on individual psychotropic agents cannot be generalized. Future studies should focus on amassing sufficient data across variables on individual agents.

REFERENCES

1. Chouinard G, Annable I. 1982. Pimozide in the treatment of newly schizophrenic patients. *Psychopharmacology* **76**: 13–19.
2. Fields IZ, Gordon JH. 1982. Estrogen inhibits the dopaminergic supersensitivity induced by neuroleptics. *Life Sci* **30**: 229–34.
3. Villeneuve A, Langlier P, Bedard P. 1978. Estrogens, dopamine and dyskinesias. *Can Psychiatr Assoc J* **23**: 68–70.
4. Chouinard G, Annable I, Steinberg S. 1986. A controlled clinical trial of fluspirilene, a long-acting injectable neuroleptic in schizophrenic patients with acute exacerbation. *J Clin Psychopharmacol* **6**: 21–6.
5. Seeman MV. 1983. Interaction of sex, age and neuroleptic dose. *Compr Psychiatry* **24**: 125–8.
6. DiMello DA, MacNeil JA. 1990. Sex differences in bipolar affective disorder; neuroleptic dosage variance. *Compr Psychiatry* **31**: 80–3.
7. Simpson GM, Yakalam KG, Levinson DP *et al*. 1990. Single dose pharmacokinetics of fluphenazine after fluphenazine decanoate administration. *J Clin Psychopharmacol* **10**: 417–21.
8. Ereshefsky L, Saklad SR, Watanabe MD *et al*. 1991. Thiothixene—pharmacokinetic interactions: a study of hepatic enzyme inducers, clearance inhibitors, and demographic variables. *J Clin Psychopharmacol* **11**: 269–301.
9. Haring C. 1977. Long term treatment of schizophrenia with penfluridol. *Med Welt* **28** (13): 639–42.
10. Dawkins K, Potter WZ. 1991. Gender differences, pharmacokinetics and pharmacodynamics of psychotropics: focus on women. *Psychopharmacol Bull* **27**: 417–26.
11. Smith JM, Kucharski IT, Oswald WT. 1979. Tardive dyskinesia: effect of age, sex, and criterion level of symptomatology on prevalence estimates. *Psychopharmacol Bull* **5**: 69–71.
12. Chouinard G. Jones BD, Annable I, Ross-Chouinard A. 1990. Sex differences and tardive dyskinesia (letter). *Am J Psychiatry* **137**: 507.
13. Smith JM, Dunn DD. 1979. Sex differences in the prevalence of severe tardive dyskinesia. *Am J Psychiatry* **136**: 1080–2.
14. Chouinard G, Annable I, Ross-Chouinard A, Nestoros JN. 1979. Factors related to tardive dyskinesia. *Am J Psychiatry* **136**: 79–83.
15. Yassar, Jeste DV. 1992. Gender differences in tardive dyskinesia: a critical review of the literature. *Psychol Bull* **18**(4): 701–15.
16. Jeste DV. 1995. *Gender and Ethnicity Differences in Pharmacology of Neuroleptics.* American Psychiatric Association Annual Meeting.
17. Banov MD, Tohen M, Friedberg J. 1993. High risk of eosinophilia in women treated with clozapine. *J Clin Psychiatry* **54**: 466–9.
18. Weissman MM, Klerman GL. 1977. Sex differences and the epidemiology of depression. *Arch Gen Psychiatry* **134**: 98–111.
19. Davidson J, Pelton S. 1986. Forms of atypical depression and their response to antidepressant drugs. *Psychiatr Res* **17**: 87–95.
20. Raskin A. 1974. Age-sex differences in response to antidepressant drugs. *J Nerv Ment Dis* **159**: 120–30.
21. Burrows G, Scoggins BA, Turecek IR, Davies B. 1974. Plasma nortriptyline and clinical response. *Clin Pharmacol Ther* **16**: 639–44.
22. Zeigler VI, Biggs JT. 1977. Tricyclic plasma levels: effect of age, race, smoking. *JAMA* **238**: 2167–9.
23. Preskorn SH, Mac DS. 1985. Plasma level of amitriptyline: effect of age and sex. *J Clin Psychiatry* **46**: 276–7.

24. Moody JP, Tait AC, Todrick A. 1967. Plasma levels of imipramine and desmethylimipramine during therapy. *Br J Psychiatry* **113**: 183–93.

25. Greenblatt DJ, Friedman H, Bernstein ES *et al.* 1987. Trazodone kinetics: effect of age, gender and obesity. *Clin Pharmacol Ther* **42**: 193–200.

26. Abernathy DR, Greenblatt DJ, Shader RI. 1984. Imipramine disposition in users of oral contraceptive steroids. *Clin Pharmacol Ther* **35**: 792–7.

27. Conrad CD, Hamilton JA. 1986. Recurrent premenstrual decline in serum lithium concentration. *J Am Acad Child Psychiatry* **26**: 852–3.

28. Kukopulos A, Minnai G, Muller-Oelinghausen B. 1985. The influence of mania and depression on the pharmacokinetics of lithium: a longitudinal single-case study. *J Affect Disord* **8**: 159–66.

29. Chamberlain S, Hahn PM, Cassan P, Reid RL. 1990. Effect of menstrual cycle phase and oral contraceptive use on serum lithium levels after a loading dose of lithium in normal women. *Am J Psychiatry* **147**: 907–9.

30. Greenblatt DJ, Allen MD, Harmatz JS, Shader RI. 1980. Diazepam disposition determinants. *Clin Pharmacol Ther* **27**: 301–12.

31. Macleod SM, Giles HG, Bengerr B *et al.* 1979. Age and gender related differences in diazepam pharmacokinetics. *J Clin Pharmacol* **19**: 15–19.

32. Smith RB, Divoll M, Gillespie WR, Greenblatt DJ. 1983. Effect of subject age and gender on the pharmacokinetics of oral triazolam and remazepam. *J Clin Psychopharmacol* **3**: 172–6.

33. Jochemsen R, Van der Graaff M, Boeijinga JK, Breimel D. 1982. Influence of sex, menstrual cycle and oral contraception on the disposition of nitrazepam. *Br J Clin Pharmacol* **13**: 319–24.

34. Divoll M, Greenblatt DJ, Harmatz JS, Shader RI. 1981. Effect of age and gender on disposition of temazepam. *J Pharm Sci* **70**: 1104–7.

35. Greenblatt DJ, Divoll M, Harmatz JS, Shader RI. 1980. Oxazepam kinetics: effects of age and sex. *J Pharmacol Exp Ther* **215**: 86–91.

36. Giles HG, Sellers EM, Naranjo CA, Greenblatt DJ. 1981. Disposition of intravenous diazepam in young men and women. *Eur J Clin Pharmacol* **20**: 207–13.

37. Ellinwood EH, Easier MP, Linnoila M *et al.* 1983. Effects of oral contraceptives and diazepam-induced psychomotor impairment. *Clin Pharmacol Ther* **35**: 360–6.

28

Gender and Ethnic Differences in the Pharmacogenetics of Psychotropics

Michael W. Smith, Ricardo P. Mendoza and Keh-Ming Lin

Harbor-UCLA Medical Center, Torrance, CA, USA

INTRODUCTION

Gender and cross-ethnic, as well as interindividual, variations in response to drug administration are the result of numerous factors. Although research into the determinants of gender variability in drug response is rudimentary, the mechanisms that underlie cross ethnic differences in drug responsiveness have come under close scrutiny during the last decade. As a result, it is now well established that mutational forces on drug metabolizing enzymes have given way to polymorphic (multiple forms of the same enzyme) variability, and ethnic-specific mutations have been clearly identified. In many cases, the differential responsiveness to the administration of pharmacologically active compounds observed among several ethnic groups is due to the presence of one of these genetically determined enzyme variants [1]. In addition, genetically determined polymorphisms of the drug-binding protein alpha-1-glycoprotein have also been identified and ethnic specificity for this protein has been demonstrated [2]. Drug binding is an important factor in drug response and alpha-1-glycoprotein is involved in the binding of many compounds used in the treatment of psychiatric disorders today [2].

Recently, factors unique to the female physiology—such as hormonal influences involved in menstruation, menopause, and pregnancy—have also been found to be important determinants of pharmacologic response. These gender-specific variations appear in many cases to be mediated through their effect on the drug-metabolizing enzymes noted above; namely, certain cytochrome P-450 (CYP) enzymes and N-acetyltransferase [1]. Gender variability in the metabolism of alcohol and the isoenzyme forms of the alcohol metabolizing enzymes has also been reported [1]. Other, more environmentally based, factors that are involved in

Cross Cultural Psychiatry. Edited by John M. Herrera, William B. Lawson and John J. Sramek.
© 1999 John Wiley & Sons Ltd.

producing gender and ethnic variations in drug response include exposure to xenobiotics, alcohol, cigarette smoke, certain dietary ingredients, and medications such as oral contraceptives. The available literature relating to how both genetic and environmental mechanisms produce gender and ethnic specific responsiveness to psychotropic medications is reviewed in this chapter.

DRUG-METABOLIZING ENZYMES AND THE METABOLIC PROCESS

Many of the medications used in the treatment of psychiatric patients are metabolized in a two-step process that renders them sufficiently water-soluble for excretion. Phase 1 of the metabolic process entails the addition of a functional group into the substrate and is predominantly carried out by CYP isozymes [3–4]. Phase 2 involves the conjugation of these agents via sulfation and glucuronidation. Genetic mutations producing structural changes can significantly alter the functional activity of the various drug-metabolizing enzymes, although it is clear that environmental factors can also exert a profound influence on enzymatic efficiency. Gender and ethnic variations in drug responsiveness are most likely to be due to a combination of these factors.

Regulation of Gender Variation in CYP Enzymes in Animals

Research that has been conducted with rodents has identified several sex-specific CYP enzyme systems, which are thought to be modulated by certain sex and pituitary hormones [5–7]. For example, data from several studies indicates that exposure to the sex hormone testosterone in the neonatal period is critical to the expression of the male-specific P-450h in rats and mice [8]. Castration during the neonatal period completely abolishes male P-450h expression; castration as an adult results in only partial reduction of its expression. The administration of exogenous testosterone in the rats castrated as neonates restores male-specific P-450h expression [5–7]. At birth, the female-specific P-450i is present in both sexes but exposure to testosterone in puberty results in its expression in females and its suppression in males [8].

Gender-specific patterns of growth hormone secretion appear to be one of the more important mechanisms underlying hormonal regulation of sex-specific CYPs by the pituitary gland [9–11]. These growth hormone secretion patterns are largely determined by neonatal and adult exposure to androgens and include the pulsatile pattern observed in males and the constant excretion pattern seen in females [12]. In hypophysectomized rats, continuous and pulsatile infusion of growth hormone can artificially re-establish the expression of the female-specific (P-450i) or male-specific (P-450h) CYPs, respectively [10, 11, 13]. Taken together, the data from these studies suggest that hormonal influences play an important role in the regulation of the CYP enzyme system.

Gender and Ethnic Variation in Human CYP Enzyme Systems

Gender and ethnic variation in the relative efficiency of the CYP enzyme system has been clearly documented using phenotyping methodologies (measurement of functional enzyme expression following administration of a probe drug). Phenotypic analysis performed in numerous populations has demonstrated that the enzymatic activity of two enzymes, CYP2D6 and CYP2C19, is bimodally distributed—that is, individuals in a given population are classified as either extensive metabolizers (EMs) or poor metabolizers (PMs) [1, 14–17]. Individuals possessing the wild-type are termed EMs while PM status indicates completely absent enzyme activity and is usually secondary to an individual being homozygotic for a specific mutation. Heterozygotes usually have a diminished or intermediate metabolic capacity and are termed slow metabolizers (SMs). An additional mutation in CYP2D6 results in the production of multiple copies of the enzyme [18]. Individuals that possess this mutation are referred to as superextensive metabolizers (SEMs). SEMs do not obtain therapeutic benefit at standard dosages from medications that are metabolized by CYP2D6 because the multiple copies of the enzyme produce an extremely high enzymatic activity and rapid substrate clearance. As phenotyping strategies are subject to environmental influences, genotyping (analysis of actual genetic structure employing molecular biological approaches) methodologies such as polymerase chain reaction and restriction fragmentation length polymorphism have been used to correlate actual gene structure with functional expression.

The information from studies of variability in drug response that have employed phenotyping and genotyping methodologies currently supports the following:

1. while there is an abundance of data supporting ethnic specific mutations, no sex-specific CYP enzyme systems or genetically determined gender-specific variations in CYP expression have been identified among humans to date [19];
2. genetic mutations are primarily responsible for much of the ethnic variability observed in the activity of the CYP2D6 and CYP2C19 enzymes, the only two possessing proven polymorphic variation; and
3. environmental factors such as diet, use of oral contraceptives, hormonal fluctuations during the menstrual cycle, and toxin exposure underlie both the gender and ethnic variations observed in two other important CYP enzymes: CYP1A2 and CYP3A3/4. Each of the enzymes displaying ethnic or gender variation will be reviewed below.

CYP2D6

Many of the drugs currently used in medicine and psychiatry today—such as antihypertensives, antidepressants and antipsychotics—are metabolized by

TABLE 28.1 Drugs subject to CYP enzyme metabolism

Cardiovascular drugs	Psychotropics	Analgesics
Alprenolol, amiflamine, bufranol, encainide, flecainide, guanoxan, indoramin, methoxyphenamine, metiamide, metropolol, N-propl-alamine, perhexilene, propafenone, propranolol, sparteine, timolol	Amitryptiline*, chlorpromazine, clozapine*, clomipramine, desipramine, fluoxetine, fluvoxamine, haloperidol*, imipramine*, methoxyamphetamine, nortriptyline, olanzapine*, paroxetine, perphenazine, risperidone, sertraline, thioridazine	Phenformin, codeine*, phenacetin, dextromethorphan

* Partially metabolized through this pathway

CYP2D6 [20–24] (see Table 28.1). Given the importance of the enzyme in the psychopharmacological management of patients it has been closely studied.

Recent reports focusing on pregnancy and the CYP system have yielded findings which point to the importance of circulating hormones in determining expression of functional CYP2D6 enzyme. In 1997, Wadelius et al. [25] reported that CYP2D6 activity is induced during pregnancy. This induction was noted in seven homozygote EMs and six heterozygote SMs, but not in the four PMs (as expected: PM status denoting enzyme function is absent) included in the study. In this study previously genotyped women were phenotyped using the probe drug dextromethorphan during late pregnancy and then 7–11 weeks after birth. The greatest induction of CYP2D6 was noted among the heterozygote group, only a moderate change being noted among the homozygote EMs. This study supports a previous report, which indicated that the clearance of the CYP2D6 substrate metropolol was four to five times higher during pregnancy than in the same women 3–6 months following delivery [26].

Although the mechanism for this induction in pregnancy remains unclear, endogenous substrates present during pregnancy are highly suspect. Among the most likely candidates for an endogenous inducer are the two steroid hormones progesterone and estrogen. During the luteal phase of the menstrual cycle, when progesterone plays a predominant role, CYP2D6 activity of debrisoquine is 25% higher than in the preovulatory phase [27]. In another study [28], clearance of propranolol, which is metabolized via ring oxidation by CYP2D6, increased when given the drug concurrently with ethinyl estradiol to female subjects.

In contrast to the sketchy and incomplete data on gender variation, cross ethnic differences in the frequency of PM phenotype of CYP2D6 are widely reported. The frequency of PMs of CYP2D6 varies from less than 1% in Mexican Americans [29] and several Asian subgroups including Chinese [30] and Japanese [31], to 3–10% in Caucasians in Europe and North America. A wider range of frequencies is found in Black Africans, with 0–8% of Saharan Africans, 1.9% of African Americans, and 19% of Sans Bushmen being classified as PMs [32].

CYP2C19

Another enzyme that displays interethnic differences in the incidence of PMs is CYP2C19. This enzyme, which is inherited as an autosomal recessive trait [33], is involved in the metabolism of benzodiazepines, imipramine, and other drugs [33–35]. Although the frequency of PMs of CYP2C19 is quite low among Caucasians, PMs are quite common in Asian populations [32]. African Americans have a PM frequency significantly higher than that in Caucasians [36] while Mexican Americans were recently noted to have a rate of 1%, similar to that reported among Caucasians [37].

No direct data to support gender variation in the CYP2C19 polymorphism have been reported; however, indirect evidence suggests that differences do exist. Both propranolol and diazepam have been reported to exhibit decreased clearance in female subjects [38–39]. The decreased clearance of propranolol in females was found to be specific to a decrease in side chain oxidation which is performed by CYP2C19 [39]. In the same study, administration of testosterone increased clearance of propranolol among female subjects, while administration of ethinyl estradiol produced the opposite results. Although we report these findings primarily to demonstrate that CYP2C19 (like CYP2D6) appears to be under sex-hormone regulation, they have additional clinical significance: both CYP2D6 and CYP2C19 are clearly involved in the metabolism of propranolol, and exposure to circulating sex hormones can produce dramatic and opposite results in the clearance of parent compound. However, because many drugs are metabolized by several CYP enzymes, inducing or inhibiting a particular pathway might not affect the overall clearance of parent compound although it may radically shift the characteristics of metabolites. These shifts in the metabolic profile can have profound implications for certain side-effects and toxicities, as well as other medical morbidities such as cancer.

CYP3A3/4

The CYP3A3/4 enzyme system is probably the most important of the CYP enzymes, accounting for more than one-half of all CYP in the body. Although no clear-cut genetically determined polymorphisms have been identified, large inter-individual variations have been reported. For example, among certain subjects there is a 30-fold difference in the amount of enzyme in the liver, and 11-fold differences have been reported in the intestine [40]. In addition, the activities of the enzymes in the two organs do not appear to be correlated with each other [40]. This could explain the differences observed in the rate of drug metabolism when the route of administration is varied [41]. CYP3A3/4 is involved in the metabolism of a variety of drugs used in medicine today, including cyclosporin, erythromycin, several cardiac drugs (quinidine, verapamil, diltiazem, and nifedipine), antihistamines (terfenadine and astemizole), and cocaine [42]. Among the psychotropic compounds metabolized by CYP3A3/4 are the benzodiazepines alprazolam, midazolam, and triazolam, as well as the antidepressants imipramine and nefazo-done [43], and the antipsychotics clozapine, quetiapine, and ziprasidone [44].

Increased CYP3A3/4 activity has been observed in both animal and human females. Lin et al. [45] suggest that gender differences in the levels of CYP3A isoforms may explain the increased metabolism of the protease inhibitor indinavir in female rats and dogs. The activity of this enzyme in humans has also been noted to be higher in women than men, with a 24% increase in the activity of the enzyme in the liver and a 45% increase in the gut [46–47]. In women this may in part explain the increased metabolism of methylprednisolone observed in females [48]. Further supporting the close relationship between CYP3A3/4 activity and hor-mone levels is the 50% increase in nefazodone concentration that has been observed in older females [49]. At variance with this finding, however, recent studies with the CYP3A substrates alfentanil and midazolam failed to demonstrate any variation due to menstrual cycle effects [50] or gender [51].

Ethnic variation in the metabolism of nifedipine, a CYP3A3/4 substrate, has been reported by several authors [52–55]. Both East Asians and Mexicans have been reported to metabolize nifedipine slower. Several initial reports of bimodal distribution of nifedipine metabolism [53–54] suggested the existence of a genetic polymorphism similar to that observed with CYP2D6 and CYP2C19. A follow-up study, however, reported a unimodal nifedipine metabolism distribution and suggested that earlier reports of variation were secondary to either small sample size or environmental influences [56].

In addition to being the most abundant CYP enzyme in the human body, CYP3A3/4 appears to be one of the most sensitive to environmental influences such as concurrent medications and diet. For example, the administration of the antimycotic agent ketoconazole can inhibit the enzyme, prolonging the half-life of triazolam by 6–7-fold [56]. Similar results have been seen with grapefruit juice [57]. Practitioners should be familiar with the recent literature concerning drug–drug and drug–diet interactions, which focuses considerable attention on CYP3A3/4 [42–43].

CYP1A2

Reports of gender and ethnic variation in the enzyme activity of CYP1A2 are sparse. However, substrates of the enzyme such as clozapine, fluvoxamine, olanza-pine, and tacrine have been demonstrated at higher concentrations in females [44, 58]. In a recent review article [44], clozapine and olanzapine concentrations were reported to be at least 30% higher in females, especially non-smoking females, than in males. These findings could be the result of hormonal influences.

Similar to CYP3A3/4, CYP1A2 exhibits increased sensitivity to environmental factors such as cigarette smoking and dietary habits. Cigarette smoking can induce the metabolism of haloperidol and olanzapine by more than 30% [44]. It induces CYP1A2 through the nitrosoamines found in the tar; these chemicals are also

TABLE 28.2 Drugs subject to acetylation

Drug	Role
Aminoglutethimide	Inhibitor of adrenal steroid synthesis
Amrinone	Positive inotropic
Caffeine	Stimulant
Clonazepam	Antiepileptic
Dapsone	Antimicrobial
Dipyrone	Analgesic
Endralazine	Antihypertensive
Hydralazine	Antihypertensive
Isoniazid	Antimicrobial
Nitrazepam	Antidepressant
Phenelzine	Antidepressant
Prizidilol	Antihypertensive
Procainamide	Antiarrhythmic
Sulfadiazine	Antimicrobial
Sulfamerazine	Antimicrobial
Sulfamethazine	Antimicrobial
Sulfapyridine	Antimicrobial

found in charcoal-cooked food and certain vegetables such as cabbage and brussels sprouts [59]. Oral contraceptives inhibit the CYP1A2 metabolism of caffeine [60].

Phase 2 Drug-metabolizing Enzymes

The data regarding the second phase of drug metabolism is meager. Synthetic sex hormones and certain psychotropics are largely eliminated from the body during the second phase of drug metabolism [61]. Although the activities of several Phase 2 enzymes such as UDP-glucuronosyltransferase, glutathione peroxidase, super-oxide dismutase and catalase have been shown to display gender differences in rodent species [62], no similar findings have been reported in humans. The available data focusing on gender and ethnic variability regarding acetylation and glucuronidation is reviewed below.

N-Acetyltransferase

Acetylation is a major route of metabolism for a large number of pharmacoactive agents, including some frequently prescribed psychotropics [63–64] (see Table 28.2). Inherited in an autosomal recessive fashion [65], *N*-acetyltransferase is primarily found in the liver and demonstrates bimodal distribution of metabolic phenotypes. PMs of drugs metabolized by *N*-acetyltransferase have been shown to be at higher risk of developing drug induced systemic lupus erythematosus, isoniazid polyneuropathy, and other hypersensitivity reactions [66], and more likely to respond to phenelzine, hydralazine, and isoniazid than EMs treated with similar doses. Acetylation status is a significant risk factor for the development of certain cancers [67].

The literature concerning gender differences and acetylation efficiency is limited to a report focusing on gender's influence on isoniazid plasma levels [68] and another report of an increased rate in the development of lupus erythematosus in hydralazine-treated women with unique tissue typing [69]. Acetylation status and its relevance to health and disease represents an active area of research [67].

With respect to ethnic considerations, the frequency of acetylator PMs ranges from 38% to greater than 50% in most Western populations [70–71], while rates in the Cuna and Ngawbe Guaymi Amerindians occur at the rate of 24% and 29%, respectively [72]. This is similar to frequencies observed in Japanese, Chinese, Koreans, and Eskimos and indicates a significant proportion of extensive metabolizers in these populations [73–74].

Glucuronidation

Another Phase 2 enzymatic process that displays both gender and ethnic variation in activity is glucuronidation. In certain animal species, males have demonstrated increased glucuronidation compared with females [74]. This is consistent with reports of decreased glucuronidation in human females [47]. In addition, isolated reports of gender variation in glucuronidation during puberty [75] and evidence for coregulation of CYP1A2 and glucuronidation [76] has recently appeared in the literature.

The issue of glucuronidation and ethnic differences was recently investigated in a series of well conducted studies by Yue and associates [77–80]. These studies demonstrated that glucuronidation of codeine was slower in Chinese as compared to Swedish Caucasians. The slower glucuronidation of codeine led to significantly higher concentrations among Chinese studied and, from a clinical perspective, appears to indicate comparable analgesic effects may be achieved utilizing lower doses of codeine when treating Chinese patients with complaints of pain.

Alcohol Metabolism

It is well recognized that gender and ethnicity are important factors influencing the manner and rate of development of alcoholism. Gender and ethnicity not only represent important social and cultural determinants; they are also important physiological factors that underlie the development of alcoholism [81]. Animal research indicates that alcohol metabolism differs between males and females [82–84], and hormonal influences appear to be involved in this variation [85–86]. Although similar research in humans has produced inconsistent results [87], hereditary influences are felt to play an important role in the development of alcoholism among humans.

Ethanol is first oxidized by alcohol dehydrogenase (ADH) to acetaldehyde, and then oxidized by aldehyde dehydrogenase (ALDH) to produce non-toxic acetate. Both ADH and ALDH are enzyme systems that demonstrate genetically determined polymorphic variation. The contribution of these enzymes to the gender and ethnic variability seen in the development of alcoholism is discussed below.

ADH

ADH isozymes are grouped in distinctive 'classes' based on their enzymatic characteristics and structural similarities [88]. The class I ADHs exhibit a high activity of ethanol oxidation, and play a major role in ethanol oxidation, in general, as well as being involved in the oxidation of neurotransmitters. They are most abundant in the liver, and are found in the lung, kidney, and other tissues. The Class II ADHs are primarily found in the liver but also exist in the stomach [89–90]. Class III ADH is found in all tissues. All ADH genes are located on chromosome 4q21–25 in humans [91].

Three different ADH enzymes, ADH_2 (β subunit), ADH_3 (γ subunit) and ADH_4 (π subunit) have been shown to be polymorphic in nature and display gender and ethnic variation. The frequency of the wild type (usual) ADH_2^1 gene exceeds 90% in Caucasians, but among Asians it is found at a frequency rate of about 30%. The more atypical ADH_2^2 genotype, on the other hand, is more common in Asians, occurring at a frequency of approximately 70%. Another atypical gene, ADH_2^3, is fairly common in Blacks. Also, two other ADH genes, the wild type ADH_3^1 gene and variant form, ADH_3^2, are commonly found in Caucasians; however, the frequency of the variant form is low in Asians [88, 91]. In addition, Yasunami $et\ al.$ [93] recently cloned and characterized the ADH_6 gene, and found that the enzyme produced by the gene exhibits Class II ADH characteristics, is expressed in the stomach, and has a hormone-responsive element.

Women appear to be more susceptible to alcoholic liver injury than men. Frezza $et\ al.$ [92] have reported that a significantly larger amount of ethanol is metabolized in the stomach of men, and that the ADH activity of stomach mucous membranes were substantially higher in men than in women. Owing to this decreased ADH activity, the amount of alcohol available for absorption in women is increased. Increased alcohol absorption, along with a decreased volume of distribution, could explain the higher peak blood alcohol levels observed in women and may be risk factors for alcoholic liver disease in women.

ALDH

Sensitivity to alcohol, or the phenomenon of 'alcohol flushing', is well recognized among Asians and is the result of ethnic-specific genetic variability at the ALDH gene locus. Certain mutations of the ALDH enzyme result in inefficient metabolism of acetaldehyde with resulting increases in circulating blood levels. Increased concentrations of acetaldehyde produce the dramatic clinical presentation of facial flushing, tachycardia, anxiety, and nausea. This phenomenon has been observed in more than 80% of Asians and about 50% of American Indians, but in less than 10% of Caucasians [94, 95].

Several ALDH isoenzymes have been identified [88]. The cytosolic liver $ALDH_1$ and the mitochondrial liver $ALDH_2$, which exhibit high activities for the oxidation of acetaldehyde, are considered to play a major role in acetaldehyde detoxification in the liver. Approximately 50% of Asians lack $ALDH_2$ activity in their livers. The deficiency of the $ALDH_2$ enzyme is due to a mutation in the $ALDH_2$ locus [96, 97]. The frequency of the variant $ALDH_2^2$ gene is about 30% in Japanese and null (or very low) in Caucasians [98]. Heterozygous $ALDH_2^1/ALDH_2^2$ individuals and homozygous atypical $ALDH_2^2/ALDH_2^2$ lack $ALDH_2$ activity in their livers—that is, the variant $ALDH_2^2$ gene is dominant in the expression of enzyme activity.

The most remarkable genomic difference between alcohol flushers and non-flushers, and between alcoholic patients and controls, is the frequencies of the wild-type $ALDH_2^1$ and the atypical Asian-type $ALDH_2^2$ genes. Virtually all Japanese alcohol-flushers are either heterozygous ($ALDH_2^1/ALDH_2^2$) or homozygous atypical ($ALDH_2^2/ALDH_2^2$) at the $ALDH_2$ locus. The genotypes associated with flushing appear to afford protection against alcoholism and, therefore, most patients with alcoholic liver diseases are homozygous; $ALDH_2^1/ALDH_2^1$ [91]. Other studies that have examined $ALDH_2$ genotypes in Japanese and Chinese alcoholics confirm the presence of wild-type status in these patients [99, 100].

Research that has focused on the alcohol drug-metabolizing enzyme system has established the foundation from which to understand the molecular biological basis of ethnic variability in the development and maintenance of alcoholism. These research findings also point to possible future research directions, such as identification of the gene(s) that may be responsible for the development of alcoholism, and study of the metabolism of certain endogenous neurotransmitters that are biotransformed by both ADH and ALDH [101, 102].

PLASMA PROTEIN BINDING

Pharmacologically active compounds are transported in the bloodstream bound to various elements in the plasma such as proteins and blood cells. Changes in the concentration and efficiency of these drug-binding proteins can have profound effects in as much as it is only the free or non-bound fraction of administered drug that is able to cross the blood–brain barrier and exert pharmacological influence [2, 103–106]. Two categories of plasma proteins—alpha-1 acid glycoproteins [107, 108] and albumins [109]—are generally regarded as most important with respect to drug binding. Of the two, alpha-1 acid glycoprotein (AAG) is felt to influence the pharmacokinetics of many psychotropic compounds, and has been demonstrated to exhibit isoenzyme variation that is genetically determined. Drugs such as imipramine, chlorpromazine, fluphenazine, loxapine, thioridazine, thiothixene, carbamazepine, and triazolam have been shown to have a higher affinity for this glycoprotein than for albumin [110–113]. Polymorphic variation has been identified in a particular S variant of AAG that is involved in the binding of nortriptyline, amitriptyline and methadone [114, 115].

Interethnic variation has been demonstrated in absolute levels of AAG, as well as in the distribution of the two variants, S (slow) and F (fast) [116–121]. Population studies reveal that Asians have an S variant frequency in the range of 15–27%, while Black and Caucasian Americans and Europeans demonstrate a range of 34–67%. Eskimos, Canadian and South American Indians have a frequency of 43–45%, which is higher than that observed among Asians. Indians from Mexico are reported to have a frequency of 54%.

Information on gender variation in protein binding is sparse. One limited study by Wilkinson and Kurata [122] suggests that in certain circumstances the protein binding of drugs is decreased in females. During pregnancy the binding of many drugs, including phenytoin and diazepam, is decreased [123], with the greatest decrease noted during the third trimester [124]. This may in part be due to the decreased levels of albumin reported during pregnancy [125].

Although no data is available on gender differences in the expression of the S variant of a AAG, alterations in AAG concentration have been reported. Kishino *et al.* [126] reported that AAG concentrations were significantly higher in men than in women. The concentration of AAG is reported to vary in conjunction with the menstrual cycle [127], and is reportedly decreased in pregnancy [128, 129]. Studies on the effect of oral contraceptives on AAG concentration reveal mixed results: one study reveals no effect of oral contraceptives [130], while three other studies noted lower concentrations of AAG in women using oral contraceptive [131–133]. It is at present unclear whether these qualitative and quantitative differences could lead to clinical effects.

CONCLUSION

The growing importance and level of sophistication of research in the field of pharmacogenetics appears to hold tremendous promise for refinements in the practice of pharmacotherapy. The main focus of investigation for pharmacogenetic researchers to date has been the drug-metabolizing enzymes. Using sophisticated analytical strategies, researchers have established that a variety of forces, both genetic and environmental, can significantly influence the efficiency of these enzymes and subsequent pharmacological response. It is now well recognized that these factors underlie the interethnic differences in drug responses that have long been reported. It is unfortunate, but presently the role that gender plays in pharmacological responsiveness remains largely unexplored—only recently have reports surfaced in the clinical literature pointing to gender variations in drug response. Early investigative attempts to gain a better understanding into the nature of these variations offer no definitive answers but indicate the need to further explore the role of hormonal influences. The available data, from both animal and human studies, suggests that hormonal regulation plays an important role in modulating the function of the CYP and other drug-metabolizing enzyme systems, as well as in determining the concentration of certain plasma proteins involved in binding psychotropic compounds. Exposure to circulating hormones during early critical developmental periods may also determine later expression of drug-metabolizing enzymes. The differences in the activity of the drug and alcohol-metabolizing enzymes noted between men and women may also be due to other, perhaps more environmentally based, factors such as diet, smoking, pollution, and other medications.

The lessons learned from the psychopharmacological management of patients from different cultures should be heeded when administering psychotropic medications to women. Genetic and environmental influences on the drug-metabolizing enzymes, as well as fluctuating hormonal influences during menstruation and pregnancy, unique to the female physiology, may place women at an increased risk of developing adverse effects and toxicity. This risk may be heightened in certain women of color since ethnic specific mutations have been identified that result in poor or absent metabolism of parent compounds and subsequent toxicity. Future pharmacological research must employ rigorous methodologies that will take into account the ethnicity, gender, and hormonal status of research subjects if progress is to be made in the area of psychopharmacotherapy, an area which is growing increasingly complicated. The dissemination of such knowledge can only assist clinicians in their efforts to individualize their pharmacological management of patients and achieve positive therapeutic outcomes.

ACKNOWLEDGMENTS

This chapter was written from the Research Center on the Psychobiology of Ethnicity and the Department of Psychiatry, UCLA School of Medicine, Harbor-UCLA Medical Center. The work was supported in part by the Research Center on the Psychobiology of Ethnicity MH47193.

REFERENCES

1. Kalow W. 1991. Interethnic variation of drug metabolism. *Trends Pharmacol Sci* **12**: 102–7.
2. Baumann P, Eap C. 1991. Plasma monitoring of antidepressants: clinical relevance of the pharmacogenetics of metabolism and of acid glycoprotein binding. *Biol Psychiatry* **29**: 75–95.
3. Clark W, Brater D, Johnson A. 1988. *Goth's Medical Pharmacology*, 12th ed. St. Louis: CV Mosby.

4. Shen W, Lin K. 1990. Cytochrome P-450 monooxygenases and interactions of psychotropic drugs. *Int J Psychiatr Med* **21**: 21–30.

5. Gonzalez F, Nebert D. 1990. Evolution of the P450 gene superfamily: animal–plant 'warfare' molecular drive and human genetic differences in drug oxidation. *Trends Genet* **6**: 182–6.

6. Nebert DW, Gonzalez FJ. 1985. Cytochrome P450 gene expression and regulation. *Trends Pharmacol Sci* **6**: 160–4.

7. Gonzalez FJ, Skoda RC, Kimura S, Umeno M, Zanger UM, Nebert DW *et al*. 1988. Characterization of the common genetic defect in humans deficient in debrisoquin metabolism. *Nature* **331**: 442–6.

8. Dannan GH, Guengerich FP, Waxman DJ. 1986. Hormonal regulation of rat liver microsomal enzymes: role of gonadal steroids in programming, maintenance, and suppression steroid-5a-reductase, flavin containing monoxygenase, and sex-specific cytochromes P-450. *J Biol Chem* **261**: 10728–35.

9. Mode A, Norstedt G, Simic B, Eneroth P, Gustafsson JA. 1981. Continuous infusion of growth hormone feminizes hepatic steroid metabolism in the rat. *Endocrinology* **108**: 2163–8.

10. Morgan ET, MacGeoch C, Gustafsson JA. 1985. Hormonal and developmental regulation of expression of the hepatic microsomal steroid 16a-hydroxylase cytochrome P-450 apoprotein in the rat. *J Biol Chem* **260**: 11895–8.

11. Pampori NA, Shapiro BH. 1994. Over-expression of CYP2C11, the major male-specific form of hepatic cytochrome P450, in the presence of nominal pulses of circulating growth hormone in adult male rats neonatally exposed to low levels of monosodium glutamate. *J Pharmacol Exp Ther* **271**(2): 1067–73.

12. Jansson JO, Ekberg S, Isaksson O *et al*. 1985. Imprinting of growth hormone secretion, body growth, and hepatic steroid metabolism by neonatal testosterone. *Endocrinology* **117**: 1881–9.

13. Kato R, Yamazoe Y, Shimada M *et al*. 1986. Effect of growth hormone and ectopic transplantation of pituitary gland on sex-specific forms of cytochrome P-450 and testosterone and drug oxidations in rat liver. *J Biochem* **100**: 895–902.

14. Gonzalez F. 1989. The molecular biology of cytochrome P450s. *Pharmacol Rev* **40**: 243–88.

15. Meyer U, Zanger U, Grant D, Blum M. 1990. Genetic polymorphisms of drug metabolism. *Adv Drug Res* **19**: 307–23.

16. Wilkinson GR, Guengerich FP, Branch RA. 1989. Genetic polymorphism of S-mephenytoin hydroxylation. *Pharmacol Ther* **43**: 53–76.

17. Wood AJ, Zhou HH. 1991. Ethnic differences in drug disposition and responsiveness. *Clin Pharmacokinet* **20**: 1–24.

18. Dahl ML, Johansson I, Bertilsson L, Ingelman-Sundberg M, Sjoqvist F. 1995. Ultra-rapid hydroxylation of debrisoquine in a Swedish population. Analysis of the molecular genetic basis. *J Pharmacol Exp Ther* **274**(1): 516–20.

19. George J, Byth K, Farrell GC. 1995. Age but not gender selectively affects expression of individual cytochrome P450 proteins in human liver. *Biochem Pharmacol* **50**(5): 727–30.

20. Dahl-Puustinen ML, Liden A, Alm C *et al*. 1989. Disposition of perphenazine is related to polymorphic CYP2D6e hydroxylation in human beings. *Clin Pharmacol Ther* **46**: 78–81.

21. Bertilsson L, Eichelbaum M, Mellstrom B *et al*. 1980. Nortriptyline and antipyrine clearance in relation to debrisoquine hydroxylation in man. *Life Sci* **27**: 1673–7.

22. Bertilsson L, Aberg-Wistedt A. 1983. The debrisoquine hydroxylation test predicts steady-state plasma levels of desipramine. *Br J Clin Pharmacol* **15**: 388–90.

23. Mellstrom B, Bertilsson L, Lou YC *et al.* 1983. Amitriptyline metabolism: relationship to polymorphic debrisoquine hydroxylation. *Clin Pharmacol Ther* **34**: 516–20.

24. Skjelbo E, Brosen K, Hallas J, Gram LF. 1991. The mephenytoin oxidation polymorphism is partially responsible for the *N*-demethylation of imipramine. *Clin Pharmacol Ther* **49**: 18–23.

25. Wadelius M, Darj E, Frenne G, Rane A. 1997. Induction of CYP2D6 in pregnancy. *Clin Pharmacol Ther* **62**: 400–7.

26. Hogstedt S, Lindberg B, Peng DR, Regardh CG, Rane A. 1985. Pregnancy-induced increase in metoprolol metabolism. *Clin Pharmacol Ther* **37**: 688–92.

27. Llerena A, Cobaleda J, Martinez C, Benitez J. 1996. Interethnic differences in drug metabolism: influence of genetic and environmental factors on debrisoquine hydroxylation phenotype. *Eur J Drug Metab Pharmacokinet* **21**: 129–38.

28. Fagan TC, Walle T, Walle UK *et al.* 1993. Ethinyl estradiol alters propranolol metabolism pathway-specifically. *Clin Pharmacol Ther* **53**: 241.

29. Mendoza R, Wan Y, Poland RE, Smith M, Lin KM. CYP2D6 Polymorphism in a Mexican American population: Relationship between genotyping and phenotyping (submitted for publication).

30. Du YL, Lou YQ. 1990. Polymorphism of debrisoquine 4-hydroxylation and family studies of poor metabolizers in Chinese population. *Acta Pharmacol Sin* **11**: 7–10.

31. Horai Y, Taga J, Ishizaki T, Ishikawa K. 1990. Correlations among the metabolic ratios of three test probes (metoprolol, debrisoquine, sparteine) for genetically determined oxidation polymorphism in a Japanese population. *Br J Clin Pharmacol* **29**: 111–15.

32. Silver B, Poland R, Lin K. 1993. Ethnicity and the pharmacology of tricyclic antidepressants. In: Lin K, Poland R, Nakasaki G, eds. *Psychopharmacology and Psychobiology of Ethnicity*. Washington, DC: American Psychiatric Press.

33. Inaba T, Jurima M, Kalow W. 1986. Family studies of mephenytoin hydroxylation deficiency. *Am J Hum Genet* **38**: 768–72.

34. Bertilsson L, Henthorn TK, Sanz E *et al.* 1989. Importance of genetic factors in the regulation of diazepam metabolism: relationship to *S*-mephenytoin, but not debrisoquine, hydroxylation phenotype. *Clin Pharmacol Ther* **45**: 348–55.

35. Meier UT, Dayer P, Male PJ, Kronbach T, Meyer UA. 1985. Mephenytoin hydroxylation polymorphism: characterization of the enzymatic deficiency in liver microsomes of poor metabolizers phenotyped in vivo. *Clin Pharmacol Ther* **38**(5): 488–94.

36. Masimirembwa CM, Hasler JA. 1997. Genetic polymorphism of drug metabolizing enzymes in African populations: implications for the use of neuroleptics and antidepressants. *Brain Res Bull* **44**(5): 561–71.

37. Smith M, Lin KM, Mendoza R, Wan Y, Poland RE. 1998. CYP2C19 Polymorphism in a Mexican American population: Relationship between genotyping and phenotyping (submitted for publication).

38. Macleod SM, Giles HG, Bengert B *et al.* 1979. Age and gender related differences in diazepam pharmacokinetics. *J Clin Pharmacol* **1**: 15–19.

39. Walle T, Walle U, Mathur RS, Conradi EC. 1992. The metabolic clearance of propranolol is regulated by testosterone in women as well as in men. *Clin Pharmacol Ther* **51**: 180.

40. Paine MF, Khalighi M, Fisher JM, Shen DD, Kunze KL, Marsh CL *et al.* 1997. Characterization of interintestinal and intraintestinal variations in human CYP3A-dependent metabolism. *J Pharmacol Exp Ther* **283**(3): 1552–62.

41. Ducharme MP, Warbasse LH, Edwards DJ. 1995. Disposition of intravenous and oral cyclosporine after administration with grapefruit juice. *Clin Pharmacol Ther* **57**(5): 485–91.

42. Lown KS, Kolars JC, Thummel KE, Barnett JL, Kunze KL, Wrighton SA, Watkins PB. 1994. Interpatient heterogeneity in expression of CYP3A4 and CYP3A5 in small bowel. Lack of prediction by the erythromycin breath test. *Drug Metab Disp* **22**(6): 947–55.

43. Greene DS, Barbhaiya RH. 1997. Clinical pharmacokinetics of nefazodone. *Clin Pharmacokinet* **33**(4): 260–75.

44. Ereshefsky L. 1996. Pharmacokinetics and drug interactions: update for new antipsychotics. *J Clin Psychiatry* **57**(Suppl 11): 12–25.

45. Lin JH, Chiba M, Balani SK, Chen IW, Kwei GY, Vastag KJ, Nishime JA. 1996. Species differences in the pharmacokinetics and metabolism of indinavir, a potent human immunodeficiency virus protease inhibitor. *Drug Metab Disp* **24**(10): 1111–20.

46. Harris RZ, Benet LZ, Schwartz JB. 1995. Gender effects in pharmacokinetics and pharmacodynamics. *Drugs* **50**(2): 222–39.

47. Gleiter CH, Gundert-Remy U. 1996. Gender differences in pharmacokinetics. *Eur J Drug Metab Pharmacokinet* **21**(2): 123–8.

48. Fletcher CV, Acosta EP, Strykowski JM. 1994. Gender differences in human pharmacokinetics and pharmacodynamics. *J Adolescent Health* **15**: 619–29.

49. Barbhaiya RH, Buch AB, Greene DS. 1996. A study of the effect of age and gender on the pharmacokinetics of nefazodone after single and multiple doses. *J Clin Psychopharmacol* **16**(1): 19–25.

50. Kharasch ED, Russell M, Mautz D, Thummel KE, Kunze KL, Bowdle A, Cox K. 1997. The role of cytochrome P450 3A4 in alfentanil clearance. Implications for interindividual variability in disposition and peri-operative drug interactions. *Anesthesiology* **87**(1): 36–50.

51. Thummel KE, O'Shea D, Paine MF, Shen DD, Kunze KL, Perkins JD, Wilkinson GR. 1996. Oral first-pass elimination of midazolam involves both gastrointestinal and hepatic CYP3A-mediated metabolism. *Clin Pharmacol Ther* **59**(5): 491–502.

52. Ashan CH, Renwick AG, Macklin B, Challenor VF, Waller DG, George CF. 1991. Ethnic differences in the pharmacokinetics of oral nifedipine. *Br J Clin Pharmacol* **31**: 399–403.

53. Kleinbloesem CH, van Brummelen P, Faber H, Danhof M, Vermeulen NPE, Breimer DD. 1984. Variability of nifedipine pharmacokinetics and dynamics: a new oxidation polymorphism in man. *Biochem Pharmacol* **33**: 3721–4.

54. Haehner BD, Gorski JC, Vandenbranden M, Wrighton SA, Janardan SK, Watkins PB, Hall SD. 1996. Bimodal distribution of renal cytochrome P450 3A activity in humans. *Mol Pharmacol* **50**(1): 52–9.

55. Schellens JHM, Soons PA, Breimer DD. 1988. Lack of bimodality in nifedipine plasma kinetics in a large population of healthy subjects. *Biochem Pharmacol* **37**: 2507–10.

56. von Moltke LL, Greenblatt DJ, Harmatz JS, Duan SX, Harrel LM, Cotreau-Bibbo MM *et al.* 1996. Triazolam biotransformation by human liver microsomes in vitro: effects of metabolic inhibitors and clinical confirmation of a predicted interaction with ketoconazole. *J Pharmacol Exp Ther* **276**(2): 370–9.

57. Hukkinen SK, Varhe A, Olkkola KT, Neuvonen PJ. 1995. Plasma concentrations of triazolam are increased by concomitant ingestion of grapefruit juice. *Clin Pharmacol Ther* **58**(2): 127–31.

58. Preskorn SH. 1997. Clinically relevant pharmacology of selective serotonin reuptake inhibitors. An overview with emphasis on pharmacokinetics and effects on oxidative drug metabolism. *Clin Pharmacokinet* **32**(Suppl 1): 1–21.

59. Kall MA, Clausen J. 1995. Dietary effect on mixed function P450 1A2 activity assayed by estimation of caffeine metabolism in man. *Hum Exp Toxicol* **14**(10): 801–7.

60. Balogh A, Klinger G, Henschel L, Borner A, Vollanth R, Kuhnz W. 1995. Influence of

ethinylestradiol-containing combination oral contraceptives with gestodene or levonorgestrel on caffeine elimination. *Eur J Clin Pharmacol* **48**(2): 161–6.

61. Kalow W. 1994. Pharmacogenetic variability in brain and muscle. *J Pharm Pharmacol* **46**(Suppl 1): 425–32.

62. Watanabe M, Tanaka M, Tateishi T, Nakura H, Kumai T, Kobayashi S. 1997. Effects of the estrous cycle and the gender differences on hepatic drug-metabolising enzyme activities. *Pharmacol Res* **35**(5): 477–80.

63. Lin K, Poland R, Smith M, Strickland T, Mendoza R. 1991. Pharmacokinetic and other related factors affecting psychotropic responses in Asians. *Psychopharmacol Bull* **27**: 427–39.

64. Mendoza R, Smith M, Poland R, Lin K, Strickland T. 1991. Ethnic psychopharmacology: the Hispanic and Native American perspective. *Psychopharmacol Bull* **27**: 449–61.

65. Lunde PKM, Frislid K, Hansteen V. 1977. Disease and acetylation polymorphism. *Clin Pharmacokinet* **2**: 182–96.

66. Rieder MJ, Shear NH, Kanee A, Tang BK, Spielberg SP. 1991. Prominence of slow acetylator phenotype among patients with sulfonamide hypersensitivity reactions. *Clin Pharmacol Ther* **49**: 13–17.

67. Weber WW. 1987. *The Acetylator Genes and Drug Responses*. New York: Oxford University Press.

68. Iselius L, Evans DAP. 1983. Formal genetics of isoniazid metabolism in man. *Clin Pharmacokinet* **8**: 541–4.

69. Batchelor JR, Welsh KI, Tinoco RM, Dollery CT, Hughes GR, Bernstein R *et al.* 1980. Hydralazine-induced systemic lupus erythematosus: influence of HLA-DR and sex on susceptibility. *Lancet* **1**(8178): 1107–9.

70. Weber WW, Hein DW. 1985. *N*-Acetylation pharmacogenetics. *Pharmacol Rev* **37**: 26–79.

71. Grant DM, Morike K, Eichelbaum M, Meyer UA. 1990. Acetylation pharmacogenetics. *J Clin Invest* **85**: 968–72.

72. Inaba T, Arias TD. 1987. On phenotyping with isoniazid: The use of urinary acetylation ratio and the uniqueness of antimodes. Study of two Amerindian populations. *Clin Pharmacol Ther* **42**: 493–7.

73. Grant DM, Tang BK, Kalow W. 1983. Polymorphic *N*-acetylation of a caffeine metabolite. *Clin Pharmacol Ther* **33**: 355–9.

74. Catania VA, Dannenberg AJ, Luquita MG, Sanchez Pozzi EJ, Tucker JK, Yang EK, Mottino AD. 1995. Gender-related differences in the amount and functional state of rat liver UDP-glucuronosyltransferase. *Biochem Pharmacol* **50**(4): 509–14.

75. Capparelli EV. 1994. Pharmacokinetic considerations in the adolescent: non-cytochrome P450 metabolic pathways. *J Adolescent Health* **15**(8): 641–7.

76. Bock KW, Schrenk D, Forster A, Griese E, Morike K, Brockmeier D, Eichelbaum M. 1994. The influence of environmental and genetic factors on CYP2D6, CYP1A2, and UDP-glucuronosyltransferases in man using sparteine, caffeine, and paracetamol as probes. *Pharmacogenetics* **4**: 209–18.

77. Yue Q, Svensson JO, Alm C, Sjoqvist F, Sawe J. 1989. Interindividual and interethnic differences in the demethylation and glucuronidation of codeine. *Br J Clin Pharmacol* **28**: 629–37.

78. Yue QY, Bertilsson L, Dahl-Puustinen ML, Sawe J, Sjoqvist F, Johansson I, Ingelman-Sundberg M. 1989. Disassociation between debrisoquine hydroxylation phenotype and genotype among Chinese. *Lancet* **2**: 870.

79. Yue QY, Hasselstrom J, Svensson JO, Sawe J. 1991. Pharmacokinetics of codeine and its metabolites in Caucasian healthy volunteers: Comparisons between extensive and poor hydroxylators of debrisoquine. *Br J Clin Pharmacol* **31**: 635–42.

80. Yue QY, VonBahr C, Odar-Cederlof I, Sawe J. 1990. Glucuronidation of codeine and morphine in human liver and kidney microsomes: Effect of inhibitors. *Pharmacol Toxicol* **66**: 221–6.

81. Mello NK. 1980. Some behavioral and biological aspects of alcohol problems in women. In: Kalant OJ, ed. *Alcohol and Drug Problems in women, Vol. 5, Research Advances in Alcoholism and Drug Problems*. New York: Plenum Press, pp. 263–98.

82. Eriksson CJP. 1973. Ethanol and acetaldehyde metabolism in rat strains genetically selected for their ethanol preference. *Biochem Pharmacol* **22**: 2283–92.

83. Eriksson K, Malmstrom KK. 1967. Sex differences in consumption and elimination of alcohol in albino rats. *Ann Med Exp Biol Fenn* **45**: 389–92.

84. Wilson JR, Erwin VG, DeFries JC *et al.* 1984. Ethanol dependence in mice: Direct and correlated responses to ten generations of selective breeding. *Behav Genet* **14**: 235–56.

85. Collins AC, Yeager TN, Leback ME *et al.* 1975. Variations in alcohol metabolism: Influence of sex and age. *Pharmacol Biochem Behav* **3**: 973–8.

86. Rachamin G, MacDonald JA, Wahid S, Clapp JJ, Khanna JM, Israel Y. 1980. Modulation of alcohol dehydrogenase and ethanol metabolism by sex hormones in the spontaneously hypertensive rat. *Biochem J* **186**: 483–90.

87. Cole-Harding S, Wilson JR. 1987. Ethanol metabolism in men and women. *J Studies Alcohol* **48**: 380–7.

88. Yoshida A, Hsu LC, Yasunami M. 1991. Genetics of human alcohol-metabolizing enzymes. *Progr Nucl Acid Res Mol Biol* **40**: 255–87.

89. Yin SJ, Wang MF, Liao CS, Chen CM, Wu CW. 1990. Identification of a human stomach alcohol dehydrogenase with distinctive kinetic properties. *Biochem Int* **22**: 829–35.

90. Moreno A, Parés X. 1991. Purification and characterization of a new alcohol dehydrogenase from human stomach. *J Biol Chem* **266**: 1128–33.

91. Yoshida A. 1983. A possible structural variant of human cytosolic aldehyde dehydrogenase with diminished enzyme activity. *Am J Hum Genet* **35**: 1115–16.

92. Frezza M, di Padora C, Pozzato G *et al.* 1990 High blood alcohol levels in women: the role of decreased gastric alcohol dehydrogenase activity and first pass metabolism. *N Engl J Med* **322**: 95–9.

93. Yasunami M, Chen CS, Yoshida A. 1991. A human alcohol dehydrogenase gene (ADH6) encoding an additional class of isozyme. *Proc Natl Acad Sci USA* **88**: 7610–14.

94. Wolff PH. 1972. Ethnic difference in alcohol sensitivity. *Science* **175**: 449–50.

95. Wolff PH. 1973. Vasomotor sensitivity to alcohol in diverse mongoloid population. *Am J Hum Genet* **25**: 193–9.

96. Yoshida A, Huang IY, Ikawa M. 1984. Molecular abnormality of an inactive aldehyde dehydrogenase variant commonly found in Orientals. *Proc Natl Acad Sci USA* **81**: 258–61.

97. Hsu LC, Tani K, Fujiyoshi T *et al.* 1985. Cloning of cDNAs for human aldehyde dehydrogenase 1 and 2. *Proc Natl Acad Sci USA* **82**: 3771–5.

98. Shibuya A, Yoshida A. 1988. Frequency of the atypical aldehyde dehydrogenase-2 gene (ALDH2) in Japanese and Caucasians. *Am J Hum Genet* **43**: 744–8.

99. Harada S. 1990. Genetic polymorphism of aldehyde dehydrogenase and its physiological significance to alcohol metabolism. *Progr Clin Biol Res* **344**: 289–91.

100. Thomasson HR, Edenberg HJ, Crabb DW *et al.* 1991. Alcohol and aldehyde dehydrogenase genotypes and alcoholism in Chinese men. *Am J Hum Genet* **48**: 677–81.

101. Agarwal DP, Hafer G, Harada S *et al.* 1982. Studies on aldehyde dehydrogenase and aldehyde reductase in human brain. In: Weiner H, Flynn TG, eds. *Enzymology of*

Carbonyl Metabolism: Aldehyde Dehydrogenase and Aldo-keto Reductase. New York: Liss, pp. 319–28.

102. Agarwal DP, Goedde HW. 1990. *Alcohol Metabolism, Alcohol Intolerance and Alcoholism.* Berlin: Springer-Verlag.

103. Crabtree B, Jann M, Pitts W. 1991. Alpha acid glycoprotein levels in patients with schizophrenia: effect of treatment with haloperidol. *Biol Psychiatry* **29**: 43A–70A.

104. DeLeve LD, Piafsky KM. 1981. Clinical significance of plasma binding of basic drugs. *Trends Pharmacol Sci* **2**: 283–4.

105. Routledge P. 1986. The plasma protein binding of basic drugs. *Br J Clin Pharmacol* **22**: 499–506.

106. Levy RH, Moreland TA. 1984. Rationale for monitoring free drug levels. *Clin Pharmacokinet* **9**(Suppl 1): 1–9.

107. Baumann P, Eap C. 1988. *Alpha-acid Glycoprotein Genetics, Biochemistry, Physiological Functions and Pharmacology.* New York: Alan R. Liss.

108. Kremer J, Wilting J, Janssen L. 1988. Drug binding to human alpha-1-acid glycoprotein in health and disease. *Pharmacol Rev* **40**: 1–45.

109. Kragh-Hansen U. 1981. Molecular aspects of ligand binding to serum albumin. *Pharmacol Rev* **33**: 1.

110. Bogra O, Piafsky KM, Nilsen OG. 1977. Plasma protein binding of basic drugs. 1. Selective displacement from α1-acid glycoprotein by *tris* (2-butoxyethyl) phosphate. *Clin Pharmacol Ther* **22**: 539–44.

111. Piafsky KM, Bogra O, Odar-Cedarlof E, Johanson C, Sloqvist F. 1978. Increased binding of propranolol and chlorpromazine in disease. *N Engl J Med* **299**: 1435–9.

112. Kornguth ML, Hutchins LG, Eichelman BS. 1981. Binding of psychotropic drugs to isolated α1-acid glycoprotein. *Biochem Pharmacol* **30**: 2435–41.

113. Kroboth PD, Smith RB, Sorkin MI, Rault R, Garry M, Juhl RP. 1984. Triazolam protein binding and correlation with alpha-1-acid glycoprotein concentration. *Clin Pharmacol Ther* **36**: 379–83.

114. Eap CB, Cuendet C, Baumann P. 1990. Binding of d-methadone, 1-methadone, and dl-methadone to proteins in plasma of healthy volunteers: Role of the variants of α1-acid glycoprotein. *Clin Pharmacol Ther* **47**: 338–46.

115. Tinguely D, Bauman P, Conti M, Jonzier-Perey M, Schopf J. 1985. Interindividual differences in the binding of antidepressants to plasma proteins: The role of variants of alpha-1-acid glycoprotein. *Eur J Clin Pharmacol* **27**: 661–6.

116. Montiel MD, Carracedo A, Blazquez-Caeiro JL, Andrade-Vide C. 1990. Orosomucoid (ORM1 and ORM2) types in the Spanish Basque country, Galicia, and Northern Portugal. *Hum Hered* **40**: 330–4.

117. Zhou H, Adedoyin A, Wilkinson GR. 1990. Differences in plasma binding of drugs between Caucasian and Chinese subjects. *Clin Pharmacol Ther* **48**: 10–17.

118. Eap CB, Bauman P. 1989. The genetic polymorphism of human alpha-1-acid glycoprotein: genetics, biochemistry, physiological functions, and pharmacology. *Progr Clin Biol Res* **300**: 111–25.

119. Fukuma Y, Kashimimura S, Umetsu K, Yuasa I, Suzuki T. 1990. Genetic variation of alpha-2-HS-glycoprotein in the Kyushu district of Japan: Description of three new rare variants. *Hum Hered* **40**: 49–51.

120. Juneja R, Weitkamp L, Straitil A. 1988. Further studies of the plasma, Alpha B-glycoprotein polymorphism: two new alleles and allele frequencies in Caucasians and in American Blacks. *Hum Hered* **38**: 267–72.

121. Umetsu K, Yuasa I, Nishimura H. 1988. Genetic polymorphisms of orosomucoid and alpha-2-HS-glycoprotein in a Philippine population. *Hum Hered* **38**: 287–90.

122. Wilkinson GR, Kurata D. 1974. The uptake of diphenylhydantoin by the human

erythrocyte and its application to the estimation of plasma binding. In: Mortselli PL, Garattini S, Cohen SN, eds. *Drug Interactions*. New York: Raven Press, pp. 289–97.

123. Dean M, Stock B, Patterson RJ *et al.* 1980. Serum protein binding of drugs during and after pregnancy in humans. *Clin Pharmacol Ther* **28**: 253–61.

124. Perucca E, Crema A. 1982. Plasma protein binding of drugs in pregnancy. *Clin Pharmacokinet* **7**: 336–56.

125. Yoshikawa T, Sugiyama Y, Sawada Y *et al.* 1984. Effect of late pregnancy on salicylate, diazepam, warfarin, and propranolol binding: use of fluorescent probes. *Clin Pharmacol Ther* **36**: 201–8.

126. Kishino S, Nomura A, Di ZS, Sugawara M, Iseki K, Kakinoki S *et al.* 1995. Alpha-1-acid glycoprotein concentration and the protein binding of disopyramide in healthy subjects. *J Clin Pharmacol* **35**(5): 510–14.

127. Parish RC, Spivey C. 1991. Influence of menstrual cycle phase on serum concentration of a-1-acid glycoprotein. *Br J Clin Pharmacol* **31**: 197–9.

128. Adams JB, Wacher A. 1968. Specific changes in the glycoprotein components of seromucoid in pregnancy. *Clin Chem Acta* **21**: 155–7.

129. Ganrot PO. 1972. Variation of the concentrations of some plasma proteins in normal adults, in pregnant women and in newborns. *Scand J Clin Lab Invest* **29**(Suppl 24): 83–8.

130. Blain PG, Mucklow JC, Rawlins MD *et al.* 1985. Determinants of plasma a-1-acid glycoprotein (AAG) concentrations in health. *Br J Clin Pharmacol* **20**: 500–2.

131. Routledge PA, Shand DG, Barchowsky A *et al.* 1981. Relationship between a-1-acid glycoprotein and lidocaine disposition in myocardial infarction. *Clin Pharmacol Ther* **30**: 154–7.

132. Song CD, Merkatz IR, Rifkind AB *et al.* 1970. The influence of pregnancy and oral contraceptive steroids on the concentration of plasma proteins. *Am J Obstet Gynecol* **108**: 227–31.

133. Walle T, Walle UK, Fagan TC, Topmiller MJ, Conradi EC. 1993. Influence of gender and sex steroid hormones on plasma binding of the propranolol enantiomers. *Clin Pharmacol Ther* **53**: 183.

29

Gender and Response to Antipsychotic Medications

Laurie Lindamer and Dilip V. Jeste

University of California, San Diego, La Jolla, CA, USA

GENDER DIFFERENCES IN SCHIZOPHRENIA

Gender differences in the clinical presentation, course of illness, and treatment response of patients with schizophrenia have been well documented [1–3]. Women, in general, tend to have a later onset of illness and better outcome. Women have been reported to exhibit more affective symptoms, primarily depressive type [4–6], more severe positive or paranoid symptoms [6–8], and less severe negative symptoms [9, 10] than men.

Gender differences have also been noted in neuroradiological and neuropsychological studies, but the results are inconsistent. Some researchers [11, 12] have reported that men with schizophrenia have significantly larger ventricles than male comparison groups while women with schizophrenia do not differ from female comparison groups. Other studies [13] have reported the opposite. Some groups have noted that male schizophrenics performed worse than female patients in cognitive functioning [14, 15], while others have found that female patients had more impaired cognitive performance than male patients [16]. More recent studies of cognitive impairment in schizophrenia have reported no gender differences [1, 17, 18].

Given the gender differences in the clinical presentation and outcome seen in schizophrenia, it could be hypothesized that other gender-related findings might be seen in the pharmacokinetics, pharmacodynamics, efficacy, and prevalence of adverse events with antipsychotic medication. This chapter will selectively review some of the literature on gender differences in pharmacokinetics and pharmacodynamics, compliance, antipsychotic dose and efficacy and antipsychotic-induced tardive dyskinesia.

Cross Cultural Psychiatry. Edited by John M. Herrera, William B. Lawson and John J. Sramek.

PHARMACOKINETICS

Gender differences in various pharmacokinetic parameters of psychotropic medications have been recently reviewed [19, 20]. Briefly, differences between men and women in body composition, weight, and ratio of fat to total body water may affect absorption, distribution, biotransformation, metabolism, and excretion of psychotropic drugs. Women secrete less gastric acid and have slower gastric emptying than men, which probably affects the absorption and bioavailability of many drugs [21]. Gender differences in the proportion of muscular and adipose tissue may influence the volume of distribution and half-lives of drugs [22]. The higher proportion of fat in women may initially lead to higher volume of distribution, and consequently to lower serum concentration for a given dose. Over time, however, more of a lipophilic drug will be stored in adipose tissue, thus increasing the half-life and producing higher serum levels of drug once steady state is achieved [19, 23]. Differences in protein binding could significantly alter the availability of drug; however [24], the few studies that have investigated gender differences in protein binding have found that the results vary with the type of protein measured [23]. There appears to be a gender-by-biotransformation interaction for hepatic metabolism: non-synthetic reactions involving hydrolysis seem to be sensitive to gender differences but synthetic reactions, such as conjugation, may not be [23, 24]. Hamilton and Yonkers [23] concluded that renal elimination is lower in women, and therefore women may have lower clearance and higher blood levels of drug that are metabolized by the kidney. With drugs metabolized by the liver most of the gender differences also increase blood levels and decrease clearance. Clearly, more studies examining differences between men and women on pharmacokinetic parameters alone and in combination are needed.

There have been reports that hormonal status influences drug metabolism. The use of oral contraceptives may attenuate, exaggerate, or reverse the pre-existing gender differences. For example, oral contraceptives have been shown to moderate some of the gender difference in gastric half-emptying and may reverse the difference in renal elimination [23]. On the other hand, oral contraceptives may further increase the proportion of free to bound drug seen in women [23]. Hamilton and Yonkers [23] hypothesized that, given the predicted effects of these mechanisms, the net bioavailability of active drug may increase for women overall, magnifying the predicted sex difference in blood levels or clearance.

There are reports that hormonal variations associated with the menstrual cycle affect gastrointestinal transit time and plasma concentrations [25]. Menstrual cycle changes in water retention may also affect drug distribution [19]. During the premenstrual phase, the overall effect of the hormonal change on pharmacokinetics may be to oppose the known gender effects [23] in women diagnosed with premenstrual syndrome. Although little is known about the normal variation of hormones with the menstrual cycle, even less in known about drug pharmacokinetics in postmenopausal women.

In summary, the data on gender differences in pharmacokinetics are sparse and little is known about the effect of hormone changes, such as occur in women taking oral contraceptives, during the menstrual cycle, or during menopause.

Given the above-mentioned gender differences in various pharmacokinetic parameters, even when antipsychotic dose is controlled different plasma levels may be expected in men and women. Studies of plasma levels of antipsychotic medications in men and women with schizophrenia have obtained inconsistent results. Simpson and colleagues [26] measured plasma levels following a single dose of fluphenazine decanoate in nine subjects (five men, four women) with chronic psychosis under the age of 45 years. The levels were significantly higher in women than in men at every time point examined (from 1 h to 26 days). There were no significant differences in weight, age, or dose between the genders. Two women were taking oral contraceptives, which may have contributed to the differing plasma levels. Ereshefsky and colleagues [27] measured plasma concentrations of thiothixene in 42 patients (mentally retarded and mentally ill) ranging in age from 21 to 76 years and found that men had a significantly higher clearance than women which could not be accounted for by body weight. In contrast, Meltzer and colleagues [28] found that women with schizophrenia had higher levels of chlorpromazine equivalents than men after receiving a fixed dose of chlorpro-mazine—however, this difference disappeared when weight was taken into account.

In the studies that have compared gender differences in plasma levels of anti-psychotic medications, there has been no consistency with regard to age, diagnosis, type of antipsychotic medication, or dosing strategy. Furthermore, while studies have taken into consideration factors such as smoking, alcohol consumption, and use of other medications, few have examined gender-related differences in these behaviors.

PHARMACODYNAMICS

In a study of gender differences in pharmacodynamics, Meltzer and colleagues [28] found that the prolactin response to a fixed dose of chlorpromazine was greater in women with schizophrenia than men, even after controlling for serum levels of antipsychotic medication. Furthermore, there was a trend for women to respond better to neuroleptics, as measured by the Brief Psychiatric Rating Scale (BPRS) [29]. Szymanski *et al.* [30] confirmed this result, demonstrating that women with first-episode schizophrenia had higher plasma prolactin levels than men over the 6-week course of treatment despite similar plasma levels of fluphenazine. Plasma levels of homovanillic acid (HVA) were also measured in this study; women had higher levels, which differed significantly from those in men after the first week. The women in this study also had higher rates of methylphenidate infusion activation than men, although this was not statistically significant. Sumiyoshi and colleagues [31] found a significant overall effect of gender, but no significant gender by diagnosis effect, when plasma HVA levels in a large group of patients with schizophrenia or schizoaffective disorder were compared with a normal group.

As Yonkers and Hamilton [20] stated, the gender differences in pharmacokinetics and pharmacodynamics may be of little clinical importance for drugs with a wide therapeutic index or for medication for which there is low correlation between plasma concentration and efficacy or side-effects, as is the case with most of the antipsychotic medications.

COMPLIANCE, ANTIPSYCHOTIC DOSE, AND EFFICACY

A major consideration in comparing medication dose or efficacy between groups is differences in compliance. A study of frequency of rehospitalizations in a sample of patients with schizophrenia, schizoaffective disorder, bipolar disorder, and major depressive disorder found that alcohol/drug problems, medication non-compliance, and male gender were related to more frequent hospitalizations. Although the interaction of gender and compliance was not examined, this study suggests that there may be an association and further research is warranted [32]. Another study of medication compliance in schizophrenic patients found that gender, as well as ethnicity, were significant predictors of extreme non-compliance. Non-compliant patients were more likely to be male, of Afro-Caribbean descent, and to have more hospital admissions [33]. In the few studies that have investigated compliance in patients with psychotic disorders, it appears that women are more compliant with medication than men: any gender differences in dose and efficacy of antipsychotic medication, therefore, should consider these differences. As none of the studies discussed below measured medication compliance, the results should be interpreted with caution.

The literature regarding gender differences in dose of antipsychotic medication for patients with schizophrenia is somewhat inconsistent. Some studies reported that younger women required higher doses of antipsychotic medication [34, 35], while others concluded that there was no gender difference [36, 37], and still others found that women needed lower doses of antipsychotic medication than men to achieve similar levels of clinical improvement [38, 39].

Zito and colleagues [34] found that there was a trend for women to have higher chlorpromazine equivalents than men (mean = 1688(±1556) mg, and 1284(±1044) mg, respectively) in a study of recently admitted patients with schizophrenia under the age of 45 who received fluphenazine, haloperidol, thiothixene, or chlorpromazine. The authors speculated that this difference might have been secondary to the disproportionately larger number of women receiving high-potency typical antipsychotics. Methodological weakness of this study included the lack of a specific measurement of symptom change and plasma antipsychotic levels.

In studies of atypical antipsychotics, women with schizophrenia have required higher doses of medication than men have. In two studies of younger inpatients with treatment-refractory schizophrenia, women have required higher doses of the atypical antipsychotic, clozapine [35, 40]. Szymanski *et al.* [40] cautioned that the women in this study were significantly older, had a longer duration of illness before starting treatment with clozapine, and were more likely to be diagnosed with disorganized or undifferentiated schizophrenia, suggesting that this sample represented a group of severely ill women. Lieberman and colleagues [35], who found similar results with a similar sample, issued the same caveat. In contrast, in a study of older patients (aged 65 or above) with a diagnosis of psychotic disorder (including agitation or psychosis related to dementia, major depression with psychotic features, bipolar with psychotic features, and schizophrenia), Zarate *et al.* [41] found that women received lower doses of risperidone (1.4(±0.9) mg) than men (2.0(±1.5) mg). When differences in body weight were controlled, however, men received slightly higher weight-corrected daily doses. Furthermore, the patients who showed most improvement were younger and male.

Several studies have found no gender difference in antipsychotic dose. In a study characterizing treatment-responsive and treatment-resistant inpatients of all ages with schizophrenia [37] along clinical, biological and neuropathological dimensions, no gender differences in response to treatment were seen. However, the sample size was quite small, which may have resulted in levels of power too low to detect group differences. In a larger study of acutely admitted younger patients with a diagnosis of psychotic disorder (schizophrenia, psychosis, not otherwise specified, major depression with psychosis, bipolar disorder with psychosis, and delusional disorder), Glick *et al.* [36] found that neither gender nor diagnosis were related to neuroleptic response when a fixed dose of haloperidol or perphenazine was administered. A recent study examined gender differences in young inpatients (24 men and 20 women) with schizophrenia or schizoaffective disorder who were similar with respect to age of onset, course of illness, prior hospitalizations, and premorbid functioning [42]. Following a washout period the patients received either placebo or typical antipsychotic medication (fluphenazine, pimozide, trifluoperazine, chlorpromazine, or thioridazine) adjusted to achieve maximal clinical efficacy under double-blind conditions. Men and women did not differ in the length of drug-free and antipsychotic treatment levels, type of antipsychotic, baseline symptomatology, antipsychotic dose, and dose by weight. The authors found no gender differences on the BPRS total [29] or the positive or negative symptom subscales following treatment.

Although some studies have found that women with a psychotic disorder, including schizophrenia, require higher or the same levels of antipsychotic medication, most work examining the gender difference in response to antipsychotic medication has found that women have a better therapeutic response. In a 2-year follow-up study of schizophrenic outpatients, Hogarty and colleagues [38] found that 63% of the men but only 37% of the women relapsed while being maintained on chlorpromazine. The dose of chlorpromazine at the end of the 2-year follow-up was, however, not reported and the authors did not state the criteria for relapse. In another study of relapse rates, Goldstein *et al.* [43] found that men with acute schizophrenia had more residual symptoms than women on high doses of fluphenazine whereas women on low doses had more residual symptoms than men on low doses. Young and Meltzer [44] compared young adult inpatients with schizophrenia requiring relatively low doses of neuroleptics (less than 200 mg chlorpromazine equivalents daily) with those requiring high doses (more than 800 mg chlorpromazine equivalents daily). The groups did not differ with respect to age, race, social status or marital status; however, there were significantly more women than men (61% versus 30%) in the low-dose group. The low-dose group also had significantly fewer hospitalizations, more prominent excitement, more specific hallucinations, shorter period between onset of symptoms and hospitalization, better family functioning, and lower readmission rates. The authors noted that the men may have required higher doses of medication due to their larger body size. In a retrospective review of gender differences of response to antipsychotics and outcome, more women than men with schizophrenia or schizoaffective disorder were classified as good responders to neuroleptics (59% versus 22%, respectively) [45]. Although plasma levels of neuroleptics and prolactin were measured in this study, no data were presented with regard to gender differences. In a comparative study of pimozide and chlorpromazine for the treatment of schizophrenic inpatients aged 18–65 years, Chouinard and Annable [39] found that female patients responded better than male patients, as measured by the BPRS [29] and Clinical Global Impression (CGI), despite similar doses of antipsychotic and regardless of the type of medication. In another study comparing therapeutic response of typical antipsychotics (fluspirilene and chlorpromazine) in newly admitted schizophrenics, the same group of investigators [46] found that men required nearly double the amount of fluspirilene than women to achieve therapeutic efficacy as determined by a physician blind to treatment condition. There was, however, no gender difference in the daily dose of chlorpromazine. The lower dose in women could not be explained by gender-related differences in initial severity of illness, previous hospitalization, weight, or side-effects. The only gender difference in psychopathology was a trend for the women to have more anxious depression factor scores on the BPRS [29]. Plasma levels of the drugs were not measured in this study. A recent study of first-episode schizophrenia patients [30] demonstrated that women had greater response to antipsychotic medication (fluphenazine) than men as measured by the Scale for the Assessment of Positive Symptoms [47] and the Scale for the Assessment of Negative Symptoms (SANS) [48], although mean serum plasma levels were similar. Full response, as defined as no positive symptoms and no rating greater than 2 on the global items of the SANS, was achieved by 87% of women and 55% of men, despite similar global psychopathology at baseline on the CGI.

Some research has demonstrated an age-by-gender interaction, with younger male and older female patients with schizophrenia requiring higher doses of antipsychotic medication. Marriott and Hiep [49] examined neuroleptic use in psychiatric patients and found that men between the ages of 21 and 40 required higher doses of neuroleptic medication (fluphenazine decanoate) than did women to achieve functional improvement as defined by the staff and family members.

Furthermore, in the 51–70-year-old group, the mean dose was reduced for male patients. The patients in this study were not well characterized with respect to diagnosis. In addition, clinical efficacy was measured by subjective ratings of improvement by staff and family. In a study designed to reduce neuroleptic medication to the lowest possible effective amount in outpatients with chronic schizophrenia, Seeman [50] found that younger women (aged 20–39) needed to be maintained on lower doses than men and that, after age 40, women required higher doses than men. However, the amounts of medication were not reported, nor were plasma levels measured. A gender-by-age interaction was observed in a large study of bipolar disorder [51]: men younger than and women greater than 40 years of age received higher doses of neuroleptics.

In general, premenopausal women with schizophrenia appear to require lower doses of neuroleptic medication than do men with schizophrenia; the reverse may be true for postmenopausal women [49, 50].

In summary, the inconsistencies in the methodology in different studies are considerable and therefore preclude definitive conclusions. Some of the variability may be due to methodological differences in terms of diagnosis and the use of diagnostic criteria, design of the study, and selection of outcome measures. In addition, studies differ with respect to sample characteristics such as age, chronicity of illness, refractoriness, and treatment itself (for example, dosing strategy, length of trial, type of antipsychotic). A number of these studies also have methodological shortcomings, such as lack of objective measurement of improvement, or absence of measurement of plasma levels of antipsychotic medications.

TARDIVE DYSKINESIA

It has been reported that women tend to suffer more adverse effects than men when age, number of drugs, and duration of hospitalization are controlled [52, 53]. Some studies have reported that women who receive antipsychotic medication are at higher risk of tardive dyskinesia (TD) [54]; others have found no significant gender differences [55, 56]. Yassa and Jeste [57], in a meta-analysis of studies of the prevalence of TD found significantly higher prevalence in women than in men (26.6% and 21.6%, respectively). There was a gender-by-age interaction, with prevalence of TD increasing with age in women but not in men. Women also reportedly tend to have more severe TD than men [57]. Two recent investigations in older patients, however, reported no significant gender differences in the incidence of TD [55–58].

The lack of studies and the inconsistency of design and methodology make it difficult to draw conclusions about gender differences in the response to antipsychotic medications. While there may be gender-related differences in some of the pharmacokinetic parameters, the clinical utility of these differences is yet to be determined. Differences between pharmacodynamic effects of antipsychotic medication are not well studied, and the results of studies investigating differences between men and women with schizophrenia and other psychotic disorders in terms of dose levels and efficacy are inconsistent at best. The inconsistencies may be related to sample characteristics, such as proportion of women to men, age differences, diagnostic heterogeneity, and variability in the severity of illness. The lack of consistency of outcome measures in efficacy studies further complicates direct comparisons. Finally, gender differences in behaviors known to affect drug doses, levels, and efficacy—such as alcohol consumption, smoking behavior, weight differences, compliance, and prescribing practices—must be considered. We believe that there is a need for well designed systematic investigations of gender differences in response to antipsychotic medications.

ACKNOWLEDGMENTS

This work was supported, in part, by NIMH grants MH43693, MH45131, MH49671–01, MH01580, Department of Veterans Affairs, and the National Alliance for Research on Schizophrenia and Depression.

REFERENCES

1. Andia AM, Zisook S, Heaton RK, Hesselink J, Jernigan T, Kuck J et al. 1995. Gender differences in schizophrenia. J Nerv Ment Dis 183: 522–8.
2. Shtasel DL, Gur RE, Gallacher F, Heimberg C, Gur RC. 1992. Gender differences in the clinical expression of schizophrenia. Schizophr Res 7: 225–31.
3. Lindamer LA, Lohr JB, Harris MJ, Jeste DV. 1997. Gender, estrogen and schizophrenia. Psychopharmacol Bull 33(2): 221–8.
4. Lewine R. 1981. Sex differences in schizophrenia: Timing or subtype? Psychol Bull 90: 432–4.
5. Lewine R. Schizophrenia: An amotivational syndrome in men. Can J Psychiatry. 1985; 30: 316–18
6. Goldstein JM, Link BG. 1988. Gender and the expression of schizophrenia. J Psychiatr Res 2: 141–55.
7. Castle DJ, Sham PC, Wessely S, Murray RM. 1994. The subtyping of schizophrenia in men and women: a latent class analysis. Psychol Med 24: 41–51.
8. Marneros A. 1984. Frequency of occurrence of Schneider's first rank symptoms in schizophrenia. Eur Arch Psychiatry Neurol Sci 234: 78–82.
9. Goldstein JM, Santangelo SL, Simpson JC, Tsuang MT. 1990. The role of gender in identifying subtypes of schizophrenia: A latent class analytic approach. Schizophr Bull 16: 263–75.
10. Arnold SE, Gur RE, Shapiro RM, Fisher KR, Moberg PJ, Gibney MR et al. 1995. Prospective clinicopathologic studies of schizophrenia: Accrual and assessment of patients. Am J Psychiatry 152: 731–7.
11. Flaum M, Arndt S, Andreasen NC. 1990. The role of gender in studies of ventricle enlargement in schizophrenia: a predominantly male effect. Am J Psychiatry 147: 1327–32.
12. Nopoulos P, Flaum M, Andreasen NC. 1997. Sex differences in brain morphology in schizophrenia. Am J Psychiatry 154: 1648–54.

13. Nasrallah H, Coffman J, Schwarzkopf S, Olson S. 1990. Reduced cerebral volume in schizophrenia. *Schizophr Res* **3**: 17.
14. The Scottish Schizophrenia Research Group. 1987. The Scottish first episode study. III. Cognitive performance. *Br J Psychiatry* **150**: 338–40.
15. Aylward E, Walker E, Bettes B. 1984. Intelligence in schizophrenia: Meta-analysis of the research. *Schizophr Bull* **10**(3): 430–59.
16. Perlick D, Mattis S, Stastny P, Teresi J. 1992. Gender differences in cognition in schizophrenia. *Schizophr Res* **8**: 69–73.
17. Goldberg TE, Gold JM, Torrey EF, Weinberger DR. 1995. Lack of sex differences in the neuropsychological performance of patients with schizophrenia. *Am J Psychiatry* **152**: 883–8.
18. Albus M, Hubmann W, Mohr F, Scherer J, Sobizack N, Franz U *et al.* 1997. Are there gender differences in neuropsychological performance in patients with first-episode schizophrenia? *Schizophr Res* **28**: 39–50.
19. Yonkers KA, Kando JC, Cole JO, Blumenthal S. 1992. Gender differences in pharmacokinetics and pharmacodynamics of psychotropic medication. *Am J Psychiatry* **149**: 587–95.
20. Yonkers KA, Hamilton JA. 1996. Sex differences in pharmacokinetics of psychotropic medications, part II: Effects on selected psychotropics. In: Jensvold MJ, Halbreich U, Hamilton JA, eds. *Psychopharmacology of Women: Sex, Gender, and Hormonal Considerations.* Washington, DC: American Psychiatric Press, Inc., pp. 43–71.
21. Yonkers KA, Kando JC, Hamilton J. 1996. Gender issues in psychopharmacologic treatment. *Ess Psychopharmacol* **1**: 54–69.
22. Dawkins K, Potter WZ. 1991. Gender differences in pharmacokinetics and pharmacodynamics of psychotropics: Focus on women. *Psychopharmacol Bull* **27**: 417–26.
23. Hamilton JA, Yonkers KA. 1996. Sex differences in pharmacokinetics of psychotropic medications, part 1: Physiological basis for effects. In: Jensvold MJ, Halbreich U, Hamilton JA, eds. *Psychopharmacology of Women: Sex, Gender, and Hormonal Considerations.* Washington, DC: American Psychiatric Press, Inc., pp. 11–42.
24. Wilson K. 1984. Sex-related differences in drug disposition in man. *Clin Pharmacokinet* **9**: 189–202.
25. Wald A, Van Thiel DH, Hoechstetter L, Egler KM, Verm R, Scott L, Lester R. Gastrointestinal transit: The effect of the menstrual cycle. *Gastroenterology* **80**: 1497–500.
26. Simpson GM, Yadalam KG, Levinson DF, Stephanos MJ, Lo ES, Cooper TB. 1990. Single-dose pharmacokinetics of fluphenazine after fluphenazine decanoate administration. *J Clin Psychopharmacol* **10**: 417–21.
27. Ereshefsky L, Saklad SR, Watanabe MD, Davis CM, Jann MW. 1991. Thiothixene pharmacokinetic interactions: A study of hepatic enzyme inducers, clearance inhibitors, and demographic variables. *J Clin Psychopharmacol* **11**: 296–301.
28. Meltzer HY, Busch DA, Fang VS. 1983. Serum neuroleptic and prolactin levels in schizophrenic patients and clinical response. *Psychiatry Res* **9**: 271–83.
29. Overall JE, Gorham DR. 1988. The Brief Psychiatric Rating Scale (BPRS): Recent developments in ascertainment and scaling. *Psychopharmacol Bull* **24**: 97–9.
30. Szymanski S, Lieberman JA, Alvir JM, Mayerhoff D, Loebel A, Geisler S *et al.* 1995. Gender differences in onset of illness, treatment response, course, and biologic indexes in first-episode schizophrenic patients. *Am J Psychiatry* **152**: 698–703.
31. Sumiyoshi T, Hasegawa M, Jayathilake K, Meltzer HY. 1997. Sex differences in plasma homovanillic acid levels in schizophrenia and normal controls: relation to neuroleptic resistance. *Biol Psychiatry* **41**: 560–6.
32. Haywood TW, Kravitz HM, Grossman LS, Cavanaugh JLJ, Davis JM, Lewis DA. 1995. Predicting the 'revolving door' phenomenon among patients with schizophrenic, schizoaffective, and affective disorders. *Am J Psychiatry* **152**: 856–61.

33. Sellwood W, Tarrier N. 1994. Demographic factors associated with extreme non-compliance in schizophrenia. *Soc Psychiatry Psychiatr Epidemiol* **29**: 172–7.
34. Zito JM, Craig TJ, Wanderling J, Siegel C. 1987. Pharmaco-epidemiology in 136 hospitalized schizophrenic patients. *Am J Psychiatry* **144**: 778–82.
35. Lieberman JA, Safferman AZ, Pollack S, Szymanski S, Johns C, Howard A *et al.* 1994. Clinical effects of clozapine in chronic schizophrenia: Response to treatment and predictors of outcome. *Am J Psychiatry* **151**: 1744–52.
36. Glick M, Mazure CM, Bowers MB, Zigler E. 1993. Premorbid social competence and the effectiveness of early neuroleptic treatment. *Compr Psychiatry* **34**: 396–401.
37. Jeste DV, Kleinman JE, Potkin SG, Luchins DJ, Weinberger DR. 1982. Ex uno multi: Subtyping the schizophrenia syndrome. *Biol Psychiatry* **17**: 199–222.
38. Hogarty GE, Goldberg SC, Schooler NR. 1974. Drug and sociotherapy in the aftercare of schizophrenic patients: III. Adjustment of nonrelapsed patients. *Arch Gen Psychiatry* **31**: 609–18.
39. Chouinard G, Annable L. 1982. Pimozide in the treatment of newly admitted schizophrenic patients. *Psychopharmacology* **76**: 13–19.
40. Szymanski S, Lieberman J, Pollack S, Kane JM, Safferman A, Munne R *et al.* 1996. Gender differences in neuroleptic nonresponsive clozapine-treated schizophrenics. *Biol Psychiatry* **39**: 249–54.
41. Zarate CA, Baldessarini RJ, Siegel AJ *et al.* 1997. Risperidone in the elderly: A pharmacoepidemiological study (abstract). *J Clin Psychiatry* **58**: 311–17.
42. Pinals DA, Malhotra AK, Missar CD, Pickar D, Breier A. 1996. Lack of gender differences in neuroleptic response in patients with schizophrenia. *Schizophr Res* **22**: 215–22.
43. Goldstein MJ, Rodnik EH, Evans JR, May PRA, Steinberg MR. 1978. Drug and family therapy in the aftercare of acute schizophrenia. *Arch Gen Psychiatry* **35**: 1169–77.
44. Young MA, Meltzer HY. 1980. The relationship of demographic, clinical and outcome variables to neuroleptic treatment requirements. *Schizophr Bull* **6**: 88–101.
45. Kolakowska T, Williams AO, Ardern M, Reveley MA, Jambor K, Gelder MG, Mandelbrote BM. 1985. Schizophrenia with good and poor outcome I: Early clinical features, response to neuroleptics and signs of organic dysfunction. *Br J Psychiatry* **146**: 229–46.
46. Chouinard G, Annable L, Mercier P, Ross-Chouinard A. 1986. A five-year follow-up study of tardive dyskinesia. *Psychopharmacol Bull* **22**(1): 259–63.
47. Andreasen NC. 1984. *The Scale for the Assessment of Positive Symptoms (SAPS)*. Iowa City: University of Iowa.
48. Andreasen NC. 1981. *The Scale for the Assessment of Negative Symptoms (SANS)*. Iowa City: University of Iowa.
49. Marriott P, Hiep A. 1978. Drug monitoring at an Australian depot phenothiazine clinic. *J Clin Psychiatry* **39**: 206–12.
50. Seeman MV. 1983. Interaction of sex, age, and neuroleptic dose. *Compr Psychiatry* **24**(2): 125–8.
51. D'Mello DA, McNeil JA. 1990. Sex differences in bipolar affective disorder: Neuroleptic dosage variance. *Compr Psychiatry* **31**: 80–3.
52. Domecq C, Naranjo CA, Ruiz I, Busto U. 1980. Sex-related variations in the frequency and characteristics of adverse drug reactions. *Int J Clin Pharmacol* **18**: 326.
53. Bottiger LE, Furhoff AK, Holmberg L. 1979. Fatal reactions to drugs. *Acta Med Scand* **205**: 451–6.
54. Kane JM, Jeste DV, Barnes TRE *et al.* 1992. *Tardive Dyskinesia: A Task Force Report of the American Psychiatric Association*. Washington, DC: American Psychiatric Association.
55. Saltz BL, Woerner MG, Kane JM, Lieberman JA, Alvir JM, Bergmann KJ *et al.* 1991. Prospective study of tardive dyskinesia incidence in the elderly. *JAMA* **266**: 2402–6.

56. Jeste DV, Lindamer LA, Evans J, Lacro JP. 1996. Relationship of ethnicity and gender to schizophrenia and pharmacology of neuroleptics. *Psychopharmacol Bull* **32**: 243–51.
57. Yassa R, Jeste DV. 1992. Gender differences in tardive dyskinesia: a critical review of the literature. *Schizophr Bull* **18**(4): 701–15.
58. Jeste DV, Caligiuri MP, Paulsen JS, Heaton RK, Lacro JP, Harris MJ *et al.* 1995. Risk of tardive dyskinesia in older patients: A prospective longitudinal study of 266 patients. *Arch Gen Psychiatry* **52**: 756–65.

30

National Institute of Mental Health: An Update on Women and Minorities in Research

Rick A. Martinez

Janssen Pharmaceutical Inc., Titusville, NJ, USA

INTRODUCTION

In 1998, the US Congress appropriated $12.9 billion to the 17 institutes that comprise The National Institute of Health (NIH). As the world's single largest biomedical research institute, the NIH supports over 30 000 research projects in heart disease, cancer, stroke, AIDS, mental illness and other diseases that threaten the public health.

Over 17 000 academic centers receive NIH funding to conduct biomedical research. These studies ultimately lead to changes in standards of care and health policy; therefore, when claims are made about the efficacy and effectiveness of new interventions, it is important to understand the nature of these effects in all patients, including women and members of minority groups. The generalizability of new research findings is a scientific concern. It is also a public policy issue that has been addressed by legislation mandating administrative efforts to improve the quality of this work. This chapter discusses NIH policy designed to address this issue and reviews information about administrative efforts to streamline NIH grants and how to plan a research career.

Although the focus of this review deals with topics concerning women and ethnic minorities, the information presented is applicable to all candidates for federal research awards, regardless of gender or ethnicity.

INCLUSION OF WOMEN AND MINORITIES IN STUDY POPULATIONS

When members of Congress asked its General Accounting Office to determine how women and minorities were represented in NIH-sponsored trials, it discovered that

Cross Cultural Psychiatry. Edited by John M. Herrera, William B. Lawson and John J. Sramek.
© 1999 John Wiley & Sons Ltd.

the NIH had 'no readily accessible source of data on the demographics of [the institute's] study populations' [1]. In addition, members of minority groups have traditionally been underrepresented in clinical trials [2–4].

Including women of childbearing age in clinical trials is not without its risks, but undue caution has caused their underrepresentation problem in important clinical trials. Concern about fetal teratogenicity is legitimate reason for concern; however, liability is the purview of proper informed consent. It is the opinion of officials at NIH that as long as warnings of potential risks are part of a woman's consent to participate in research, 'it is unlikely that she will succeed in any subsequent negligence action . . .' [5].

The research community's lack of outreach to minority populations is addressed by NIH policy, but suspicion of the healthcare system among people of color is another dimension to this problem.

According to Annette Dulla the lack of trust is 'justified' given the history of ethical violations in medicine—such as various state involuntary sterilization projects and the infamous Tuskegee Syphilis Project [6]. Yet this suspicion does not serve minority groups well and a lack of knowledge about the effects of new treatments is harmful to the public health. Nor should these types of sentiments deter investigators from approaching ethnic populations. In a review of factors influencing participation in research, Arean and Gallagher-Thompson found that belonging to an ethnic group was not associated with responding to or dropping out of a study. They did find that 'the recruitment and retention strategies, do differ [between white and non-white subjects]' [7]. Direct contact with community leaders, health education efforts, travel and caregiver reimbursement are useful strategies for engaging ethnic minority populations [8].

In 1993, the US Congress addressed the historical underrepresentation of women and minorities in clinical treatment trials with the National Institutes of Health Revitalization Act (section 492B of Public Law 103–43) [9]. The new law authorized the NIH Offices of Research on Woman's Health and Minority Health to develop guidelines that would apply to all grants submitted after June 1, 1994. The new policy contains some provisions that differ substantially from the 1990 rules.

Overall, the guidelines reflect the spirit of the law, which is intended to relieve problems of sample bias in federally funded clinical studies. Except in situations where the trials are inappropriate with respect to the health of the subjects or purpose of the research (for example, a prostate cancer trial would exclude women), each institute must ensure that women and minorities are included in all clinical research studies. In particular, phase III clinical trials must include both groups in treatment studies. The law also prohibits the use of cost as a consideration for excluding members of each group from such trials.

IMPACT OF THE NIH REAUTHORIZATION ACT

In response to the legislation, NIH has been compiling data on the number of women and minorities enrolled in intramural and extramural sponsored trials. The fiscal year 1995, the first full year of guideline implementation, serves as the baseline for future comparisons. Interestingly, the data show that women and minorities have been enrolled in substantial numbers. In fiscal year 1995, approximately 61% of subjects in NIH-sponsored trials were women. Native, Hispanic, Asian, and African Americans were 2%, 8%, 9% and 12% of the subjects enrolled [10].

Institutional review boards (also known as study sections) have the primary responsibility for ensuring that these guidelines are implemented in their review of research applications. The formal peer-review process is actively engaged in evaluating grant applications under the new guidelines. NIH has prepared a handbook (*NIH Outreach on the Inclusion of Women and Minorities in Biomedical and Behavioral Research*) to address investigators' questions about the new rules. The booklet contains general information about the guidelines as well as advice on how to enhance outreach efforts to improve recruitment and retention of women and minority subjects. This booklet can be obtained by writing to the Office of Research and Women's Health at NIH, Building 10, Room 201, 9000 Rockville Pike, Bethesda, MD 20892 or by fax. (301) 402–1798.

THE (REORGANIZED) NATIONAL INSTITUTE OF MENTAL HEALTH

In 1998, the US Congress appropriated over $750 million to NIMH. Each year, the bulk of the institute's budget is spent maintaining a national academic infrastructure designed to advance the treatment and prevention of mental illness. Funding for extramural research occurs through three of its five divisions. In 1997, the three divisions were reorganized from a disorders-based to a neuroscience/intervention-based administrative structure. This reorganization created the divisions of Basic and Clinical Neuroscience Research, Services and Intervention Research and Mental Disorders, Behavioral Research and AIDS.

NIMH GRANTS AND AWARD MECHANISMS

The Application Packet

The Public Health Service 398 form is required for all new, revised competing continuation, and supplemental research submissions to NIH. This application packet was revised in May 1995 and is available on request from the Center for Scientific Review (formerly the Grants Information Office, Division of Research Grants), National Institutes of Health, 6701 Rockledge Drive, Room 1040, MSC 7710, Bethesda, MD 20892–7710; phone (301) 435–0714 (you may download applications and other NIH publications from the Internet at http://www.nih.gov). Investigators should anticipate that NIH would eventually be able to accept electronic submission of grants; information about this development will be published in the NIH Guide.

The Crisis in Clinical Research and Career Development

Most US house officers complete their clinical training with almost no formal coursework or hands-on experience in research methodology. The pipeline of new clinical researchers is threatened by a number of other constrictions including high medical school debts and low salaries for fellows. In addition, academic health centers located in areas of high managed care penetration have experienced a relative decline in NIH extramural awards [11]. These factors, along with the perception that NIH peer review is biased in favor of supporting PhD basic science researchers over MDs has contributed to what many consider a crisis in clinical research [12].

The research project award (RO1) is the pre-eminent federal grant awarded to an independent investigator. However, there are other NIH research award mechanisms that are organized by career level, the type of previous training, and whether a mentor is required.

To address the pressing need in clinical research training and career development, NIH Director Harold Varmus announced the creation of three new training and career awards in 1998. The Mentored Patient-Oriented Research Development Award (K23), the Mid-Career Investigator in Patient-Oriented Research Development Award (K24) and an Institutional Curriculum Award (K30) were created to bridge the gap between the bench and bedside. The first two are designed to free up the clinician's time from direct patient care in order to obtain didactic training (K23) or to dedicate time for research and mentoring (K24). The K30 is designed for institutions to develop high-quality courses in biostatistics, epidemiology, study design and ethics [13].

These awards are offered in addition to NIH's usual grant mechanisms for new investigators who need additional training and mentoring before they are ready to compete for an independent research project grant. In 1995, six career development awards replaced 14 previous career development mechanisms. Individuals with health-professional degrees who need support to obtain an intensive, supervised research experience may apply for the Mentored Clinical Scientists Development (K08) Award. This replaces four older mechanisms, including the former Scientist Development Award for Clinicians (K20). Specific details about these and other changes can be obtained from the NIH Guide [14].

NIMH Minority and Women's Supplements

In the autumn of 1993, NIH announced an 'emphasis' on the use of administrative supplements to attract underrepresented minorities into biomedical and behavioral research [15]. The supplemental funding, made available to a parent grant, is designed for junior researchers (graduate and postgraduate) but includes high school and undergraduate minority individuals. The principal investigator initiates the actual application process on behalf of the minority investigator. The application packet is submitted to the NIMH program staff, not the Center for Scientific Review. NIH has also moved forward with efforts to increase the number of women researchers, with modified versions of the administrative supplement. Principal investigators are advised to contact program staff before initiating this award mechanism.

PLANNING A RESEARCH CAREER

Formulating a Research Question

The competitive nature of applying for federal research grants and the myriad of award mechanisms available may at first seem intimidating, but candidates must consider several options in planning an academic career. In most cases, junior investigator exposure to research occurs during the clinical research fellowship. After completing the fellowship the new faculty member must determine an area of research interest, collect pilot data and endeavor to publish in the area of interest. This process helps to focus the young investigator's questions, refine methodology, and generate hypotheses for systematic study. Some junior researchers spend a great deal of time anticipating which topics or ideas for research are the most 'fundable' and assume that agency staff possess some secret knowledge about research ideas. The truth is, ideas for projects come from the field, not NIMH staff. Agency and institute priorities emerge from scientific perspectives that are crafted and developed in public forums such as scientific meetings, consensus conferences, and medical journals. This body of scientific information is the best source of information for generating hypotheses for investigation.

Finding Mentors

Finding a mentor is an important step in career planning. A senior faculty member who has successfully competed for federal (and non-federal) research money is an invaluable resource to the beginning researcher. Ideally, counsel from an experienced mentor can help the researcher to organize an academic career by providing advice on scientific topics and tips on preparing a federal award application. NIMH program staff can also make useful contributions in terms of discussing ideas for possible studies, reviewing draft proposals, and providing general technical assistance around a particular research project or idea.

Choosing the Right Award Mechanism

Once potential researchers have decided to commit time to a research career, applicants can take advantage of entry-level NIH career development awards.

These provide significant portions of investigators' salaries, to relieve them of clinical responsibilities that can draw them away from research activities. The Mentored Clinical Scientist Award (K08), mentioned earlier, provides salary and up to $50 000 for research development support for tuition, fees, supplies, and equipment. For the candidate with a research doctorate (and in some cases a health-professional doctorate) a comparable mentored experience is provided with the Mentored Research Scientist Development Award (K01). After 3–5 years of support from the mentored awards, investigators will have had sufficient time to accumulate pilot data and enough research experience that should one day make them competitive for an RO1 award as an independent investigator.

CONCLUSION

NIH seeks to address the underrepresentation of minorities and women in research. The strategy has two fronts—to increase their numbers in clinical trials and among the ranks of investigators who receive federal funding. Recent legislative efforts have partially remedied the situation. However, the field of biomedicine must pursue these goals with the same rigor with which it pursues all scientific questions.

Planning an academic research career in medicine, regardless of gender or ethnicity, is no simple matter. The commitment in time, effort, and patience extracts a great deal from individuals who choose to balance clinical responsibilities and data generation with other important personal obligations. Getting started requires supportive department chairs and deans who can help launch an academic career. This is crucial because obtaining funding usually takes several submissions before it finally receives funding. As a result, maintaining this career requires that new faculty must become sophisticated consumers of NIH programs and federal (and non-federal) funding mechanisms.

REFERENCES

1. Nadel MV. 1990. National Institutes of Health: Problems Implementing Policy on Women in Study Populations. US General Accounting Office, testimony before the Subcommittee on Health and the Environment, Committee on Energy and Commerce, US House of Representatives, 18 June.
2. Thomas C, Pinto H, Roach M et al. 1994. Participation in clinical trials: is it state-of-the-art treatment for African-Americans and other people of color? *J Natl Med Assoc* **86**: 177–81.
3. Svensson CK. 1989. Representation of American Blacks in clinical trials of new drugs. *JAMA* **261**: 263–5.
4. El-Sadr W, Capps L. 1992. The challenge of minority recruitment in clinical trials for AIDS. *JAMA* **267**: 954–7.

5. Hayunga EG, Rothenberg KH, Pinn V. 1996. Women of childbearing potential in clinical research: Perspectives on NIH policy and liability issues. *Food Drug Med Device Law Dig* **13**: 7–11.
6. Dulla A. 1994. African American suspicion of the healthcare system is justified: What do we do about it? *Camb Quart Healthcare Ethics* **3**: 347–57.
7. Arean PA, Gallagher-Thompson D. 1996. Issues and recommendations for the recruitment and retention of older ethnic minority adults into clinical research. *J Consult Clin Psychol* **64**: 875–80.
8. Harris Y, Gorelick PH, Samuels P et al. 1996. Why African-Americans may not be participating in clinical trials. *J Natl Med Assoc* **88**: 630–4.
9. *Federal Register* March 28, 1994; reprinted in *NIH Guide for Grants and Contracts*, March 18, 1994, vol. 23, no. 11.
10. Communication from the Office of Women's Health, Office of the Director, National Institutes of Health.
11. Shine K. 1997. Some imperatives for clinical research. Commentaries. *JAMA* **278**: 245–6.
12. Thompson JN, Moskowitz J. Preventing the extinction of the clinical research ecosystem. *JAMA* **278**: 241–5.
13. National Institute of Health. 1998. Clinical Research Curriculum Award. National Institute of Health Guide (on-line), http://www.nih.gov/grants/guide/rfa-files/RFA-OD-98-007.html
14. National Institute of Health. 1995. Mentored Clinical Scientist Development Award. National Institute of Health Guide (on-line), 24(15). http://www.nih.gov/grants/guide/1995/95.04.28/pa-mentored-clinical010.html
15. National Institute of Health. 1993. Research Supplements for Underrepresented Minorities. National Institute of Health Guide (on-line), 22(3). http://www.nih.gov/grants/guide/1993/93.11.26/notice-research-supp003.html

Children and Adolescents

31

Interethnic Psychopharmacologic Research in Children and Adolescents

James J. Hudziak and Lawrence P. Rudiger

University of Vermont, Burlington, VT, USA

INTRODUCTION

It is estimated that up to 8 million children currently suffer from some type of severe emotional and behavioral or mental disorder [1]. Despite the demand for treating this group and the ever-increasing number of psychopharmacologic agents available, there has been little scientific evidence to support the use of most psychopharmacologic compounds in children. For those agents for which pharmacodynamic data are available the research has been almost exclusively limited to studies of a single ethnic group. Vitiello and Jensen state, 'Because of the lack of knowledge in this area [pediatric psychopharmacology], physicians and families are forced to make difficult choices, based upon extrapolating information concerning safety and efficacy from studies of adults with similar conditions' [1]. This lack of basic information and a scarcity of empirically sound developmental psychopharmacologic approaches has led some to refer to the child psychiatric patient as a 'therapeutic orphan' [2], and to pediatric psychopharmacologic research as a 'methodologic orphan' [3].

Much of what is known about interethnic pediatric psychopharmacology comes from recent research, but most of these studies were conducted on adults. A brief review of this literature, combined with the broader needs of pediatric psychopharmacology, will allow us to discuss specific issues of pharmacoepidemiology, pharmacokinetics, pharmacodynamics, and developmental psychopharmacology. In addition, we will consider drug efficacy and effectiveness as they relate to comorbidity and compliance from an interethnic perspective.

Cross Cultural Psychiatry. Edited by John M. Herrera, William B. Lawson and John J. Sramek.
© 1999 John Wiley & Sons Ltd.

INTERETHNIC CHILDHOOD EPIDEMIOLOGY AND PHARMACOEPIDEMIOLOGY

Rates of childhood psychopathology in all ethnic groups command considerable interest among researchers and clinicians. The National Institute of Mental Health has recently launched a broad-based general epidemiologic study of childhood psychopathology—the Use, Need, Outcomes, and Costs in Child and Adolescent Populations (UNO-CAP) [4]. This has three broad goals. First, it will bring rigorous diagnostic and methodological measurements to the field. Second, it will report on the prevalence of mental disorders among children of all ethnic groups. Finally, it will provide data on service utilization associated with childhood emotional and behavioral problems. Until this information is made available, little will be known about the general rates of psychopathology in childhood.

Although a number of studies have reported rates of individual disorders, many have been confounded by ascertainment bias and methodological questions. Costello and colleagues [5] reported epidemiologic rates of childhood psychopathology from the primary care perspective. Their study has served as a benchmark for the field, but it falls short of the general epidemiologic research needed to understand interethnic differences [5]. In the only large-scale general population-based study of childhood psychopathology reported to date, race did not account for an appreciable amount of variance of rates of psychopathology [6]. In addition, other scholars using similar methodology have reported on base rates and impairment of psychopathologic conditions in other countries. These reports have contributed to current knowledge about national differences in the rates of psychopathology [7]. However, none of these studies reported on DSM diagnosis rates and therefore they may not be generalizable to studies that use categorical diagnostic systems. However, in spite of this limitation they will serve as a basis of comparison for the UNO-CAP and other reports on interethnic rates of psychopathology. While the appropriate methodological approach to general epidemiologic studies of children remains unclear (for example in children aged 3–6), it is hoped that the UNO-CAP study will demonstrate interethnic differences in rates of childhood psychopathology. However, it is clear that an understanding of how psychiatric disorders vary in their presentation and prevalence within different populations will help clinicians respond to the needs of diverse groups.

Interethnic Pharmacoepidemiology

Porta and Hartzema [8] describe pharmacoepidemiology as 'the application of epidemiologic knowledge, methods, and reasoning to the study of the effects (beneficial and adverse) and uses of drugs in human populations'. The use of pharmacoepidemiology in childhood psychopharmacology has been addressed by Costello and associates [9], who reported on differential prescribing techniques used for children and adolescents. Pharmacoepidemiology is of special importance to child psychiatry because, as Geller [10] and Zito and Riddle [11] have pointed out, there are significant distinctions between adult and pediatric psychopharmacology. Zito and Riddle [11] outline the importance of addressing drug evaluation questions 'from an epidemiologic research perspective' that would 'extend the current research model by ensuring that knowledge of drug use prevalence is routinely made available'. They point out that the study of pharmacoepidemiology may also help researchers measure long-term effectiveness and develop systematic methods for assessing drug safety. These techniques should also help to explain interethnic variations in children's responses to medications. Such an understanding is important because of the potential pharmacogenetic, pharmacokinetic, and sociologic variations among different ethnic groups.

INTERETHNIC PHARMACOGENETICS

Interethnic pharmacokinetics has received increased attention over the past 15 years. Progress has been made in understanding ethnic differences in response to various medications [12–16]; however, the importance of these findings has been compromised by various methodological problems. Strickland and colleagues [17] attribute these shortcomings to diagnostic misclassification, the treatment of various ethnic groups in a homogeneous and undifferentiated manner, failure to control for age and gender, and minimal consideration for chronicity of illness. Nevertheless, a number of authors have been able to report interethnic pharmacokinetic differences in populations of adult Asians, Hispanic, African Americans, Native Americans, and Caucasians [15–20]. Pharmacogenetics, with its ability to both identify specific alleles and pinpoint activity at these alleles, can be particularly informant of interethnic pharmacokinetics. It is important to note that, regardless of a sample's ethnicity, pharmacogenetic variability is often reported in within-race pharmacokinetic studies [21]. Such variability should be expected in all ethnic groups.

An example of the impact of pharmacogenetics on pharmacokinetics is the recent discovery of the genetic polymorphisms identified in the human cytochrome P450 (CYP) system. It is known that each CYP isoenzyme is the product of a separate gene, and a number of these genes have multiple alleles that result in genetic polymorphisms. As DeVane summarizes [22], both CY2D6 and CYP2C gene families are polymorphic. A number of the polymorphisms result in dysfunctional enzymes and may thus directly affect drug metabolism [23]. The CYP2D6 polymorphism, debrisoquine hydroxylase, is found on the long arm of chromosome 22. This polymorphism is associated with a poor or slow metabolizer group and an extensive metabolizer group [24, 25]. Interethnic differences in the rates of these polymorphisms have been reported, with the slow metabolizer group found in 5–8% of Whites, 2–10% of African Americans, and 2–10% of Asians. Other researchers have observed intraethnic variability. For example, Masimirembwa reported differences between frequency rates of slow metabolizers in African Americans (2–10%) and in a Black Zimbabwean population (1.8%) [26].

Striking differences have also been found in other putative neurotransmitter allele frequencies. Comings and co-workers reported that 46% of American Caucasians with attention deficit/hyperactivity disorder (ADHD) had the CYPD2R allele while only 20% of those without ADHD had the same polymorphism [27]. Much excitement ensued about a possible association between this polymorphism and ADHD. This finding was then contrasted with interethnic variations. Barr and Kidd conducted a general population study complete with interethnic subtyping and found the Al allele in 75% of American Muskoke Indians [28]. While the importance of this discovery is not yet clear, it once again demonstrates the importance of identifying interethnic and intraethnic genetic differences at those genes and receptors involved in pharmacodynamics.

As with all non-mendelian genetic studies (those that do not attend to autosomal dominant, autosomal recessive, or sex-linked patterns of inheritance), it is important to recognize that the effects of genes are highly interrelated with interactions with other genes and environmental influences. As Lin and colleagues point out, pharmacokinetic studies should 'be designed not only to ascertain differences in drug responses, but also to examine genetic and environmental (e.g., diet, exposure to enzyme inducers) factors that may contribute to these differences. Pharmacogenetic probes could be used in combination with studies examining pharmacokinetic and pharmacodynamic issues for such purposes' [30]. Because these results are culled from interethnic pharmacogenetic studies of adults it is important to conduct similar investigations in children that might account for unique developmental pharmacokinetic effects.

INTERETHNIC PHARMACOKINETICS AND PHARMACODYNAMICS

Both pharmacokinetics and pharmacodynamics may vary among children from different ethnic groups. Although pharmacodynamic effects may be influenced by some of the pharmacogenetic distinctions and similarities outlined above, developmental processes may also influence pharmacokinetic variability. For descriptions of pharmacokinetics in children and adolescents we refer the reader to a pair of review articles on this subject [10, 29]. Drug absorption, first-pass effect, distribution, metabolism, and excretion properties all change during childhood and this variability can be modulated by pharmacogenetic differences. Once again, a number of interethnic variations have been reported in the adult literature. When aminoglycoside pharmacokinetics were compared no differences were found among Asian, Hispanic, and Caucasian adults [20]. However, Lin and colleagues [30] reported that when comparing Asian and non-Asian subjects 'pharmacokinetic differences have been consistently found with haloperidol and some benzodiazepines while results of studies focusing on tricyclic antidepressants have been inconclusive' [18]. Mendoza and colleagues noted that, while there is ample evidence for differences in drug response and disposition among certain ethnic groups, we know relatively little about

Latino and Native American populations [16]. Strickland and associates reported that, although differences have been observed for African Americans, the research findings have been inconsistent, largely due to methodological limitations [17]. In general, there is a paucity of solid interethnic research on psychopharmacokinetics even in adults, and certainly in children and adolescents. As Rudorfer writes: 'Ethnic background can significantly influence the metabolism and the pharmacodynamics of a variety of drugs' [12]. Other researchers have pointed out that a 'fundamental understanding of developmental pharmacokinetics is a necessary prerequisite to the safe, effective administration of psychotropic medications to children and adolescents' [29]. What is not yet known is the degree to which ethnicity might influence pharmacokinetics and dynamics in children and adolescents.

INTERETHNIC STUDIES OF EFFICACY VERSUS EFFECTIVENESS

For a review of the importance of post-marketing studies in pediatric psychopharmacology relating to effectiveness we refer the reader to Zito and Riddle [11]. Subjects engaged in drug trials tend to be homogeneous. Compared with a general population they are likely to have few rather than multiple psychiatric disorders, typical rather than atypical presentations, an absence of coexisting medical conditions, and less severe social and family problems. Therefore, the issue of efficacy and effectiveness is particularly important in studies of interethnic psychopharmacology.

It is not yet clear which cultural biases might influence how patients take psychiatric medications. In addition, prescribing practices are not consistent across countries [31, 32]. Other reports indicate that there are cultural variations in the diagnosis and treatment of childhood psychopathology, such as ADHD [33–37]. Moreover, because children from these populations may be more likely to drop out of studies the impact of selective subject loss should be considered [38]. Finally, socioeconomic status must be accounted for, as children from lower socioeconomic strata of all races will have higher rates of psychopathology and may be less likely to receive psychiatric treatment [39].

Studies of drug safety and efficacy involving children from various ethnic groups need to be conducted, along with post-marketing effectiveness research to determine how medications perform where there is ethnic, socioeconomic, and family constellation variability. These data could enhance clinicians' ability to make more informed decisions regarding issues of efficacy and effectiveness in a full range of diverse populations.

SUMMARY

Interethnic pediatric psychopharmacology is essentially unstudied. It will be informed by large-scale epidemiology studies (such as UNO-CAP) to establish rates of psychopathology at sequential developmental levels; it will be advanced by pharmacokinetic studies of children from many ethnic groups at the major developmental stages; it will benefit from future pharmacogenetic studies to establish genetic and environmental contributions to pharmacodynamic phenomena. Finally, research is needed that considers not only the efficacy but also the effectiveness of new agents within and across ethnically diverse populations.

REFERENCES

1. Vitiello B, Jensen P. 1995. Developing clinical trials in children and adolescents: Developmental perspectives in pediatric psychopharmacology. *Psychopharmacol Bull* **31**: 75–81.
2. Shirkey H. 1968. Therapeutic orphans. *J Pediatr* **72**: 119.
3. Bonati M. 1994. Epidemiologic evaluation of drug use in children. *J Clin Pharmacol* **34**: 300–5.
4. UNO-CAP. 1994. *Use, Need, Outcomes, and Costs in Child and Adolescent Populations.* Department of Health and Human Services, Public Health Service, National Institutes of Health, and National Institute of Mental Health.
5. Costello EJ, Costello AJ, Edelbrock C. 1988. Psychiatric disorders in pediatric primary care: Prevalence and risk factors. *Arch Gen Psychiatry* **45**: 1107–16.
6. Achenbach TM, Howell CA, McConaughy SH, Stanger C. 1995. Six year predictors of problems in a national sample of children and youth: III. Transitions to young adult syndromes. *J Am Acad Child Adolesc Psychiatry* **34**: 658–69.
7. Ferdinand RF, Verhulst FC, Wiznitzer M. 1995. Continuity and change of self-reported problem behaviors from adolescence into young adulthood. *J Am Acad Child Adolesc Psychiatry* **34**: 680–90.
8. Porta MS, Hartzema AG. 1987. The contribution of epidemiology to the study of drugs. *Drug Intell Clin Pharm* **21**: 741–7.
9. Costello EJ, Burns BJ, Angold A. 1993. How can epidemiology improve mental health services for children and adolescents? *J Am Acad Child Adolesc Psychiatry* **32**: 1106–14.
10. Geller B. 1991. Psychopharmacology of children and adolescents: Pharmacokinetics and relationships of plasma/serum levels to response. *Psychopharmacol Bull* **27**: 401–9.
11. Zito JM, Riddle MA. 1995. Psychiatric pharmacoepidemiology for children. *Child Adolesc Psychiatr Clin North Am* **4**: 77–95.
12. Rudorfer MV. 1993. Pharmacokinetics and psychiatric drugs. *J Clin Psychiatry* **54**: 50–4.
13. Wood AJ, Zhou HH. 1991. Ethnic differences in drug disposition and responsiveness. *Clin Pharmacokinet* **20**: 350–73.
14. Moussaoui D. 1992. Transethnic and transcultural psychopharmacology. *Clin Neuropharmacol* **15**: 485A–6A.
15. Lin KM, Shen WW. 1991. Pharmacotherapy for Southeast Asian psychiatric patients. *J Nerv Ment Dis* **179**: 346–50.
16. Mendoza R, Smith MQ, Poland RE, Lin KM, Strickland TL. 1991. Ethnic psychopharmacology: The Hispanic and Native American perspective. *Psychopharmacol Bull* **27**: 449–61.
17. Strickland TL, Ranganath V, Lin KM, Poland RE, Mendoza R, Smith MW. 1991. Psychopharmacologic considerations in the treatment of Black American populations. *Psychopharmacol Bull* **27**: 442–8.
18. Lin KM, Han CY, Lin BK, Hardy S. 1993. Slow acetylator mutations in the human

polymorphic *N*-acetyltransferase gene in 786 Asians, Blacks, Hispanics, and Whites: Application to metabolic epidemiology. *Am J Hum Genet* **54**: 827–34.

19. Shimoda K, Minowada T, Noguchi T, Takahashi S. 1993. Inter-individual variations of desmethylation and hydroxylation of clomipramine in an Oriental psychiatric population. *J Clin Pharmacol* **13**: 181–8.

20. Jhee SS, Burm JP, Gill MA. 1994. Comparison of aminoglycoside pharmacokinetics in Asian, Hispanic, and Caucasian patients by using population pharmacokinetic methods. *Antimicrob Agents Chemother* **28**: 2073–7.

21. Evans DA, Mahgoub A, Sland TP. 1980. A family and populations study of the genetic polymorphism of debrisoquine oxidation in a White British population. *J Med Genet* **17**: 102–5.

22. DeVane CL. 1994. Pharmacogenetics and drug metabolism of newer antidepressant agents. *J Clin Psychiatry* **55**: 38–45.

23. Nelson DR, Kamataki T, Waxman DJ. 1993. The P450 superfamily: Update on new sequences, gene mapping, accession numbers, early trivial names of enzymes, and nomenclature. *DNA Cell Biol* **12**: 1–51.

24. Brosen K. 1990. Recent developments in hepatic drug oxidation: Implications for clinical. *Clin Pharmacokinet* **18**: 220–39.

25. Cholerton S, Daly AK, Idle JR. 1992. The role of individual human cytochromes P450 in drug metabolism and clinical response. *Trends Pharmacol Sci* **13**: 434–9.

26. Masimirembwa CM, Johansson I, Hasler JA. 1993. Genetic polymorphism of cytochrome P450 CYP2D6 in Zimbabwean population. *Pharmacogenetics* **3**: 275–80.

27. Comings DE, Muhleman D, Dietz G, Shahbahrami B. 1991. The dopamine D2 receptor locus as a modifying gene in neuropsychiatric disorders. *JAMA* **266**: 1793–1800.

28. Barr CL, Kidd KK. 1993. Population frequencies of the A1 allele at the dopamine 2 receptor locus. *Biol Psychiatry* **34**: 204–9.

29. Clein PD, Riddle MA. 1995. Pharmacokinetics in children and adolescents. *Child Adolesc Psychiatr Clin North Am* **4**: 59–75.

30. Lin KM, Poland RE, Smith MW, Strickland TL, Mendoza R. 1991. Pharmacokinetic and other related factors affecting psychotropic responses in Asians. *Psychopharmacol Bull* **27**: 427–39.

31. Granat M. 1977. Inter-Nordic variations in sales of medicines. *Nordic Statistics on Medicines: Parts I and II*. Uppsala: Nordic Council on Medicines, pp. 21–24.

32. Trott GE, Wirth S, Badura F, Firese HJ, Nissen G. 1993. Use of drugs by 7 to 14 year-old children: Results of a parental survey (English translation). *Z Kinder Jugenpsychiatr* **21**: 148–55.

33. Hiltbrunner B. 1990. Attention deficit disorder in Switzerland. In: Conners K, Kinsbourne M, eds. *Attention Deficit Hyperactivity Disorder*. Munich: Medizin Verlag Munchen.

34. Anderson J. 1990. Attention deficit disorder in New Zealand. In: Conners K, Kinsbourne M, eds. *Attention Deficit Hyperactivity Disorder*. Munich: Medizin Verlag Munchen, pp. 162–71.

35. Sauceda JM, de la Vega E. 1990. Attention deficit disorder in Mexico. In: Conners K, Kinsbourne M, eds. *Attention Deficit Hyperactivity Disorder*. Munich: Medizin Verlag Munchen.

36. Luk SL. 1990. Childhood hyperactivity in a Chinese population. In: Conners K, Kinsbourne M, eds. *Attention Deficit Hyperactivity Disorder*. Munich: Medizin Verlag Munchen, pp. 177–81.

37. Cartwright JD. 1990. Attention Deficit Disorder in South Africa. In: Conners K, Kinsbourne M, eds. *Attention Deficit Hyperactivity Disorder*. Munich: Medizin Verlag Munchen.

38. Gould MS, Shaffer D, Kaplan D. 1985. The characteristics of dropouts from a child psychiatry clinic. *J Am Acad Child Adolesc Psychiatry* **24**: 316–28.
39. McLoyd VC. 1988. Socioeconomic disadvantage and child development. *Am Psychol* **53**: 185–204.

32

Psychopharmacology of Children and Adolescents

Diane Buckingham
Truman Medical Center, Overland Parks, KS, USA

INTRODUCTION

While there is continuous controversy regarding the efficacy of medication used in children and adolescents, there exists only a limited amount of literature pertaining to studies of children and even less on children of color [1]. In the past, children of color have been found to have had a higher likelihood of being diagnosed with schizophrenia than European Americans. With the lack of available clinical study literature, underlying issues, cultural variation, and diagnosis all need to be examined when trying to assess psychiatric symptoms in children and adolescents. In this chapter, our efforts are to review the use of algorithms to guide psycho-pharmaceutical treatment in children and adolescents. The algorithms are based on DSM-IV criteria and will illustrate options in the treatment of various childhood psychiatric disorders.

Overall, physicians often strive to treat conditions without medication, with special consideration taken towards children and adolescents. This is because considerable controversy persists regarding medication in young patients [2, 3]. Even so, physicians do sometimes elect to use psychotherapeutic medications on children and adolescents. Those medications that are normally used are listed in the following classes: antidepressants, antipsychotics, mood stabilizers, anxiolytics, and psychostimulants.

As one reviews the potential drug reaction implications and research, it should be kept in mind that psychopharmacological investigations have not been performed on children and adolescents. As such, the primary approved indications of these medications do not normally cover how the clinician typically uses them in practice on children and adolescents. The attached algorithms may be used by the clinician in guiding the decision to use medication. This clinical decision should also be based on the review of the problem list (symptoms, comorbid conditions), symptom intensity, symptom frequency, and symptom duration. A detailed evaluation should

Cross Cultural Psychiatry. Edited by John M. Herrera, William B. Lawson and John J. Sramek.

include screening for physical, psychophysiological, family, and social history. Clarify with the child the symptoms that interfere with home, school, and social life. Find out the time of onset and duration of the symptoms and review the interventions that have already been taken to reduce the symptoms. It is also important to screen the ability of the child and family to be receptive and understand each other and to understand your recommendation. When educating the child or adolescent, note their ability to retain information. The capability to recollect information is important in deciding how to treat the condition. Screening the patient for medical conditions, environmental and developmental issues will also provide a better understanding of the potential for prognosis and remission and thus guide psychotropic intervention strategies.

ALGORITHM USAGE IN CHILDREN AND ADOLESCENTS

Algorithm decision-making is based on reviewing the risks and benefits of a medication. The first step of this process is to review the targeted symptoms of the child or adolescent. The next step is to review their past responses to medication and adverse events profile. Third, a realistic response to the targeted symptoms with the medication step must be determined. Be sure to review the option of monotherapy: this is usually attempted but sometimes ineffective. Also remember to review the therapeutic response and blood levels, issues of chasing adverse effects, tolerance response to medication versus the impact of the environment, and any rebound response effect.

ANTIDEPRESSANTS

Psychotherapy continues to be effective in the treatment of depression in children and adolescents but often needs to be augmented with antidepressants due to the impairment of home, school and social life. The efficiency of the use of antidepressant medication in children and adolescents remains controversial. Even so, a few studies have noted some improvement of depressive symptoms with medication [4]. The best method to adopt when prescribing antidepressants is to start with a low dose and gradually increase the dose until the required therapeutic level is obtained.

Major depression can be treated with various medications such as the selective serotonin reuptake inhibitors (SSRIs), tricyclic antidepressants, selective dopamine reuptake inhibitors, $5HT_2$-receptor antagonists, and selective serotonin norepinephrine reuptake inhibitors (SSNRIs). The SSRIs include fluoxetine, sertraline, paroxetine, and fluvoxamine. Few adverse effects are associated with these medications. With all SSRIs, however, caution must be maintained not to induce a hyperexcitable adolescent to a hypomanic or manic-type state. The first line of treatment usually taken in major depression of children and adolescents is fluoxetine, sertraline, or paroxetine. These drugs are also useful for the treatment

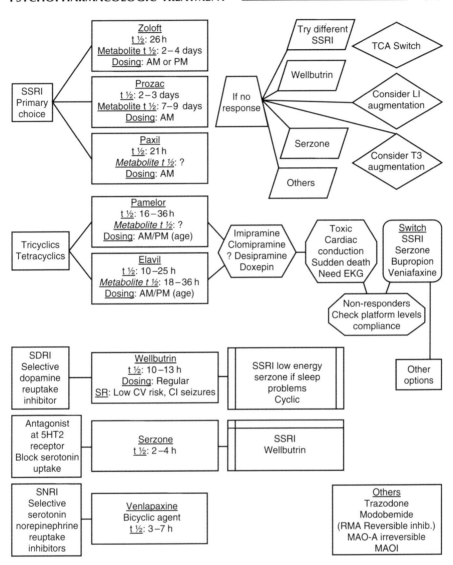

FIGURE 32.1 Major depression: medication decision tree

of panic disorder, obsessive-compulsive disorder, and Tourette syndrome. Of these medications, fluoxetine has a longer half-life and is perhaps more useful for non-compliance. Sertraline, which sometimes has a shorter half-life, also has a calming type of effect on the more irritable, angry, depressed adolescents. Paroxetine has been reported to be more useful for those adolescents that have more problems with anxiety and sleep while fluvoxamine has been recommended as a treatment for obsessive-compulsive disorder.

The second line of treatment for depression in children and adolescents is the use of Wellbutrin (bupropion hydrochloride), which has undergone some limited control studies in children and adolescents, although no reportable studies have reviewed the efficacy in children and adolescents of color. Wellbutrin has been shown to be useful in children with comorbid depression and attention deficit hyperactivity disorder (ADHD). Serzone, a triazolopyridine, is also recommended in the treatment of adolescents with sleep problems. SSNRIs such as venlafaxine have not been studied in children of color, though some studies have shown these medications to be useful in children with mood disorder and ADHD. Another course of action is to use tricyclic antidepressants, the efficacy of which in the treatment of children with depression has not been proven, but which have been useful in the treatment of ADHD with some mood symptoms.

MOOD STABILIZERS AND TREATMENT OF BIPOLAR AFFECTIVE DISORDER

Historically, lithium has been the first choice for the management of acute mania [5]. Lithium is usually provided in conjunction with antipsychotics and/or benzodiazepine. However, concerns now prevail regarding the use of lithium in younger children. There should be even more consideration if enuresis or thyroid disease is evident in the child: prescreening of thyroid, heart and kidney function is imperative in this matter. Depakote, an anticonvulsant, should be considered in the first line of treating mania episodes. Carbamazepine, another anticonvulsant, is also effective in the acute treatment of manic episodes. Caution must be maintained if carbamazepine is used with a tricyclic, because the latter are structurally similar to imipramine. Two other medications that are sometimes used, gabapentin and lamotrigine, have not been studied in people of color.

ATTENTION DEFICIT HYPERACTIVITY DISORDER (ADHD)

The first line of medication for ADHD is generally methyphenylate hydrochloride (Ritalin); however if Ritalin fails to initiate a sustained therapeutic response, there is a 50–70% response rate with the second-line drug, Dexedrine (dexamphetamine sulfate). Clinicians have also slowly started moving towards Adderall (an amphetamine mixture made up of amphetamine sulfate, amphetamine aspartate, dextroamphetamine saccharate, and dextroamphetamine sulfate) as a first-line drug, although careful alteration of the dosing needs to be heeded with this medication. On the other hand, if a child or adolescent has substance abuse problems and ADHD, Wellbutrin, clonidine or Tenex (guanfacine hydrochloride) should be considered. Cylert (pemoline) is no longer used as a first-line drug due to the number of deaths related to liver disorder. If the first lines of medication do not

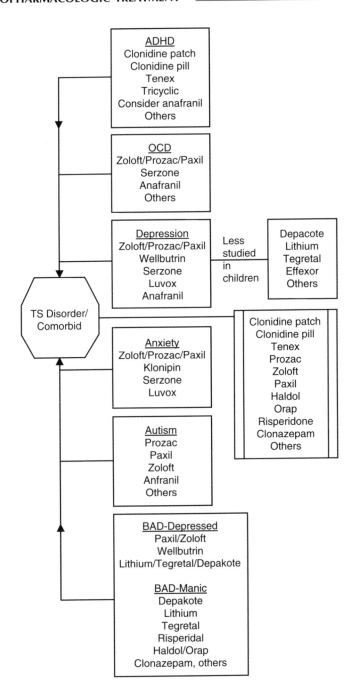

FIGURE 32.2 Medication for Tourette syndrome/comorbid disorder: decision tree

work, there are many alternatives: venlafaxine is sometimes used, although there are no controlled studies for this medication with people of color; Pamelor (nortriptyline hydrochloride) still remains useful, especially with comorbid ADHD mood, sleep symptoms, and anxiety; beta-blockers also continue to be alternatives for children that do not have severe asthma.

Historically, ADHD with enuresis has been treated with imipramine or Pamelor [6]. The efficacy is generally sufficient while the medication is in the system, but once the drug is discontinued, there is a risk of exacerbation. If a child or adolescent has comorbid ADHD and depression, they must be stable on medication for the attention condition. If they are, and the depressive symptoms are not drug induced, an SSRI such as fluoxetine, sertraline or paroxetine may be administered. If they are not taking stimulants, Wellbutrin may be considered for the comorbid ADHD and depression. If the child or adolescent has ADHD with comorbid anxiety that is not medication induced, an SSRI may be administered with the stimulant. Pamelor should be considered, but this medication carries cardiovascular risk. When treating comorbid Tourette syndrome and ADHD, clonidine or Tenex should be considered as first line. Ritalin and Dexedrine continue to be used with children and adolescents with tics that are being treated for ADHD, but the tics should be closely observed during the treatment. Tenex might be more useful for the patient with inattention ADHD symptoms. Clonidine should be considered useful for the impulsive, excitable, hyperactive symptoms. The first line of treatment for comorbid substance abuse and ADHD is clonidine or Tenex. For comorbid autism and ADHD symptoms the stimulants clonidine, Tenex, or Pamelor should be used.

ANXIOLYTICS

Buspirone has proven efficacious in the treatment of generalized anxiety disorder for aggressive children and adolescents. Diphenhydramine and hydroxyzine have also been used to treat anxiety. The benzodiazepines have a high abuse potential and thus should be prescribed with caution to adolescents.

While assessing and treating aggressive behavior, certain information needs to be ascertained about the patient: the underlying behavioral symptoms before the aggressive act; whether the behavior is an expression of underlying depression, injury from abuse, fear or explosive tendencies; whether the behavior is related to mood liability or sexual misconduct. This information should be used to strengthen the youth's ability to cope and manage their frustration. This is imperative when decreasing the behavior of medication.

ANTIPSYCHOTICS

In recent years, use of olanzapine and risperidone for treatment of psychotic illness or acute mania has increased. These atypical antipsychotics require lower doses

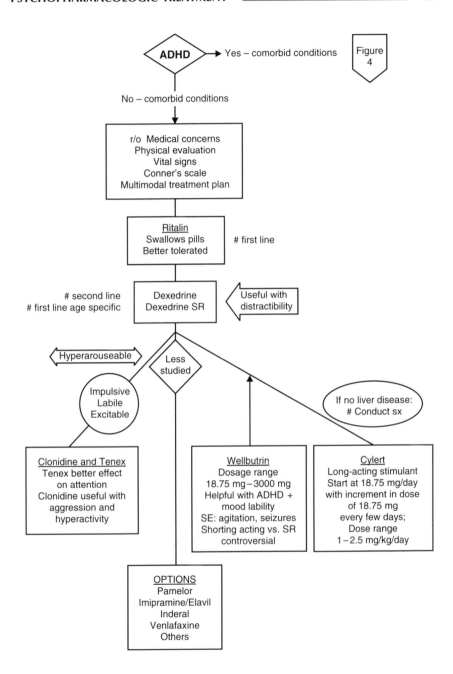

FIGURE 32.3 Medication for ADHD: decision tree

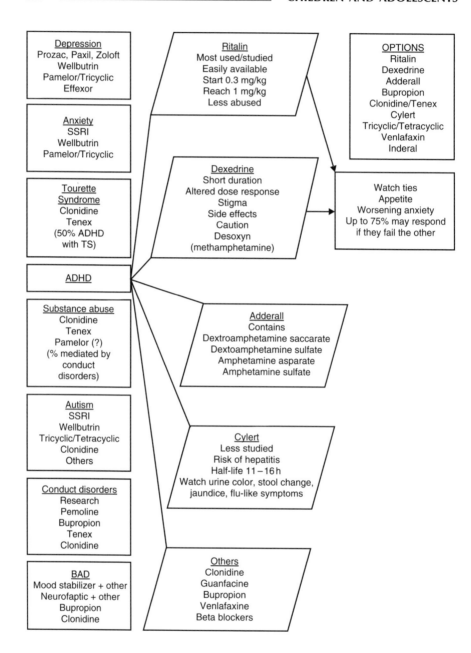

Depression
Prozac, Paxil, Zoloft
Wellbutrin
Pamelor/Tricyclic
Effexor

Anxiety
SSRI
Wellbutrin
Pamelor/Tricyclic

Tourette
Syndrome
Clonidine
Tenex
(50% ADHD
with TS)

ADHD

Substance abuse
Clonidine
Tenex
Pamelor (?)
(% mediated by
conduct
disorders)

Autism
SSRI
Wellbutrin
Tricyclic/Tetracyclic
Clonidine
Others

Conduct disorders
Research
Pemoline
Bupropion
Tenex
Clonidine

BAD
Mood stabilizer + other
Neurofaptic + other
Bupropion
Clonidine

Ritalin
Most used/studied
Easily available
Start 0.3 mg/kg
Reach 1 mg/kg
Less abused

Dexedrine
Short duration
Altered dose response
Stigma
Side effects
Caution
Desoxyn
(methamphetamine)

Adderall
Contains
Dextroamphetamine saccarate
Dextoamphetamine sulfate
Amphetamine asparate
Amphetamine sulfate

Cylert
Less studied
Risk of hepatitis
Half-life 11–16 h
Watch urine color, stool change,
jaundice, flu-like symptoms

Others
Clonidine
Guanfacine
Bupropion
Venlafaxine
Beta blockers

OPTIONS
Ritalin
Dexedrine
Adderall
Bupropion
Clonidine/Tenex
Cylert
Tricyclic/Tetracyclic
Venlafaxin
Inderal

Watch ties
Appetite
Worsening anxiety
Up to 75% may respond
if they fail the other

FIGURE 32.4 Medication for comorbid ADHD: decision tree

and have a lesser risk of causing tardive dyskinesia. Risperidone has also increasingly been used for the treatment of Tourette syndrome. Use of high-potency antipsychotics continues although, while the high-potency antipsychotics are initially effective, the efficiency declines with continuous usage.

CONCLUSION

Mention must be made of long-term treatment. When using any medication for an extended period, it is crucial to evaluate teratogenic effects because the risk of adolescent pregnancy is high in these patients. It is also vital to remember that Asian-American children have an increased sensitivity to alcohol and increased sensitivity to neuroleptics. It is also important to remember that the parents or guardian may attempt to use alternative treatment approaches for their child's behavioral problems. Dietary alteration may be attempted, and vitamin, herbal, and other supplements given. The success of management depends on the overall compliance of the family or guardian as well as the patient. The clinician should check who is giving the medication. Compliance in taking medication is sometimes higher if verbal and educational information about the medication is provided. The response to medication should be continuously monitored, using adverse-effect screening forms for children and constant review of the behavioral and emotional response and changing environmental issues.

REFERENCES

1. Hudziak JJ, Geller B. 1996. Interethnic psychopharmacologic research in children and adolescents. *Psychopharmacol Bull* **32**: 259–63.
2. Campbell M, Cueva J. 1995. Psychopharmacology in child and adolescent psychiatry: a review of the past seven years. *J Am Acad Child Adolesc Psychiatry* **34**: 1262–72.
3. Vitiello B, Jensen P. 1995. Developmental perspectives in pediatric psychopharmacology. *Psychopharmacol Bull* **31**: 75–81.
4. DeVane C, Salle F. 1996. Serotonin selective reuptake inhibitors in child and adolescent psychopharmacology: A review of published experience. *J Clin Psychiatry* **57**: 55–66.
5. Tohen M, Zarate CA Jr. 1998. Antipsychotic agents and bipolar disorder. *J Clin Psychiatry* **59**(Suppl 1): 38–48.
6. Bramble DJ. 1995. Antidepressant prescription by British child psychiatrists: practice and safety issues. *J Am Acad Child Adolesc Psychiatry* **34**: 327–31.

Index

Note: Page references in **bold** refer to Tables; those in *italics* refer to Figures

Index compiled by Annette Musker